IN THE EYE'S MIND

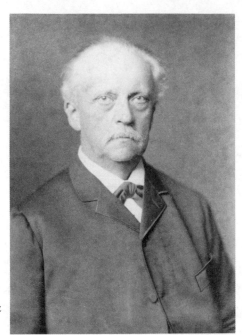

Hermann Ludwig
Ferdinand von Helmholtz
(1821–1894).

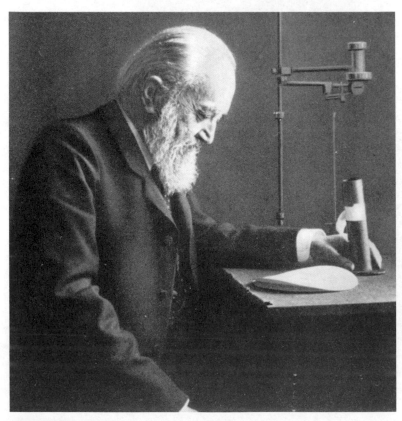

Karl Ewald Konstantin Hering (1834–1918).

IN THE EYE'S MIND

VISION AND THE HELMHOLTZ–HERING CONTROVERSY

R. Steven Turner

PRINCETON UNIVERSITY PRESS   PRINCETON, NEW JERSEY

Copyright © 1994 by Princeton University Press
Published by Princeton University Press, 41 William Street,
Princeton, New Jersey 08540
In the United Kingdom: Princeton University Press,
Chichester, West Sussex
All Rights Reserved

Library of Congress Cataloging-in-Publication Data
Turner, R. Steven (Roy Steven), 1944–
In the eye's mind : vision and the Helmholtz-Hering controversy /
R. Steven Turner.
p.   cm.
Includes bibliographical references and index.
ISBN 0-691-03397-8
1. Visual perception—History—19th century.   2. Helmholtz,
Hermann von, 1821–1894.   3. Hering, Ewald, 1834–1918.   I. Title.
[DNLM: 1. Helmholtz, Hermann von, 1821–1894.   2. Hering, Ewald,
1834–1918.   3. Visual Perception.   4. Vision—physiology.
5. Research—history.   WW 105 T951i 1994]
QP491.T87   1994   612.8′4—dc20
DNLM/DLC   for Library of Congress   93-37258

This book has been composed in Adobe Sabon

Princeton University Press books are printed
on acid-free paper and meet the guidelines
for permanence and durability of the Committee
on Production Guidelines for Book Longevity
of the Council on Library Resources

Printed in the United States of America

1   3   5   7   9   10   8   6   4   2

For Glenda and Laura

Contents

List of Figures and Tables   xi

Preface and Acknowledgments   xiii

PART ONE: INTRODUCTION   1

Chapter One
Introduction   3

   The Eye's Mind   3
   The Story and Its Themes   5

Chapter Two
Physiological Optics from Wheatstone to Helmholtz   10

   The Unification of Physiological Optics   11
   The Stereoscope and the Problem of Visual Space   13
   Binocular Vision in the 1850s   17
   Light and Color before Colorimetry   26

PART TWO: THE PROTAGONISTS   33

Chapter Three
Helmholtz on Spatial Perception   35

   From Potsdam to Heidelberg   35
   The Olympian Displayed   38
   Intellectual Commitments   40
   The Hunting of the Horopter   41
   The Defense of Listing   48

Chapter Four
Hering on Spatial Perception   54

   Ewald Hering   54
   Again, the Horopter   58
   Hering and the Theory of Identity   60
   The Theory of Retinal Space Values   63

Chapter Five
The Nativist-Empiricist Controversy Begins   68

   The Reform of Physiological Optics   68
   The Dispute over Spatial Localization before the Handbuch   69

The Dispute over Spatial Localization in the Handbuch   73
The Refutation of Hering   80
The Rhetorical Achievement of the Handbuch   87
Hering and Die Lehre vom binocularen Sehen *(1868)*   89
Conclusion   93

Chapter Six
Helmholtz on Light and Color   95

Helmholtz on Color Mixing, 1852–55   95
Clerk Maxwell and the Origins of Colorimetry   99
Young's Theory and the Handbuch *(1860)*   104
Simultaneous Contrast   108
Conclusion   113

Chapter Seven
Hering on Light and Color   115

The Reception of Young's Theory in Germany, 1860–75   115
Hering on the Organism   120
The "Spiritualistic" Direction in Physiology   121
Simultaneous and Successive Light Induction   123
Hering on Black   126
A Theory of the Visual Substance   128
The Opponent Process Theory of Color Vision   130
Reprise: The Unification of Physiological Optics   134

PART THREE: THE WIDER CONTROVERSY   137

Chapter Eight
Core Sets and Partisans   139

The Core Set   139
Significant Partisans: Hering   142
Significant Partisans: Helmholtz   145
Styles of Scientific Leadership: Hering   149
Styles of Scientific Leadership: Helmholtz   151
The Nonaligned   153
Conclusion   154

Chapter Nine
The Nativist-Empiricist Debate, 1870–1925   156

The Main Protagonists   156
Developmental Issues   159
The Stability of Retinal Depth Values   162
The Evidence of the Clinic: Anomalous Correspondence   168
The Ascendance of Nativism   172

Chapter Ten
Color Vision Controversies, 1875–90   176

Foundations   176
Debates over Color Blindness during the 1870s   177
The Evidence of the Unilaterals   179
The Defense of Young, circa 1880   180
Hering Takes the Offensive   184
Hering versus Kries   189
Helmholtz on Hering   193

Chapter Eleven
Color Vision Controversies, 1890–1915   196

König, Response Curves, and the Fundamental Sensations   197
The Specific Brightness of Colors   202
Rods, Cones, and Visual Purple   206
The Duplicity Theory of Vision   211
The Duplicity Theory and the Larger Controversy   214

Chapter Twelve
The Roots of Incommensurability   218

Incommensurabilities of Program   219
The Problem of Brightness   220
Semantics and Incommensurability   224
Schools as Linguistic Communities   231
The Limits of Incommensurability   233

Chapter Thirteen
Controversy and Disciplinary Structure   235

The Disciplinary Basis of Vision Studies   235
The Physics of Sensation   237
Colorimeters and Experimental Practice   240
German Physiologists and the Vision Debates   243
The Institutionalization of Ophthalmology   247
Visual Perception and the New Psychology   251
Conclusion: The Fragmentation of Vision Studies   256

PART FOUR: CONCLUSION   259

Chapter Fourteen
In Search of Denouement: The Twentieth Century   261

The Internationalization of Vision Studies   261
Zone Theory Established   265
Contrast and Stereopsis   271

Perception Theory in the Twentieth Century   273
Conclusion: Consensus and Controversy   276

Appendix   281

Notes   289

References and Abbreviations   299

Index   329

List of Figures and Tables

Figures

2.1	Wheatstone's stereogram	16
2.2	Nagel's hypothesis of projection spheres	20
2.3	Newton's color circle	27
3.1	Patterns of corresponding retinal meridians	45
3.2	Helmholtz's demonstration of the horopter	46
3.3	Helmholtz's afterimage experiment	49
5.1	Rotation of the frontal plane around the core point of visual space	83
5.2	Helmholtz's elaboration of Figure 5.1	83
5.3	Localization of half-images of an object lying in the median plane	85
5.4	Hering's retinal depth value experiment	85
5.5	Hering's law of equal innervations	90
6.1	Helmholtz's sketch of the spectral locus	99
6.2	Maxwell's rotating color wheel	100
6.3	Maxwell's sketch of the spectral locus	103
6.4	Maxwell's color triangle	104
6.5	Helmholtz's sketch of the spectral frequency response curves for Young's processes	106
6.6	Helmholtz's spectral locus	292
7.1	Hering's afterimage experiment	124
7.2	Hering's equilateral color triangle	131
9.1	Empirical longitudinal horopter	165
11.1	König's "elementary sensation" response curves for two dichromats and one monochromat	198
11.2	König's "elementary sensation" response curves for two normal trichomats and one anomalous trichomat	199
11.3	König's "fundamental sensation" response curves for two normal trichomats, one anomalous trichomat, and four dichromats	201
11.4	König's color triangle	201
11.5	König's determination of the spectral absorption curve of visual purple	208
13.1	König–Helmholtz spectral colorimeter	241
13.2	Hering spectral colorimeter	242
14.1	Svaetichin's schematic representation of spectral response curves	268
14.2	Hurvich–Jameson opponent process chromatic response curves	270

Tables

8.1	The Core Set of the Helmholtz–Hering Controversy	141
8.2	Factors in the Success or Failure of Research Schools	144

_____ *Preface and Acknowledgments* _____

THIS BOOK is the result of a long and evolving interest in the career of Hermann von Helmholtz, the institutional determinants of science in nineteenth-century Germany, and the nature of scientific controversy. Some of the material it contains has been previously published in different forms. Parts of Chapters Two, Three, and Five have appeared in "Consensus and Controversy: Helmholtz on the Visual Perception of Space," in *Hermann von Helmholtz and the Foundations of Nineteenth-Century Science*, ed. David Cahan (Berkeley/Los Angeles: University of California Press, 1993; copyright © 1993 by the Regents of the University of California). Parts of Chapter Eight have appeared in "Vision Studies in Germany: Helmholtz versus Hering," *Research Schools*, ed. Frederic L. Holmes and Gerald L. Geison (OSIRIS, vol. 8; Chicago: University of Chicago Press, 1993; copyright © 1993 by History of Science Society. All rights reserved.) Other material, including the tables in the Appendix, appeared in "Paradigms and Productivity: The Case of Physiological Optics, 1840–94," *Social Studies of Science* 17(1987): 35–68 (copyright © 1987 SAGE Publications Ltd.). This material is reproduced by the courtesy of the University of California Press, the University of Chicago Press, and SAGE Publications Ltd.

Many individuals have helped me in various ways during the preparation of this work. I am especially indebted to Mitchell Ash, Gary Bowden, Thomas Broman, David Cahan, Sabine Fahrenbach, Gerald Geison, Gary Hatfield, Godelieve van Heteren, Frederic Holmes, Dorothea Jameson, John Krauskopf, Richard Kremer, Peter Lundgren, John Mollon, Peter Nolte, Lynn Nyhart, Gert Schubring, William Woodward, and my colleagues in the Department of History at the University of New Brunswick for their invaluable advice and assistance. They are not, of course, responsible for the errors and shortcomings of this book. Parts of the research were done while I was a Fellow of the Alexander von Humboldt Stiftung and a guest of the Abteilung für Gesichtswissenschaft und Philosophie of the University of Bielefeld. The research and writing were supported by the Social Sciences and Humanities Research Council of Canada (Grants No. 410–85–0515 and 410–91–0032). I am grateful to these institutions, as well as to the Zentrales Archiv der Deutschen Akademie der Wissenschaft (Berlin), the University Museum Utrecht, and the Interlibrary Loan Office of the University of New Brunswick. I am particularly indebted to Dr. Günther Hering and the Hering family for their cooperation in this project and their kindness to me.

The photo of Karl Ewald Konstantin Hering is from the *Wissen-schaftliche Abhandlungen von Ewald Hering*, ed. Sächsische Akademie der Wissenschaft zu Leipzig, 2 vols. (Leipzig: Georg Thieme, 1931), fron-tispiece, and is reproduced courtesy of the Georg Thieme Verlag. The photo of Arthur König is from Arthur König, *Gesammelte Abhandlungen zur Physiologischen Optik* (Leipzig: J. A. Barth, 1903), frontispiece. It is reproduced courtesy of Barth Verlagsgesellschaft mbH. The photo of Johannes von Kries is from L. R. Grote, ed., *Die Medizin der Gegenwart in Selbstdarstellungen*, 4:124–87 (Leipzig: Meiner, 1925), 124, and is re-produced courtesy of Felix Meiner Verlag GmbH. The photo of Francis-cus Cornelis Donders is from a portrait of Donders painted by Abra-hamina Hubrecht. Copyright © University Museum Utrecht. It is repro-duced by courtesy of the University Museum Utrecht. I am indebted to the Hering family for permission to reproduce photos of Franz Hillebrand, Armin von Tschermak-Seysenegg, and Ernst Heinrich Siegfried Garten from originals in their possession.

Most of all I am grateful to Glenda, for her unfailing patience and support throughout this long project, and to Laura, who supplied the book's title and endured endless dinner table talk about minds and eyes.

R. *Steven Turner*
Fredericton, New Brunswick
June 24, 1993

Part One

INTRODUCTION

CHAPTER ONE

Introduction

THE EYE'S MIND

The strawberries went untended in Ewald Hering's garden during the summer of 1918. The old man was dead. He had remained active to the end of a long scientific career that had made him one of the most imposing figures in German physiology and also one of the discipline's most feared polemicists. Hering had cultivated the gardens of his scientific institutes with the same devotion and meticulous intensity he lavished upon the cadres of research students who passed through those institutes. Especially in the study of visual sensation and perception, he and his students had warred implacably against what they branded as the scientific orthodoxy of their day, and in so doing had inflamed one of the most notorious scientific controversies of the nineteenth century. The issues of the dispute had dictated the basic directions of vision research in Germany for almost forty years, yet few if any of them had been resolved at Hering's death.

The particular bitterness and the extravagant notoriety that surrounded this controversy sprang in part from the fact that Hering's chief opponent had been one of the most famous scientists of the nineteenth century. Hermann von Helmholtz (1821–94) had formulated the principle of the conservation of energy at age twenty-six, invented the ophthalmoscope at age thirty-one, and gone on to lay the foundations of modern physiological optics and acoustics in a series of monumental syntheses published in the 1850s and 1860s. He had then abandoned physiology for electrodynamics and finished his career as the doyen of German physics. Hering and Helmholtz had exchanged polemics directly in the 1860s, and thereafter Hering and his students warred with scientists they regarded as Helmholtz's disciples and surrogates, notably Adolf Fick, Arthur König, and Johannes von Kries.

Helmholtz, Hering, and their schools disagreed on many issues, chief among them being the proper sense in which the eye may be said to possess and to require a mind with which to see. On this issue they disputed the basis of the human capacity to visually perceive space and to localize objects in that visual space. Is this capacity innate and present at birth (the nativist position), or is it gradually acquired through learning and individual experience and mediated by inferential processes (the empiricist position)? The question of the eye's mind impinged upon the two schools' disagreement about the probable receptor mechanisms that underlie color vision. Do these consist of three mechanisms producing respectively the sensations of three fundamental colors, which are then psychologically mixed to produce the full range of color experience? Or do they consist of three sets of antagonistic receptors, producing respectively the sensations black-white, red-green, and yellow-blue? Can the eye's mind, in choosing among these alternatives, veridically assess the primitive or compound nature of its sensations? Do experience and inferential processes underlie the phenomena of contrast and adaptation, or are these produced by direct physiological mechanisms in the retina? These issues ramified into other lines of controversy: the interpretation of optical illusions, color constancy, eye movements, and adaptation; and the nature of retinal correspondence, with its implications for ophthalmological practice. The schools' antagonistic interpretations of all of these phenomena grew out of deep and divergent methodological commitments and ultimately out of disparate conceptions of the nature of life and of organic function.

Hering's death did not bring the dispute over these questions to an immediate end. His militant students kept the controversy alive for another decade, and textbooks preserved the memory of the dispute far longer, usually in pseudohistorical accounts served up for pedagogical or didactic purposes. Nevertheless, many contemporaries must have felt with relief that Hering's death had closed a chapter on an episode that had been uniquely unsettling among the scientific controversies of the nineteenth century. The persistence of the dispute, its pervasiveness, its resistance to compromise, the deep differences of methodological and philosophical principle that had divided its protagonists had challenged perceptions of scientific method and progress. By 1920 the controversy had already begun to pass into disrepute, ridiculed as scientific obscurantism par excellence and held up as a cautionary example against the uncontrolled proliferation of speculative theories.

Those same features make the history of the Helmholtz–Hering controversy a dramatic story and a revealing episode about the larger role of controversy in modern science. This book tells that story, from the initial confrontation of Helmholtz and Hering in the 1860s to the dissolution of Hering's school in the 1920s. Like the controversy itself, this narrative account of it sprawls across the history of a half-dozen academic disciplines over more than five decades and ramifies into accounts of many subproblems. Much, inevitably, has had to be neglected, and some arbitrary limits have been imposed upon the story in the interests of narrative cogency.

One of those limits is geographical and cultural. The account here deals almost exclusively with the Helmholtz–Hering controversy in Germany, where it began and was always most acute. The account largely ignores the reverberations of the dispute outside Central Europe, as it does the many developments in the larger science of vision that did not divide the two warring schools. The other limit is temporal. Despite the rhetoric of repudiation that was widespread after 1918, and despite the fact that the nature of the controversy changed decisively in the 1920s, the dispute itself has in one sense never ended. The broad issues of the Helmholtz–Hering controversy persist today and in some areas still structure the research front in problems of vision. That fact challenges both our conventions of historical narration and our understanding of how unresolved controversies affect the long-term development of science. This account touches upon these problems, but both lie outside its main focus on the decades from the 1860s to the 1920s.

THE STORY AND ITS THEMES

The narrative that follows opens with a general overview of vision studies in the two decades prior to the scientific debuts of Helmholtz and Hering. Chapter Two argues that the period between 1842 and 1867 marked a basic discontinuity in the venerable European tradition of vision research. Those years saw the creation of most of the new syntheses, methodologies, and integrating theories that were to dominate the field well into the twentieth century. Of course, the work of that period drew heavily upon past traditions and older research, but in consolidating and integrating them so successfully it simultaneously reduced them to largely historical interest. Helmholtz and Hering were two of the leading contributors to that midcentury integration of vision studies. Ironically their later dispute presupposed the elements of consensus which that integration generated; their controversy was to prove bitter and intractable in part because they agreed about so much.

The study goes on in Part Two to examine the careers, personalities, and programs of the two chief protagonists. It traces their initial clash over the issues of spatial and color perception, how their polemical exchanges mutually shaped the early development and presentation of their ideas, and how their competing ideas were received by contemporaries. Rhetorical analysis figures significantly in that discussion. Both protagonists were masters of the techniques of scientific argumentation, and they exploited those techniques consciously for programmatic ends. Rhetorical strategies included not only the usual forms of verbal argument, but also the visual and graphical techniques by which the two men represented concepts like color space and visual projections.

Those chapters insist, as historian Martin Rudwick has also done, on the "constitutive" nature of controversy in scientific change (Rudwick 1985). They contend that controversy does not act primarily in selectionist fashion to eliminate research programs and theoretical alternatives; it actively shapes outcomes. On this view, facts must be considered "controversy-laden" as well as "theory-laden"; theory itself may often be the product of tacit "negotiation" carried on as a crucial subtheme of polemical exchanges. Accordingly, the disputes between Helmholtz and Hering deeply shaped their own understanding and presentation of their respective scientific programs. Chapter Five argues in particular that the origins of the infamous nativist-empiricist controversy can only be understood fully in light of the respective programs and personal antagonisms of Helmholtz and Hering.

Part Three turns from the protagonists to their schools and traces the progress of the controversy from the late 1870s into the early twentieth century. It opens with a prosopographical examination of the most significant participants in the controversy and applies to the dispute the core set analysis advocated by Harry Collins and Martin Rudwick (Collins 1979, 1981, 1985; Rudwick 1985). From the 1870s this controversy was above all else a dispute between scientific schools. The school structure strongly polarized the core set into two opposed groups of partisans. At least before the early twentieth century, only a few "nonaligned" contributors participated significantly in the dispute. Partisans of both schools courted these nonaligned participants very intensely, yet their small numbers limited their ability to influence, compromise, or moderate the debate.

Chapter Eight measures the schools of Helmholtz and Hering against the factors that determine the success of research schools, including leadership style, recruitment, and advancement of the sociodisciplinary interests of participants. It also emphasizes the role of what might be called "affective interests" in the dynamics of research schools: the ties of duty, fidelity, love, and inspiration that coexist alongside material and cognitive determinants. That kind of analysis is particularly crucial for understanding the academic world of nineteenth-century Germany, with its strong tradition of research schools, its powerful patriarchs, its hierarchical traditions, and the pervasive insecurity of the careers it afforded. The coherence and persistence of Hering's group in the face of substantial opposition especially reflect the real power of the emotional ties that sometimes bound members of a research group to the master and one another.

Subsequent chapters present the narrative history of the controversy, emphasizing the perception of light and color and the nativist-empiricist dispute. They exploit the long baseline of the controversy to trace how alliances within the core set altered, how the terms of the dispute underwent subtle changes of meaning, and above all, how the constellation of focal problems that constituted the dispute shifted over time. The most important of these shifts occurred in the 1890s, when the study of achromatic sensation replaced that of chromatic sensation and color blindness as the principal focus of dispute. Another shift, occurring at roughly the same period, was the growing appeal to clinical evidence and to the study of strabismus as arbiters in the dispute over spatial perception.

That discussion carries on the central theme of controversy as a constitutive element in scientific change. It demonstrates how polemical papers served a double purpose: that of refuting the opposition and winning the allegiance of outsiders, as well as that of negotiating potential compromises or terms of closure with the opposition. The two programs used controversy as a tool, and that tool in turn affected their mutual development. The duplicity theory of vision, the specific brightness of colors, the empirical horopter as the locus of apparent equidistance—all represented ideas introduced by one school or the other to serve specific strategic and polemical ends. All, however, fundamentally altered the research programs into which they were introduced in ways that the partisans scarcely foresaw.

Part Three concludes with two more analytical discussions. One of these introduces the notorious concept of incommensurability, which Thomas S. Kuhn believed should always attend episodes of deep change in science. Chapter Twelve argues that the Helmholtz–Hering controversy was rife with incommensurable perspectives, and that they can be traced on programmatic, perceptual, and linguistic levels. The last of these levels displayed Kuhnian incommensurability most vividly. Perhaps more than in any other scientific controversy of the century, this dispute was a struggle for semantic control, specifically in this case over the language in which visual experience would be described and analyzed. That discussion also contends that incommensurability can be strategic and deliberate. It can result from strategies of communication pursued by one or both parties to a controversy, and those strategies in turn from the sociodisciplinary interests of the group (Biagioli 1990).

That discussion also notes that incommensurability can adhere in the different ways in which competing groups of scientists bring together the different resources of objects, instruments, ideas, and persons in the day-to-day activity of investigating what are ostensibly the same problems. The schools of Helmholtz and Hering differed in the kinds of experiments that they performed and to which they gave most credence, in the forms of graphical and mathematical analysis they pursued, in the representations they gave of their results, and in the type of experimental subject they favored for study. The very instruments that they constructed reflected their different theories of human vision and in turn reinforced those differences.

Disciplinary interests and investments bore upon the Helmholtz–Hering controversy in ways that are analyzed in Chapter Thirteen. That controversy was fought out within the professionalized and bureaucratized framework of the German university system, and the parameters of that institutional world and the career paths it defined influenced the controversy at every turn. The dispute cut across several fields that were after 1850 just in the process of establishing themselves as institutionalized and autonomous disciplines. These included physiology, ophthalmology, and experimental psychology; physics, with a more venerable institutional tradition, was also a disciplinary center of vision research. The chapter discusses how Helmholtz, Hering, and their respective programs appealed to these various disciplinary perspectives and examines the changing involvement of these fields with the controversy and its central issues.

Historians' accounts of scientific controversies deal on the one hand with the men and women who conduct scientific disputes: their interests, institutions, compulsions, visions of nature, and their own consciousness of their enterprise. On the other hand these accounts also treat the theoretical ideas in dispute, and these can acquire an autonomous and historically legitimate existence apart from the personalities that created and shaped them. They come to be preserved in textbook accounts and in the collective memory of the community; ideas that have been rejected or ignored at a cognitive level often retain a tacit embodiment in instruments, presuppositions, and research practices. The historian aims wherever possible at a seamless joining of these potentially separate accounts.

In the history of the Helmholtz–Hering controversy, that narrative join proves impossible to sustain much past 1930. As a school controversy or as one susceptible to core set analysis, the dispute was largely over by that date, even though few of the key issues had been resolved or compromised and little consensus had been achieved. But if the history of the dispute in one sense had closed by 1930, in another sense it had just begun. The perspectives formerly represented by the two schools continued to inform the practice of vision research deep into the twentieth century, and in the 1950s and 1960s many of the original terms of the dispute seemed vehemently to reassert themselves. The story of the controversy, which (on this telling) has such a decisive beginning at the middle of the nineteenth century, threatens to have no single, unambiguous ending at all in the twentieth. Chapter Fourteen looks briefly at the survival of the issues of the dispute after 1930 and their place in the international study of vision. It suggests that within the framework of the historical evidence and the conventions of narration, several different endings might legitimately be applied to the story of the Helmholtz–Hering controversy. Each possible ending affords a subtly different perspective on the narrative significance of this account of the eye's mind and the rivalries among those who struggled to comprehend it.

CHAPTER TWO

Physiological Optics from
Wheatstone to Helmholtz

BETWEEN 1885 AND 1894 Hermann Helmholtz and his protégé Arthur König labored over the successive installments for a second edition of Helmholtz's *Handbuch der Physiologischen Optik*. The task presented many difficulties. Helmholtz had abandoned physiology for physics around 1870, and his relative unfamiliarity with the burgeoning recent literature made hopeless any prospect of endowing the second edition with the scope or synthetic power of the epic first edition. To compensate in part for the inevitable limitations and omissions, König annexed to the second edition a massive bibliography of almost eight thousand items, listing (in principle) all the works published on the science of vision to 1894, the year of Helmholtz's death.

This massive bibliography did not solve the problems foreseen by Helmholtz and König; the second edition of the *Handbuch* had little impact. In compiling the bibliography, however, König was inadvertently creating an indispensable historical tool for modern historians attempting to trace the development of vision studies during the nineteenth century. Tables 1 and 2 in the Appendix present a quantitative breakdown of König's bibliographical information. For the period 1840–94, Table 1 shows changing levels of literature output in each of the seventy-seven literature categories or research lines into which König had grouped the scientific literature. The table expresses literature output over five-year intervals and as a percentage of all the literature items recorded for the interval. Table 2 shows König's categories combined into six supercategories or problem-complexes. On the assumption that relative levels of literature output mirror the current scientific interest attached to a given problem and the investment of resources in it, then Tables 1 and 2 "map" the intellectual topography of vision studies over five decades of development.[1] Coming chapters of this study will trace the contours of that topography in some detail.

Tables 1 and 2 show a small scientific field with a modest literature output in the 1840s; a period of explosive growth occurred during the late 1850s and early 1860s. When recalculated to moving averages, they show that the literature on physiological optics grew in a roughly exponential fashion between 1840–44 and 1880–84 with a doubling time of about ten years. The early years of exponential growth were associated with the rapid expansion of the proportion of German-language literature, which reached norms of 85 percent in some literature categories. That in turn reflected the "takeoff" of German natural science in the 1840s, the rapid growth of the German university system with its strong research orientation, and the successive establishment of physiology and ophthalmology as autonomous disciplines within those universities.

THE UNIFICATION OF PHYSIOLOGICAL OPTICS

Other evidence, less immediately obvious from the data of Tables 1 and 2, suggests that the middle decades of the nineteenth century brought still deeper changes to physiological optics. The study of vision possessed, of course, a venerable and dynamic tradition reaching back to antiquity. Yet before this period it had scarcely constituted a unified scientific field. Vision study was fragmented into many disconnected problems that were usually dealt with by different researchers, and it possessed few overarching theories that were both widely known and accepted and also capable of integrating the field. Controversies were widespread, and that controversy was endemic, disjointed, irresolute, and many-sided. The field lacked a well-defined research front, and in the absence of a research front older and newer literature possessed an equal relevance to the ongoing debates. In all these respects vision study closely resembled what Thomas S. Kuhn called the "pre-paradigm state" through which, on his model, scientific fields normally pass (Kuhn 1962, 10–22; 1970, 272).

Between 1840 and 1870, however, vision study in Europe experienced a transition that endowed the field with a methodological and theoretical integration it had not possessed previously. Certain classical problems about vision were either solved or lost much of their former interest during this period, and a series of new problems emerged to focus research on new areas. Research traditions began to crystallize around new experimental methods and new instruments. Several unexpectedly powerful theories emerged that integrated previously disparate phenomena. These developments were rapidly synthesized into a unified textbook tradition that obliterated the older, classical literature of the field in the very act of incorporating it. What emerged scarcely constituted a Kuhnian paradigm, but it did forge the scientific study of vision into roughly its modern form. The theoretical structure of vision studies in 1940 was only a complex elaboration of that which existed in 1867, while that of 1867 differed fundamentally from that of 1840 (Dodwell 1975, 57).

Research on the dioptric functioning of the eye was one of several lines that illustrate this critical midcentury turn. In 1845 Göttingen physicist

J. B. Listing adapted to the human eye Gauss's general theory for a centered optical system of arbitrarily many refracting surfaces, and in 1854 he set out a definitive mathematical treatment (Listing 1845, 1854). Helmholtz adopted and expanded the Gauss–Listing theory in his *Handbuch* volume of 1856 (*PO5* 1:57–120). These developments by no means definitively settled the vexed and venerable problems of the eye's dioptrical function, but Table 1 shows that they promptly deflected the research energies of contemporaries into other channels. Research lines 9, 10.1, and 10.2 had been active fields in the 1840s and 1850s, yet they attracted only the most spasmodic research interest later, after the definitive work of Listing and Helmholtz. In the same way both Helmholtz and Dutch ophthalmologist Antonie C. Cramer offered proofs that accommodation is achieved through a change in form of the crystalline lens (Cramer 1855, *WAH* 2:280–82, no. 28). In 1855 Helmholtz introduced the ophthalmometer, a device that allowed him to measure the curvature of refracting surfaces in the living eye (*WAH* 2:283–345, no. 39). How the change of form of the lens is brought about in accommodation remained intermittently controversial for decades. Nevertheless, relative levels of research interest in accommodation promptly collapsed in the wake of the papers by Cramer and Helmholtz, as research line 12.3 in Table 1 shows.

As classical problems were settled in this transitional period, new research lines were opened up. In 1856 Würzburg anatomist Heinrich Müller demonstrated a neural connection between the rods and cones (first distinguished by Kölliker as separate structures) and the radial nerve fibers in the more anterior parts of the retina (*PO5*, 2:29–31, 43–44; 1:212–22). He also claimed to prove by the method of entoptical shadows that posterior layers of the retina, probably the rod-cone layer, must be the light-sensitive ones. Just what elements in the complex microscopic anatomy of the retina were light-sensitive was then an open and controversial question, but backed by Kölliker, Müller's views found quick acceptance. Helmholtz immediately incorporated Müller's result into the *Handbuch*, although as late as 1860 he was still skeptical that rods as well as cones are light-sensitive elements (H. Müller 1856, *PO5* 1:212–22; 2:29–31, 43–44).

Definitive acceptance of the rods and cones as sensitive elements opened up a flood of new research lines in physiological optics. They included study of the anatomical basis of visual acuity, the difference between rods and cones and their function, and in general the physiological, comparative-anatomical, and chemical and physical properties of rods and cones. Literature on the retina and the optic nerve had been comparatively insignificant in the 1840s, but Table 1 shows that it averaged 2.5 percent of the total literature of the field from the 1850s on. This development typified changes occurring across the whole research front of physiological optics during this crucial midcentury period of transition and integration. Old problems were (at least temporarily) settled or abandoned, important new research lines were opened up, new instruments and research techniques were introduced, and anatomical structure was successfully related to physiological function on a broad front. Similar developments also occurred in the study of visual spatial perception.

THE STEREOSCOPE AND THE PROBLEM OF VISUAL SPACE

For all its philosophical ramifications, the problem of visual spatiality is primarily one of localization: when an external object makes a visual impression on our retinas, what physiological and psychological processes mediate our determination of the *direction* of the object with respect to the central planes of our bodies and our fields of vision? What processes mediate our determination of how far the object lies from us (depth perception) or its distance relative to other objects in the visual field (the perception of relief)?

These issues had a venerable history within philosophy and speculative psychology, though some had seemed more pressing than others (Hatfield 1990; Leary 1982; Boring 1942, 221–311). The fact that the monocular visual image (from either of the two eyes alone) appears spatially extended in two dimensions, for example, had always seemed relatively unproblematic to most theorists. After all, the two-dimensional image that we see with one eye alone conforms closely—although not exactly—to the two-dimensional image physically formed upon the retina by the dioptrical apparatus of that eye. Writers typically explained this conformity by assuming that each retinal point is connected to the sensorium by a separate and independent nerve fiber, so that the order of points in the physical image on the retina is preserved in its transfer to the sensorium. Others merely noted that the conformity of the retinal and visual images pointed to some innate and inborn arrangement (Gehler 1796, 12; Volkmann 1846, 317).

Because the retina is not extended in the third dimension, however, our capacity for depth perception had always seemed more paradoxical. It had been taken for granted at least since the time of George Berkeley (1685–1753) that this capacity rests on learned, monocular cues such as the superposition of objects in the visual field, the visual angle subtended by familiar objects, atmospheric perspective, or the perceived sharpness of a seen object. Other cues that allow us to estimate the distance of objects visually were thought to depend upon our subliminal awareness of tension in the ocular muscles: the degree of accommodation necessary to fixate on an object, and the degree of convergence of the visual axes of the two eyes. Most theorists speculated that we have learned what these cues mean about the distance of objects by associating them with perceptions of distance built up from the more primitive spatial sense that resides in the sense of touch; visual space was often regarded as derived from tactile space. Nearly all theorists distinguished between raw sensations and our conscious perceptions of objects in depth, but they disagreed as to whether the processes that connect sensations and perceptions are "judgmental" in nature and proceed from the faculty of the understanding, or are "associational" in nature and more closely related to basic sensory processes (Hatfield 1990, 32–45).

At the end of the eighteenth century, Immanuel Kant attempted to endow spatiality with a profoundly different epistemological and ontological status. Kant insisted that space was a "concept" or a "pure intuition"—something imposed upon sensory data by the understanding rather than discovered in the world by the visual *or* the tactile sense. In the nineteenth century the legion of theorists who reacted to Kant frequently interpreted (or misinterpreted) this claim as a *psychological* one, and as such they debated its meaning and correctness. But Kant did not regard our ability to visually *localize* objects within this intuitional space (at least in the third dimension) as innate or a priori; his views on the empirical psychology of vision scarcely differed from those of his contemporaries. Kantian doctrine, therefore, did not directly affect the proximate, empirical issues involved in visual spatiality.[2]

What did transform these proximate issues was Charles Wheatstone's epic invention in 1838 of the stereoscope or opticon, a device that took Victorian parlors and psychology laboratories alike by storm (Wheatstone 1838). The stereoscope is an instrument for presenting separately to the eyes two different photographs or line drawings of a single object or scene that have been made from separated points in space. The slight disparity between the two flat fields presented to each eye is resolved in the fused binocular field into a vivid, sometimes stunning perception of the object or scene in three-dimensional relief. Before 1838 the significance of binocularity and the slight disparity of the two monocular fields for the perception of relief had scarcely been appreciated. Experiments with simple stereograms, however, showed that binocular disparity alone suffices to invoke the perception of relief when the familiar empirical cues are completely absent.

Wheatstone's discovery raised the question of how the mechanism of perception translates the two flat monocular fields into a combined, binocular field that shows objects in relief. The first response to this theoretical challenge was the attempt by Sir David Brewster and others to generalize to the binocular situation the old "theory of projection" that had long been applied to monocular vision. Imagine the two eyes fixated on an external point-object; the object then images on the two foveas. If the eye's mind "knows" the interocular distance and the angle of convergence of the two eyes (the latter presumably through the tension in the ocular muscles) then the direction of the object and its distance from the body are fully specified. The two visual images of the object could then be thought of as "projected" outward along the visual direction lines from the foveas to their point of intersection and then "seen" as one at the proper distance and direction from the body. When generalized to the direction lines proceeding from all retinal points, this theory explained the whole binocular visual field as an outward projection of the two monocular fields along the lines of visual direction to their individual points of intersection. Stereogram drawings induce the eye to carry out such a projection, even though no real objects exist in space at the points to which the projections are extended.[3]

In advancing accounts like this, projection theorists did not necessarily claim to be describing the *actual* physiological or psychological processes that mediate depth perception; what they offered was a quasi-mathematical understanding of how *in principle* depth perception was possible. Their approach—studying vision through the geometrical analysis of rays and direction lines intervening between the object and the eye—linked them to a tradition in optics that was as old as Euclid.

Wheatstone's invention affected more directly a second venerable theory of binocular vision, one widely associated with German physiologist Johannes Müller. According to Müller, the retinas possess pairs of "corresponding" or "identical" points, each pair feeding the visual sensation of *one* point in the unified visual field. An external point-object located in space so that it images on a pair of corresponding points of the two retinas will always be seen single in the combined binocular field. Another small object, located at an external point in space from which its images fall on noncorresponding points, will be seen indistinctly, in double images and hence in two different directions at once. We are normally unaware of the multitude of double images in the combined visual field, but practice and introspection bring them readily to awareness. Müller suspected that the retinal correspondence was organic, and he pointed to the partial crossover of nerves in the optic chiasma as confirmation (Müller 1840, 351–85).

Müller's theory faced two problems. First, it did not explain enough. Although it explained why some external objects are seen single and some double, the theory per se did not explain why those seen single were seen in visual relief. Second, even as an explanation of single and double vision it seemed inconsistent with the evidence of the stereoscope, as Wheatstone charged in 1838. Wheatstone's instrument showed undeniably that points and lines that did not image on corresponding retinal points (and hence showed binocular disparity) could nevertheless be seen fused and single if the contour relationships were appropriate and the images neither too different nor too disparate. Indeed, it was precisely the fusing of slightly disparate and hence noncorresponding images that gave rise to the perception of binocular relief. In ordinary visual experience, Wheatstone pointed out, we routinely see small, real objects in the binocular field single; yet on the rigorous theory of identity at most only a series of points can be seen single at one time, never a real macroscopic object. Thus, Wheatstone believed that he had proved that objects not imaging on corresponding retinal points *can* be seen single in the binocular field (Wheatstone 1838, 88–90).

Worse still for Müller's theory, Wheatstone also claimed to have proved that point-objects that do image on corresponding retinal points need not invariably be seen single. He presented the readers of his 1838 treatise with the notorious stereogram shown in Figure 2.1. When this stereogram is placed in a stereoscope, Wheatstone claimed that most viewers will be able to fuse the two strong lines S_l and S_r, so that they see a single strong line in three-dimensional relief, the top of the line inclined backward. The faint line F_l presented to the left eye only will be seen vertical in the binocular field and passing through the midpoint of the strong line S_l-S_r. Wheatstone reasoned about the result as follows. Because F_l and S_r are symmetrically positioned on the stereogram, they must fall onto corresponding rows of points of the left and right retinas respectively. Hence they ought to be seen fused in the binocular field. But they are not; S_r fuses with S_l, not F_l, and the two monocular images are seen at different positions in the binocular field. Wheatstone concluded that "this experiment affords another proof that there is no necessary physiological connection between the corresponding points of the two retinae,—a doctrine which has been maintained by so many authors" (p. 83).

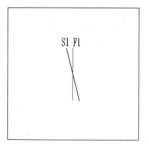 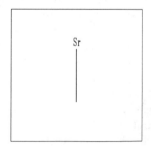

Fig. 2.1 Stereogram by Charles Wheatstone, purporting to refute the theory of retinal identity. *Source*: Wheatstone 1838, 386 (redrawn); cf. Wade 1983, 83.

BINOCULAR VISION IN THE 1850s

Tables 1 and 2 in the Appendix show clearly the intense scientific interest in problems of binocular vision, depth perception, and eye movements that Wheatstone's stereoscope triggered. In the early 1850s, especially, interest in these problems soared. Major figures like Friedrich von Recklinghausen, Alexander Rollet, Wilhelm Wundt, A. W. Volkmann, Peter Ludwig Panum, Albrecht von Graefe, Georg Meissner, and Albrecht Nagel moved aggressively into the field, and in the early 1860s they were joined by Helmholtz and Hering. In 1850–54 the literature on binocularity, depth perception, and related topics constituted 24.5 percent of the total scientific literature on vision, and it reached 29.2 percent in 1855–59.

Contributors to the literature on binocularity—predominantly Germans—frequently described the field as confused and chaotic. Young Albrecht Nagel complained in 1861 that despite an emerging plethora of new observations, "the most esteemed researchers defend to this hour diametrically opposite claims . . . [and] the most divergent views prevail over the whole theory of spatial vision" (Nagel 1861, 3). Within the general confusion, dispute coalesced around three issues in particular. One dispute pitted projection against the theory of identity.

Projection versus the Theory of Identity

Johannes Müller's student Ernst Brücke had leaped to defend the theory of retinal identity against Wheatstone's attacks. When we look at a small object, he argued in 1842, our eyes perform rapid movements in which they converge and reconverge while focusing successively on different points of the object. Our fused, stereoscopic image of an object is a composite perception, built up from this rapid succession of subliminal impressions. Thus, small objects may be seen single even if all their points do not simultaneously image on corresponding points, and points on stereograms like Figure 2.1 may be seen double even if they do. Similarly, Brücke taught that our judgment of the distance of the object and the relief of its parts is also an almost instantaneous summation, based upon kinesthetic cues. In response to Brücke, physicist H. W. Dove then viewed stereograms during spark exposures sufficiently brief (he claimed) to neutralize eye movements. He nevertheless observed visual relief in the stereograms, which supported Wheatstone and told against the theory of identity. But much uncertainty remained, and throughout the 1850s Brücke's eye movement hypothesis was widely accepted as the best explanation of binocular fusion and depth perception consistent with the theory of identity.

Like Brücke, Halle physiologist A. W. Volkmann regarded Wheatstone's attack upon the theory of retinal identity as "threatening the complete overthrow of the theory of vision" (Volkmann 1859, 3). But he regarded Brücke's line of defense as severely compromised by Dove's experiments. Volkmann therefore turned to an alternate explanation of stereoscopic fusion. Around the middle of the 1850s Volkmann began to publish detailed experimental studies to show that the binocular fusion of disparate images is a learned, "psychological" capacity. Thus, slightly disparate images of similar colors and similar contours are most easily fused, as are images of familiar objects or line drawings that can be interpreted as familiar geometrical shapes. We have learned to see familiar objects single even when they image on slightly disparate retinal points because we have acquired an idea (*Vorstellung*) of them as simple (ibid.). Volkmann continued to regard the retinal correspondence as innate and organic; psychology explained how noncorresponding images may be fused, but physiology alone sufficed to explain the fusion of corresponding images (p. 88). Volkmann did not, however, offer a fully developed theory of binocular depth perception to complement his explanation of binocular fusion. Many contemporaries, therefore, adhered to Brücke's theory of convergent eye movements to explain binocular depth perception, while accepting with Volkmann the broad influence of psychological factors in fusion.

Peter Ludwig Panum, professor of physiology at Kiel (later Copenhagen), disagreed with Volkmann on several points. He derided what he called the prevailing preference for "psychical" explanations of perception and insisted that the fusion of disparate retinal images follows fixed laws that must be innate and physiological in origin. The retinas possess not "corresponding points" but corresponding "sensory circles" (*Empfindungskreisen*). Neural anatomy guarantees that similar contours falling on corresponding sensory circles will be fused in the binocular image. The dimensions and exact contours of the sensory circles (they need not be true circles) may be deduced from experiments on binocular fusion carried out with the stereoscope (Panum 1859a, esp. 94).

As for binocular depth perception, Panum agreed with Volkmann that Brücke's eye movement hypothesis was untenable, but unlike Volkmann he took recourse to the theory of projection (ibid.). Every sensory circle possesses an innate "projection energy" that allows us to "perceive" the orientation of the direction lines from those circles to the external object being observed as well as the binocular parallax of those lines, and to localize that object in space at the intersection of those direction lines. Volkmann and Panum also rejected Wheatstone's crucial experiment purporting to show that objects imaging on corresponding points could sometimes be seen in different directions in the binocular field. Both objected to the original stereogram, to Wheatstone's report of its results, and to the logic of his argument. By 1860 acceptance or rejection of Wheatstone's stereogram had become the acid test of adherence to the rigorous theory of identity.

In 1861 Albrecht Nagel, privatdozent at Bonn and a former student of Helmholtz, published the first frontal attack on the theory of identity since Wheatstone's critique more than twenty years before (Nagel 1861). Nagel insisted that since no anatomical demonstration of a connection between corresponding retinal points can be given, the theory is both unnecessary and redundant. Correctly localizing an object in space requires seeing it single; once we have analyzed the conditions for single vision it is superfluous to postulate identical retinal points. Nagel attempted to demonstrate, in geometrical detail and with the use of the latest data of ocular dioptrics, that the hypothesis of projection will explain all the known phenomena of binocular fusion, stereoscopy, and depth perception. He admitted the problems that attended Wheatstone's crucial stereogram, but introduced new stereograms of his own to establish the same point.

Nagel also dealt with what some considered the Achilles' heel of projection theory: its inability to account for double images. In principle projection provides the eye's mind with the all the data necessary to visually construct the three-dimensional scene before the eyes with perfect accuracy and sharpness. Why, then, do we see most external objects indistinctly and in double images, rather sharp and single? To meet this problem Nagel introduced the notion of a surface of projection.

Nagel maintained that corresponding foveal images are fully projected out along the foveal direction lines to their external point of intersection, which we call the point of fixation (P_f). But the direction lines from extrafoveal half-images, he hypothesized, are not necessarily projected to their point of intersection, but only as far as an imaginary surface passing through the point of fixation. The half-image from each eye is "seen" at the point where its direction line intersects that surface, which results in double images of the same object. As for the form of this surface, Nagel contended that it consisted of two spheres, each centered at the pupillary center of its respective eye and passing through the point of fixation. Thus in Figure 2.2, if a is the point of fixation, then the object m should be seen in double images at m' and m'', and object n should be seen in double images at n' and n'' (p. 99; Hering 1862, 4). This ingenious suggestion allowed Nagel to reconcile the theory of projection to the reality of double images, and it indicated that the apparent distance of the half-images need not be same as the apparent distance of the point of fixation or the

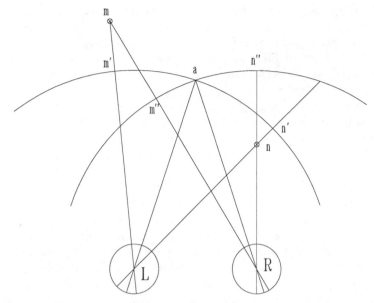

Fig. 2.2 Albrecht Nagel's hypothesis of projection spheres to explain the existence and localization of double images. *Source*: Nagel 1861, Plate III, Figure 22.

object casting them. Nagel's argument, therefore, made the localization of double images a matter of considerable theoretical importance.

Nagel was not the only theorist seeking to revive the theory of projection during the early 1860s. Ophthalmologist August Classen in Lübeck attacked the theory of identity in 1863 from a projectionist standpoint, and, much more important, Helmholtz's assistant at Heidelberg, the young Wilhelm Wundt, turned to the issue simultaneously with Nagel. Wundt did not reject the theory of retinal identity per se, but he stressed the many phenomena that prove that the binocular image is not a simple summation or blend of the two monocular images. Wundt fully accepted the validity of Wheatstone's crucial experiment and cast his own explanations of fusion and depth perception largely in projectionist terms (Wundt 1862, 5:234).

Wundt's work suggests that the fragile consensus about the theory of retinal identity was under heavy attack in Germany by the 1860s, despite the prestige of Johannes Müller that stood behind it. But there was little agreement about the relationship of binocular fusion and binocular depth perception, or even about whether projection and identity were mutually exclusive alternatives. As for Wheatstone's crucial experiment, there were as many different opinions about it as writers who examined the issue. By the early 1860s, when Helmholtz and Hering turned to these questions, projection versus identity had become an important and controversial issue, but also one that was itself highly confused and that scarcely offered clear alternatives.

The Horopter and the Theory of Eye Movements

The venerable problem of the horopter locus similarly offered no clear alternatives at the end of the 1850s, nor was it certain that the problem, although centuries old, could still be meaningfully defined. Under the influence of the theory of identity, the horopter had come by the 1850s to be regarded as the spatial locus of all external point-objects that image on corresponding retinal points (and are therefore seen single) when the eyes are fixated on a given point. Deducing the form of the horopter for a given point of fixation reduced to a mathematical problem that required assumptions about how the corresponding points are distributed across the retinas, and whether the two retinas (and so the patterns of retinal points) are rotated with respect to one another for particular points of fixation.

In the decades before 1850, Alexandre Prévost, Gerhard U. A. Vieth, Johannes Müller, and others had investigated the horopter for a horizontal point of fixation lying in the median plane and deduced it to consist of (or at least to include) a circle passing through the point of fixation and the optical centers of the eyes, plus a straight line intersecting the circumference of that circle. These deductions had been based upon the assumption that the corresponding points are distributed regularly and symmetrically about the two foveas, and that the vertical meridians of the two spherical retinas remain vertical.

But what *is* the horopter? Nagel pointed out that the usual contemporary definition could not be rigorously correct, since the stereoscope plainly showed that objects not imaging on corresponding points, and hence by definition not on the horopter, could be seen single. Considered in this way the horopter was "only a mathematical diversion" of no physiological or psychological interest (Nagel 1861, 166). Alternately, Nagel noted, the horopter could be cut loose from the theory of corresponding retinal points and redefined as the *empirically determined* locus of all external points seen single for a given set of eyes. Georg Meissner and a few others had attempted to investigate the horopter empirically by observing double images, but these determinations were considered notoriously difficult and variable from observer to observer (Meissner 1854; Wundt 1862, 5:240–52).

A third possible redefinition of the horopter, Nagel noted, is to treat it as the three-dimensional locus of points in space onto which double images are projected (it will then include all points seen single). On Nagel's theory this means the two projection spheres, but the more influential treatment in this vein was that provided by Friedrich von Recklinghausen, a young Berlin pathologist, in 1859. Recklinghausen dismissed the traditional horopter concept, claiming that for it "no physiological significance is known" (Recklinghausen 1860, 75). He rather defined a so-called normal surface as the imaginary surface in space on which all straight lines must lie if they are to be seen single, pass through the point of fixation, and appear in binocular vision perpendicular to the mean direction of vision. Recklinghausen gave this hypothetical projection surface a detailed, and subsequently influential, mathematical treatment (Recklinghausen 1859, 147–56; 1860, 71–78; POS 3:326–30, 344–50). But the uncertain relationship of this work to the classical horopter problem shows how, within a decade, that problem had become amorphous and possibly irrelevant within the new context set by Wheatstone's stereoscope.

A general solution to the horopter problem requires some assumptions about the rotation of the eyes at various positions, and this tied the horopter problem directly to the question of eye movements. Normally three coordinates are necessary to describe fully the position of one eye in the head. Two of these specify the elevation and horizontal rotation of the line of sight from the true horizontal and vertical, or from a reference setting usually called the "primary" position of the eye. The third coordinate, later called by Helmholtz the "torsion" of the eye, specifies the rotation of some reference plane (thought of as fixed to the eyeball) from its initial orientation when the eye is in the primary position. How this third coordinate, the torsion, varies with the movement of the eye is partly a convention, because its values depend upon the sequence of movements into which the net movement is analyzed.

Obscure as the whole issue of eye movements was in 1860, most writers accepted the empirical principle formulated by Dutch ophthalmologist Frans Donders and later known as Donders' law. This principle states that the angle of torsion, however measured, is uniquely determined by the angles of elevation and horizontal rotation. For every position of the eye, no matter how the eye has moved to reach that position, it assumes a unique degree of torsion. Donders (and Volkmann after him) had confirmed this principle by observing the angular departure of afterimages from vertical and horizontal orientations after the eyes had been moved to various positions. They also found the torsion to be zero at "secondary" positions (those reached by purely horizontal or vertical movements from the primary position of the eye), but nonzero at all other, "tertiary" positions.

Donders' principle still left completely obscure the question of why the eye assumes at any tertiary position the particular angle of torsion that it does. The only hypothesis purporting to solve this problem had been informally proposed (but never published) by Göttingen physicist Johann Benedikt Listing. He speculated that the eye assumes at any tertiary position just the angle of torsion it would have had, had it moved to that position out of the primary position, through a rotation around an axis through the center of the eye and perpendicular to the initial and final positions of the lines of sight. Rotations around such an axis (a "Listing axis") produce no rotation around the line of sight, that is, the eye does not "roll" during the motion, or perform (in modern terminology) a cyclorotation. If the eye moves to the tertiary position from some other initial position than the primary one, that movement will normally involve a true cyclorotation, but the degree of torsion reached at the end will always be *as if* the eye had reached the position through a Listing rotation out of the primary position.

Listing's proposal had a checkered history. Georg Meissner had originally rejected the idea, but later became its champion on the grounds of its simplicity (Meissner 1854). His attempts to test the principle empirically, however, produced wildly anomalous results (p. 97). Recklinghausen obtained similar discordant results in 1859, and he dismissed Listing's hypothesis out of hand (Recklinghausen 1859, 173–79). Wundt also criticized Meissner's support of Listing's principle, and argued on the basis of his own experiments that all eye movements produce a rolling or cyclorotation (Wundt 1862a, 4:138–41). Yet no clear alternative to Listing's hypothesis existed, and as in other areas of physiological optics the question of eye movements produced claim and counterclaim and little agreement as to the direction in which the field should move.

Physiology versus Psychology

In the confused exchanges of this period, writers also differed on whether the capacity for binocular fusion and depth perception is innate and physiological in essence, or is an empirical, acquired, "psychological" capability. This question, which Helmholtz and Hering would later elevate to the central issue of physiological optics, had been loosely prefigured in the old debate as to whether the process of depth perception was associative or judgmental in nature. In a still looser sense it was prefigured in the debate over the precise meaning of Kant's claim that spatiality is an a priori form of the intuition. As late as the 1850s, however, the arena of controversy had been limited by the tacit (though by no means universal) consensus that two-dimensional spatiality is "given" in the retinal image, while on the contrary the localization of objects in depth (if not always the intuition of depth itself) is an empirical and acquired capacity.

The stereoscope, of course, radically altered thinking about all these problems. The striking immediacy of stereoscopic relief, possible in the absence of all empirical cues except possibly convergence, defied explanation on the assumption that stereoscopic depth perception was an acquired facility mediated by judgment. On the other hand, the evidence that noncorresponding retinal images could be seen fused and single in the binocular field, and the certainty that at least *some* psychological factors influence fusion, mitigated against purely physiological explanations. Volkmann, although he regarded depth perception as an acquired capacity, still tried to strike a cautious note in his 1846 review:

> All the writers on the theory of vision have recognized that the perceptions derived from our visual sense are two-fold. One part of our optical experience not only derives from pure sensation, but depends on absolutely nothing more than the visual organ; color perception is of this nature. Other parts of our visual experience are to be had only through the interaction of other organs and functions, as for example our perception of the distance of an object seen. But it is controversial, which processes belong to pure sensation and which to the mediated. The physiology of the eye can set itself no more important problem, than to clarify the uncertainty surrounding this issue. (Volkmann 1846, 310)

In the late 1850s this "important problem" found itself modestly instantiated in the dispute between Volkmann and Panum over binocular fusion. Volkmann had contended that fusion is "an act of the soul, which presupposes experience with the real unity of the object seen, and to which we attain only through the training of the visual sense" (Volkmann 1859, 86). Panum had countered that "many perceptions which have usually been attributed to psychic activities, are to be derived from pure sensuality and from specific nerve energies," and had vowed "the conquering of a terrain for physiology which until now had been defended by psychology" (Panum 1858, 2). Throughout their lively experimental exchange, however, both men agreed on the innate spatiality of the monocular field and of the retinal correspondence itself, and both agreed that the binocular fusion of corresponding images was organic and obligatory. Albrecht Nagel usually pursued a careful middle ground as well. But in his more programmatic discussions he vigorously denounced physiology's recourse to entities like "specific nerve energies" and "brain functions" and he explained all depth perception as the result of inference and experience.

Nagel's discussion also hinted at a further important development in ideas about spatial perception. The mid-nineteenth century brought a flurry of speculation that the capacity for visual localization in two-dimensional space is not innate, as the textbook consensus still assumed, but rather is acquired through experience from aspatial visual and kinesthetic sensations (Hatfield 1990, 128–71). Theorists in this tradition usually had recourse to the hypothesis of "local signs": nonspatial and usually nonsensory qualities associated with particular retinal points that allowed the eye's mind to distinguish between identical sensations arising from the stimulation of different retinal points. From the local signs, and from the different degrees of muscular exertion required to bring peripheral visual sensations onto the fovea, we gradually acquire knowledge of the ordering of the various local signs on the retina, and we represent this ordering to ourselves in the visual image as a two-dimensional, spatial distribution. Perhaps the most influential of such theorists was philosopher-psychologist Hermann Lotze, who developed his theory of vision between 1846 and 1865, and who influenced Wundt and Helmholtz to develop similar ideas (Woodward 1978).

Theorists employing "local signs" in this way purported to explain how retinal images get localized as to direction, not how the spatial sense per se arises. One might regard the spatial sense as presupposing an a priori intuition of space, as did Lotze, or as a "psychic synthesis" emerging de novo in the ordering process as did Wundt, or as the adaptation to vision of a spatial sense already present in the sense of touch, as Helmholtz occasionally suggested. In any case, these genetic and psychological explanations of visual direction could be readily generalized to account for the perception of visual depth. They held that both monocular visual fields were originally present somehow in consciousness, but that we have learned how to superimpose these fields and to interpret the disparity of half-images as a cue to the distance from our bodies of the object responsible for them. These accounts could readily be cast in terms of the projection theory *or* the identity theory. On accounts of the latter type the retinal identity itself becomes an acquired correspondence, built up from the local signs and our experience of objects in space. All such genetic accounts (empiricist accounts, Helmholtz would later call them) place all three dimensions of spatial awareness on the same epistemological footing, as capacities acquired through experience.

One of the earliest and most famous of these genetic accounts was given by the young Wilhelm Wundt in his *Beiträge zur Theorie der Sinneswahrnehmungen*, published between 1858 and 1862. There Wundt not only reviewed the entire problem field of visual perception, but also developed his account of how the mind synthesizes its experience of the local signs, kinesthesia effects associated with convergence movements, and distance perceptions of retinal arcs passed over, in order to generate simultaneously the emergent faculty of two- and three-dimensional spaciality. "The awareness of the entire visual field as a spatially extended entity," he wrote, "is not already given in the fixed anatomical ordering of the sensory elements. Rather a psychical process is already present in that awareness. This process can . . . be nothing other than an inferential process, and, to be specific, a process of unconscious inference" (Wundt 1862a, 5:95). Thus, inferential processes and associations mediated the emergence of our spatial awareness (presumably in childhood), and they continue to mediate our localization of visual sensations in that space.

Wundt regarded an inferential theory of spatial perception as vital to his program for a scientific psychology. Such a theory would prevent the study of sensation from falling into the dangerous trap of subjective idealism represented by Fichte, Schelling, and Hegel, or succumbing to the scarcely less dangerous threat of physiological reductionism represented by Johannes Müller and Panum (Wundt 1862, 4: 116–45). Yet for all that, physiological and psychological accounts of stereopsis scarcely constituted clear alternatives to one another. They were not sharply distinguished in practice, and their confrontation found experimental expression only in the Panum–Volkmann dispute. In this sense the issue resembled the contending claims about eye movements and the horopter and the confrontation between projection and identity. The debates evinced little consensus over fundamentals, few clear choices, and endemic, many-sided controversy.

LIGHT AND COLOR BEFORE COLORIMETRY

The study of light and color perception resembled the debate over binocular vision in many respects. During the first half of the nineteenth century, scientific understanding of color and color perception drew from three distinguishable traditions. One was the empirical, craft tradition of mixing colored pigments to produce paints and dyes. Fundamental to this tradition was the belief in "primary colors"—usually taken to be red, yellow, and blue—from which all other color can be mixed. Painters obtained green from a mixture of yellow and blue, and black (really dark gray) from a proper mixture of all three primaries. European writers commonly demonstrated the properties of pigment mixing diagrammatically, typically in a color triangle with the three pigment primaries located at the vertices. Every point within the triangle represented a hue that could be mixed from these primaries, and the distances of the point from the three vertices or their opposite sides represented the respective proportions of the three primaries in the mix. Other schemes expanded the color triangle to a color solid, in order to exhibit variations in brightness (Sherman 1981, 65–71; Kremer 1993a).

Knowledge of colors also derived from the epic work of Newton. Newton had shown, of course, that white light is a mixture of many rays of different refrangibility. When white light is passed through a glass prism (or, later, a diffraction grating), the component rays are separated out according to their refrangibilities. The fact that the prismatic spectrum thus created displays the familiar rainbow sequence of colors suggests that the physical property of a light ray that determines its refrangibility (with the coming of the wave theory, its wavelength) also determines, or at least contributes to, the color sensation that the ray produces when it enters our eye (Sherman 1981, 60–63). Writers typically grouped the many perceptible shades of the spectrum into six colors: reds, oranges, yellows, greens, blues, and violets. Many writers, including Newton, interpolated a color called "indigo" between blue and violet, in order that the visible spectrum would have eight steps, like the musical octave.

Newton also turned his hand to a diagrammatic representation of colors and color mixing (Newton 1730, 155). He imagined the prismatic spectrum bent into a circle, so that violet and red were joined and all the intervening colors were displayed along the circumference (Figure 2.3).

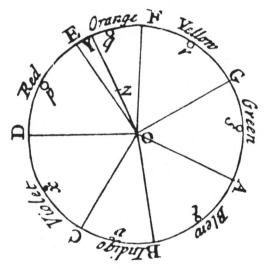

Fig. 2.3 Newton's illustration of his color circle (1704). *Source*: Newton 1730, 155. Reproduced with permission of Dover Publications, Inc.

A mixture of any two colors represented by points on the circumference would be a point lying somewhere on the straight line joining those points. Suppose we imagine the quantity of light of the first of the two hues entering into the mixture (crudely, its brightness) as a weight suspended at the end point of that straight line, and make the same assumption for the second mixture component. Then, Newton hypothesized, the color of the mixture itself will be represented by the center of gravity of the straight line joining the two color points, the line now thought of as a lever arm to which those weights are attached. The center point of Newton's color circle must be white, since white light is a mixture of all the spectral colors. Color points around the center must appear pale and unsaturated, since they are heavily diluted with white light.[4] Various writers after Newton noted and struggled with the apparent anomaly created by his color theory: the center of gravity of the spectral color circle must be white, while the center of the pigment-primary color triangle (which can be thought of inscribed somewhere inside the circle) is gray or black.[5]

A third tradition from which the scientific understanding of color phenomena drew was the accumulation of multifarious observations on subjective visual phenomena: color contrast, colored afterimages, adaptation, entoptical phenomena, perception of brightness, pressure phosphenes, the relationship of brightness to color, the effect of illness, injury, and certain drugs upon color perception, and many others. Germany in particular possessed a strong tradition of introspective observations on phenomena like these, with Goethe, Johannes Müller, and Evangelista Purkinje among the foremost names. During the 1840s studies of this type constituted almost 30 percent of the field's output (problem-complex VI in Table 2).

One particular phenomenon that rapidly became important was color blindness. John Dalton first studied that visual deficiency systematically, after discovering it in his own vision, and the condition was widely known as Daltonism in the first half of the nineteenth century. The most comprehensive study, however, was carried out by a German gymnasium instructor, August Seebeck, later director of the technical high school in Dresden. More clearly than any researcher before him (and many after him), Seebeck realized that Daltonism cannot be investigated by asking subjects to name colors; his own method called on his subjects (found in his gymnasium classes) to order series of colored papers to conform with the spectrum as they saw it, or by increasing brightness. In 1837 he reported that afflicted individuals (five of forty-one in his sample) consistently confused reds, yellows, and greens. Seebeck also distinguished two classes of color blind individuals: one that found the reds dark or colorless, and one that found them brighter but still indistinguishable from greens and yellows. Seebeck's work seems to have been unappreciated outside Germany, even though color blindness was soon to become the most confused and yet most crucial topic in the theory of color vision.[6]

Physiological optics had traditionally focused upon anatomical studies on the one hand and the geometrical-dioptrical analysis of rays on the other. Because color vision could not fruitfully be approached from either perspective, it had never been a major part of physiological optics. For example, Volkmann's authoritative survey of the topic in 1846 devoted only six pages to color vision. It did, however, include a highly critical analysis of two new theories of color vision.[7] The first theory correlated hue sensations with the degree of "physiological energy" present in the optic nerve. As the energy in a highly stimulated nerve gradually diminished, it could be expected to excite sequentially the whole spectrum of color sensations including white and black. Volkmann sniffed that this hypothesis explains chromatic fading (the so-called *Abklingen* of colors in an afterimage) but nothing else. And if hue is associated with the degree of "physiological energy" in the nerve, then with what physiological entity is the intensity or brightness of a color sensation to be associated (Volkman 1846, 313)?

Volkmann also examined and rejected a second theory of color perception. "On repeated occasions," remarked Volkmann, "the supposition has been expressed that the various color sensations are mediated through the function of specific fibres, an hypothesis which presupposes the doctrine of specific irritability" (p. 314). The model postulated three sorts of retinal nerve endings, which when stimulated produced respectively three specific color sensations, usually taken to be red, yellow, and blue. All our other color sensations are "psychological mixes" of these three primary sensations.

Although Volkmann ignored the history of this idea, the hypothesis was, in fact, that suggested by Thomas Young in 1801 and again in 1802 (Hargreave 1973; Kremer 1993a; Sherman 1981, 1–18). Its advantage lay in explaining how the same color sensation can be stimulated by many different physical lights or mixtures of lights: all that matters is that the net physical stimulus activate the three retinal receptors in the same ratio. Its appeal also lay in its explanatory economy, its apparent harmony with Johannes Müller's law of specific nerve energies, and—above all—the fact that it internalized or "psychologized" people's universal experience with pigment primaries and their mixes. Young in 1802 had taken his physiological primaries to be red, green, and violet, but most later writers rebuked him for this eccentric choice and returned to red, yellow, and blue on analogy with the pigment primaries.

Volkmann was unimpressed by these advantages of Young's theory. He wrote that the theory "creates more difficulties than it eliminates" (Volkmann 1846, 314). Volkmann seemed prepared to doubt Müller's principle that "qualitatively different sensations must derive from different organs"; and even if that law were true, he insisted, there would still be no justification for postulating particular colors as primaries over any others. If each of the receptor-types is to be regarded as a retinal element with a finite area of sensitivity, then the hypothesis conflicts with the data on visual acuity for colored and white stimuli. The physiologist Volkmann thus evaluated Young's suggestion primarily as a physiological hypothesis about the retina, not as a model to explain color mixing.

As a physiologist in Germany, Volkmann may have been unaware in 1846 of one important, additional theory of color that the indefatigable Sir David Brewster had proposed in 1822. Experiments on absorptive media had convinced Brewster that light rays of the same refrangibility can undergo a change of color when passed through properly chosen colored filters. To account for this observation, Brewster proposed that the visible spectrum of white light is actually a superposition of three coterminal spectrums. All the rays in one of these spectrums are red, in another yellow, and another blue, and each contains these colored rays in all degrees of refrangibility. These three spectrums "add" in appropriate proportions to make the other spectral colors (notably orange and green) and also white (Sherman 1981, 20–42). Thus, while Young's theory psychologized the idea of primary colors, Brewster's theory physicalized them, in that it identified the classical pigment primaries with three distinct, physical kinds of light (Kremer 1993a; Sherman 1981, 20–42; Hargreave 1973).

A clear sign of the quickening European interest in vision study is the fact that Brewster's theory, after attracting relatively little opposition for twenty-five years, suddenly became the focus of intense debate in the late 1840s. Directly or indirectly, the furor over Brewster's theory led to three developments in the mid-1850s that were to revolutionize the study of color vision. One was the development of refined experimental techniques for isolating and mixing high-intensity and highly saturated beams of monochromatic light. A second consisted of entirely new colorimetry techniques for measuring color perceptions quantitatively. A third development saw a much closer integration of the three classical traditions from which knowledge of colors was drawn and broad acceptance of a single model of vision that claimed to explain at least the principal phenomena from all three traditions.

These developments of the 1850s were to do for the study of color vision what other developments reviewed in this chapter did for other branches of physiological optics during the pivotal period between 1842 and 1867. They were to bring to an end the characteristics of scientific practice that prevailed earlier in vision studies: a fragmented and largely descriptive experimental literature, a lack of consensus about fundamentals, and endemic controversy continuing in the absence of clear theoretical alternatives or sharp alignments. In many areas of physiological optics this pivotal period resolved classical controversies and opened up entirely new lines of investigation. It certainly did not impose calm and consensus—as the later Helmholtz–Hering controversy attests—but it fundamentally changed the *nature* of the controversies in the field.

Part Two

THE PROTAGONISTS

CHAPTER THREE

Helmholtz on Spatial Perception

HERMANN HELMHOLTZ, the chief architect of the new physiological optics of the mid-nineteenth century, grew up in the city of Potsdam, the
royal retreat of the Prussian kings, just west of Berlin (Kremer 1990, xiv–
xv). His father had served in Prussia's war of liberation against Napoleon
and then studied classical philology and philosophy at the newly founded
University of Berlin before accepting a teaching post at the elite Viktoria-
Gymnasium in Potsdam (Königsberger 1902–3, 1:1–8). The profession of
gymnasium *Oberlehrer* to which Ferdinand Helmholtz belonged had
been created in the early nineteenth century with the reform of Prussia's
secondary school system. It had rapidly replaced the Lutheran pastorate
as the principal threshold of social mobility into the so-called *Bildungsbürgertum*, that influential and self-conscious element of Germany's middle class that owed its social standing not to wealth or commerce, but to
its quasi-monopoly of elite education and the access to the professions
and to the civil service that followed. From the *Oberlehrer* threshold,
upwardly mobile members of this middle class launched their sons into
careers in law, medicine, the higher civil service, and the university pro-
fessoriate (Conze and Kocka 1985; Turner 1980a). This was the course
that Ferdinand Helmholtz planned for his sickly but superbly intelligent
son Hermann, born in Potsdam on August 21, 1821.

FROM POTSDAM TO HEIDELBERG

In all but its exceptional celerity, Helmholtz's career largely followed the
familiar course of academic careers in Germany's newly professionalized
and institutionalized world of university science (McClelland 1980;
Turner 1971, 1980b).[1] Helmholtz graduated from the Viktoria-Gymna-
sium in 1838, a product of an elite educational system that stressed German literature and the classical languages, but also provided a solid
mathematical foundation (Kraul 1984; Jeismann 1974; Schubring 1983,
esp. 37–84). Helmholtz's interests had already turned to natural science,
but his father directed him to medicine, where there existed the opportunity for financial assistance for university study. Following a competitive

examination, Helmholtz was accepted into the Medicinisch-chirurgisches Friedrich-Wilhelms-Institute in Berlin, where Prussia educated its military surgeons. Students in the Friedrich-Wilhelms-Institute trained in the university medical faculty on the same footing as private students, and for the M.D. degree Helmholtz elected dissertation research under anatomist and physiologist Johannes Müller. He was thereby drawn into the circle of Müller's prominent students and assured the patronage of one of Prussia's most influential advisors in scientific matters.

After obtaining his M.D. degree in November 1842, and serving a one-year internship at the Charité hospital, Helmholtz began eight years of obligatory military service as staff surgeon, conveniently with units stationed in his native Potsdam. There he gained practical medical experience and still had time for scientific studies and research. He had become close friends with Müller's students Emil du Bois-Reymond and Ernst Brücke, and through them had become a member of the Berlin Physikalische Gesellschaft and contributor to this group's journal, the *Fortschritt der Physik*. To this society in 1847, Helmholtz presented his famous treatise on the conservation of energy, a concern closely related to his physiological interest in muscle metabolism and energy expenditures in the living organism (Bevilacqua 1993; Olesko and Holmes 1993).

The fame that this scientific work earned Helmholtz, plus the patronage and support of Johannes Müller and the aged but still redoubtable Alexander von Humboldt, secured for him a ministerial release from his remaining military obligation and, in October 1848, appointment as Müller's assistant in the Berlin Anatomical Museum and lecturer on anatomy at the Academy of Arts. In May 1849 this was followed by an appointment as associate professor of anatomy and physiology at the University of Königsberg, a position just vacated by Brücke. Helmholtz celebrated this first, real position by marrying Olga von Velten (1826–59), to whom he had been engaged since 1847.

As professor in Königsberg Helmholtz continued his research on muscle metabolism and the velocity of the nerve impulse. His interests, however, gradually began to shift toward sensory physiology. In the fall of 1851 he announced his invention of the ophthalmoscope, a diagnostic tool that rapidly became indispensable to the burgeoning medical specialty of ophthalmology. Its invention probably did more even than his treatise on the conservation of energy to establish Helmholtz as the *Wunderkind* of German science and medicine (Tuchman 1993a).

Although the Königsberg years were happy and productive ones for Helmholtz, his wife's fragile health suffered in the bitter northern climate and the institution was far from the most prestigious or lucrative. On the strength of his fame and the patronage he enjoyed in the Ministry of Education, Helmholtz was called in 1855 to the University of Bonn as professor of physiology and medicine. There he published the first volume of the *Handbuch der Physiologischen Optik*, which dealt with the dioptrics of the eye, and extended his research into physiological acoustics. Still, Helmholtz was never satisfied at Bonn. He found the facilities poor, complained that his colleagues were recalcitrant or hostile to him, and smarted under allegations made to the ministry that he favored physiology and delivered incompetent lectures on anatomy. Opportunely, the government of Baden approached him in 1857 about an appointment in physiology (not to include anatomy) at the University of Heidelberg. Liberal Baden was at this time rapidly seizing the leadership among the German states in promoting natural science and technology (Tuchman 1986, 1993b; Riese 1977; Borscheid 1976). Loyal Prussian that he was, Helmholtz hesitated, but when negotiations for a new anatomy building at Bonn stalled, he accepted the Baden offer and moved to Heidelberg in 1858. The political humiliation of losing Helmholtz rankled in Prussia until 1871, when he was triumphantly brought back to take the chair of physics at Berlin.

Helmholtz's work on sensory physiology culminated during his thirteen years at Heidelberg (1858–71). There he published the second volume of the *Handbuch* in 1860, the third and last in 1866, and in 1862 produced his classic study of physiological acoustics, *Die Lehre von den Tonempfindungen als physiologische Grundlage für die Theorie der Musik* (Vogel 1993). During his career Helmholtz had never ceased to publish on physics, and this field became more and more important as his attention turned to electrodynamics during the later Heidelberg years. Likewise, he continued to produce elegant, widely read popular lectures on various scientific topics, including lucid restatements of the philosophical and epistemological position he had first announced during the early 1850s in Königsberg.

The Heidelberg years also brought changes to Helmholtz's personal life. In 1859 Olga von Velten died, leaving Helmholtz with two small children. In 1861 he married Anna von Mohl, the daughter of a noted Heidelberg professor and political theorist. Younger than Helmholtz, Anna von Mohl was wealthy, cultivated, gregarious, and socially ambitious. In Heidelberg and later at Berlin their home became an intellectual salon, and she introduced Helmholtz to a broader social and political world (Cahan 1989, 61). After his return to Berlin in 1871 Helmholtz increasingly assumed the role of doyen of German natural science. This role was vastly enhanced by his appointment in 1887 as president of the Physikalisch-technische Reichsanstalt for research in the exact sciences and precision technology, a project to which Helmholtz's close friend, industrialist Werner von Siemens, contributed half a million marks (ibid., 1–126).

THE OLYMPIAN DISPLAYED

The versatility and productivity of Helmholtz's work astounded his scientific friends no less than other contemporaries. The genial Emil Brücke wrote to du Bois-Reymond in 1853, "The real state of affairs is this: you work *multum* but not *multa*, Helmholtz works *multum* and *multa*, and I work neither *multa* nor *multum*" (Wiesflecker 1978, 55). They regarded him as a reserved, placid individual. Brücke commented in 1849 that Helmholtz "would certainly get along well in Königsberg, because with the small number of students there his phlegmatic ways won't matter so much" (ibid., 25–26). Du Bois-Reymond wrote cattily to Carl Ludwig in 1852 that as much as he marveled at Helmholtz's immense and apparently effortless output, he was sure that Helmholtz's placid nature would bar him from the highest transports of scientific satisfaction (du Bois-Reymond 1927, 111–13). By the end of his career, however, his students and colleagues had reinterpreted that placid reserve, so as to portray it as the lofty, Olympian detachment thought suitable to an individual whose intellectual range over natural science, philosophy, and art had been equaled only by Leibnitz and Goethe.

Helmholtz's surviving correspondence yields a personal portrait much more nuanced than the Olympian stereotype.[2] It reveals the young Helmholtz as a well-adjusted, industrious, curious young man, happily launched upon a promising career and enmeshed in an extended network of family and friends who opened their parlors and dining rooms to him. Though not normally outgoing, he possessed a sociable and even jaunty side, and could twit du Bois-Reymond for being reclusive and shy "toward everyone who is not a physiologist" (Kirsten 1986, 85, no. 11). During his Potsdam years, especially, the pleasures of Biedemeier culture—art, theater, music, walking tours, parlor theatricals, and drawing room soirees—figure large in his consciousness (Kremer 1990, xi–xxvi). Helmholtz was already an accomplished pianist when he left the gymnasium, and he took his piano with him to the rooms he occupied in the Friedrich-Wilhelms-Institute, to the delight of his friends and the displeasure of those who roomed below him (Cahan 1993a, 43–48 [no. 5]). His exquisite ear and knowledge of music theory served him well in his later acoustical experimentations, as his familiarity with painting did in his optical work. Throughout his life Helmholtz had a passion for travel, and in particular a devotion to Alpine rambles spent largely in search of sublime vistas (Kremer 1990, xxv). Aesthetic concerns like these and the relationship of science to art figured prominently as themes in his popular scientific lectures (Hatfield 1993).

In this cultured and domestic Biedemeier world Helmholtz met and courted Olga von Velten. The surviving letters from the courtship paint an amusing and often touching portrait of a shy young man so extravagantly in love that no cliche could be too syrupy for the object of his affection (Kremer 1990). Before her death von Velten acted frequently as a research assistant and sometimes as a subject in perception experiments, much to the envy of her husband's scientist-friends. Domestic affairs and the well-being of family members figure large in Helmholtz's correspondence with his intimate friends such as du Bois-Reymond and Brücke, and are prominent in his correspondence with scientific acquaintances such as Frans Donders and A. W. Volkmann (Donders 1856–88; Volkmann 1856–71).

At odds with the Olympian image, Helmholtz also reveals himself, as Richard Kremer has noted, to be an ambitious man who knew his own value and gave serious thought to the techniques of career building (Kremer 1990, xix–xxvi). In the 1840s scientific fame offered Helmholtz the only avenue out of the military, and he self-consciously pursued it as such, just as in the 1850s he publicized the newly invented ophthalmoscope widely and took it on tour among physiologists and ophthalmologists to ensure it the maximum impact. Later, at the peak of his fame, he proved a tough negotiator for those who wanted his services, and was especially given to extravagant salary demands (Cahan 1989, 68–69).

Neither Helmholtz's public statements nor his private correspondence make much reference to political matters, although some evidence suggests that he did not wholly escape the revolutionary enthusiasm of 1848 (Königsberger 1902–3, 2:76; Kremer 1990, xvi–xviii).[3] A reputation for political reliability seems to have enhanced the patronage he enjoyed in the Prussian Ministry of Education and, on at least one occasion, led to his preferment over politically suspect rivals. The political inclinations of the mature Helmholtz leaned toward the "mandarin" position sketched by historian Fritz Ringer as typical of Prussian intellectuals in the Wilhelmine era: mildly liberal (in the sense of German *Bildungsliberalismus*), simultaneously nationalistic and monarchical, and distinctly scornful of party politics. Also like Ringer's mandarins, Helmholtz saw German preeminence in science and scholarship as a vital part of Germany's cultural mission (Ringer 1969, 15–42, 102–27; Cahan 1993c). Unlike those intellectuals Ringer studied, most of whom were humanists and social scientists, Helmholtz was no opponent of industrialization or technological change. Still, Helmholtz's commitment to the conservative ideals of the *Kulturstaat* can be seen in his defense of the classical and Real-gymnasium against modernist reformers (Pyenson 1983, 38–51). It also revealed itself in the pure scientific and precision-technological orientation that Helmholtz (and Siemens) imposed upon their Physikalisch-technische Reichsanstalt, an orientation German engineering associations and some branches of German industry vigorously opposed (Cahan 1989, 45–58).

Helmholtz's life, of course, was dominated by his work. His correspondence with his professional friends abounds with appointment intrigues, complaints about administrative burdens, and professional gossip. The central themes of that correspondence, however, are papers exchanged, differences tentatively and cautiously explored, and bare progress reports of research projects begun, completed, frustrated, or newly published—in short, science as production, work, and career. With some exceptions Helmholtz seems not to have discussed the details of his research in physiological optics with his scientific friends, nor used them as sounding boards for his views on theoretical issues and controversies. Although he later suffered badly from migraines and tension due to overwork, the correspondence gives little indication of angst, or of spiritual or philosophical quandaries. The Olympian stereotype was not entirely false.

INTELLECTUAL COMMITMENTS

The range of Helmholtz's intellectual interests is reflected in a remark to his father from 1839, that during a break from medical studies he was "filling in the time" by reading Homer, Byron, Biot, and Kant (Cahan 1993a, 55–56 [no. 8]). His reference to Biot recalls Königsberger's claim that Helmholtz pursued the extracurricular study of physics and analytical mechanics all through his years in medical school. The reference to Kant recalls the significant philosophical influences that acted on the young Helmholtz. Immanuel Hermann Fichte, the son of Johann Gottlieb Fichte, was a close friend of Helmholtz's father and perhaps a source of Helmholtz's attested interest in the thought of the elder Fichte and Kant. Later historians of philosophy tended to group Fichte, Schelling, and Hegel as subjective idealists against Kant and the critical philosophy. In the 1840s and 1850s, however, it was more common to stress the similarities between Kant and Fichte and to set them apart from the idealism of Schelling and Hegel (Köhnke 1986, 90–104, 151–57). Helmholtz was also influenced by the "psychological readings" of Kant, which were prominent in the period. These conceived the categories of the understanding as "faculties" and drew pregnant parallels between the manner in which the categories determine possible experience and how specific nerve energies determine our possible sensation and perception.[4] Both were important to Helmholtz's thought and figure prominently in the epistemological implications of his sensory physiology that he began to develop in the 1850s.

As Helmholtz fell increasingly under the sway of du Bois-Reymond, Brücke, and Carl Ludwig, he became more and more committed to their program to reform contemporary physiology in the direction of an "organic physics." This program had two explicit tenets: philosophically, to reject all belief in, and explanatory appeals to, "vital forces" within the living organism; and, methodologically, to recreate physiology as an experimental science dependent upon the investigatory techniques of physics and chemistry. The program radically deemphasized the significance of developmental questions in physiology (Caneva 1993). Its advocates contrasted organic physics to two alleged varieties of traditional physiology that they opposed. One variety they described in stereotypical terms as a speculative and idealistic physiology still under the influence of *Naturphilosophie*; the other, as an archaic, descriptive, natural-historical approach based on morphology and anatomy. Historians of science have become increasingly aware that the program of organic physics, despite its rhetorical successes, was but one of several methodological streams competing for prominence in German physiology between 1850 and 1865.[5] Helmholtz's espousal of that program was not independent of his academic ambitions, for organic physics was the most self-conscious and best publicized methodological current in a science on the brink of rapid institutional expansion (Ben-David 1960; Ben-David and Zloczower 1962; Zloczower 1972).

THE HUNTING OF THE HOROPTER

Several factors motivated the gradual shift of Helmholtz's research interests from nerve and muscle physiology to sensory perception during his Königsberg years. In Königsberg he found himself out of the immediate orbit of his friend du Bois-Reymond, who had first interested him in nerve and muscle physiology. He was obliged to lecture regularly there on sensory physiology, and so was introduced to the field and its problems. His decision in 1852 to attack Brewster's triple-spectrum theory of colored light probably did not originally represent a decision to embark upon a major program to investigate the perception of light and color. Once begun, however, the work led Helmholtz to the vexed problems of simultaneous contrast, to the experimental determination of complementaries that would test Newton's theory and Young's hypothesis, and to the correction of his earlier work in the face of criticisms by Grassmann (see Chapter Six).

At least as important as these factors was his invention—almost by chance as he described it—of the ophthalmoscope. Not only did this instrument bring him instant fame and professional credibility in medical circles; it also led him immediately to a pivotal discovery. In June 1851 Helmholtz announced excitedly to du Bois-Reymond that with the help of the instrument he had shown that the optic nerve itself, exposed at the point where it enters the retinal wall, is insensitive to light (Kirsten 1986, 115, no. 27). In his treatise on the ophthalmoscope he called this "an important physiological consequence" and a "paradox" since other kinds of stimuli such as pressure and electrical current readily excite the optic nerve (*WAH* 2:229–60, no. 14). The relevance of these facts to Johannes Müller's law of specific nerve energies and the epistemological questions they raised held center stage in the popular lecture, "Ueber die Natur der menschlichen Sinnesempfindungen," which Helmholtz delivered the following year (*WAH* 2:591–609, no. 20). The observation piqued Helmholtz's interest in sensory processes and further sharpened his conviction that the sensory nerves played merely passive roles in perception and act only to transmit a physiological stimulus between the end organs and the sensorium.

All through the early 1850s Helmholtz's letters to du Bois-Reymond refer disparagingly to his work on physiological optics and visual perception, perhaps to reassure his friend that he had not wavered from their common commitment to studying electrical action in nerves and muscles. In the spring of 1853, however, Helmholtz agreed to prepare a major survey of physiological optics to be part of the multivolume *Allgemeine Encyclopädie der Physik*, edited by his former acquaintance from Berlin, Gustav Karsten (Karsten 1851–53, no. 3 [6.2.1853]). That survey became the *Handbuch der Physiologischen Optik*, and Helmholtz's commitment to it signaled publicly that physiological optics and sensory perception had become his main research focus. The first volume of the survey, published from Bonn in 1856, dealt with the anatomy and dioptrics of the eye. The second volume, delayed by Helmholtz's move to Heidelberg and the death of Olga von Velten, appeared in 1860. It dealt with the sensations of light: color vision, afterimages, adaptation, and contrast. Helmholtz may have originally intended to produce only two volumes, but after a considerable delay he published a third on the issue of spatial perception in 1866, and reissued the entire set with minor additions in 1867. Each volume was preceded by published articles in which Helmholtz announced new results from his research; these results were then incorporated in more detailed and synthetic form into the *Handbuch*.

By 1860 Helmholtz had become the foremost German authority on physiological optics, but he had written little to that point on the problems of binocularity and depth perception and still seemed unaware of the controversies and complexities that surrounded them. His popular lectures of 1852 and 1855, as well as shorter scientific papers on stereoscopic luster and the binocular instrument he called the "telestereoscope," had treated the topics of stereopsis and visual space as largely unproblematic (*VuR* 1:85–117; *WAH* 2:591–609, no. 20; 2:484–91, no. 50; 3:4–6, no. 41; cf. Kirsten 1986, 173, no. 63). They contained, for example, little about the nature and origin of the retinal correspondence, differences between two- and three-dimensional spatial perception, or relative versus absolute distance localization.

These papers from the mid-1850s do show, however, that Helmholtz already thought of the processes of vision in inferential and constructivist terms. Gently pressing on the temporal side of the eyeball produces a pressure phosphene, which is nevertheless perceived on the *nasal* side of the visual field. Why? Because long visual experience has taught us that objects, the light from which images on the temporal side of the retina, are always located in external space on the nasal side of the visual field. When we experience retinal stimulation on the temporal side, we *infer* from that stimulation (falsely, in this case, since the stimulation arises from pressure and not from light) the existence of an object on the nasal side. We project (*verlegen*) the visual sensation outward in that direction on the visual field. Helmholtz thus argued that the perception of direction is achieved through a sequence of inferential judgments, which, though built up from visual experience, are nevertheless unconscious and usually impervious to control by the will (*VuR* 1:101, 110). As to the perception of relief, "we continually construct for ourselves the spatial relationships of the objects around us out of the two different perspective views of them, which come from both our eyes" (p. 105). Views like these, however, were common at the time, and they scarcely bore upon the truly controversial issues in binocular vision.

Helmholtz's commitment to Karsten's encyclopedia project determined the general nature as well as the timing of his work on physiological optics. It compelled him to undertake a synthesis of the entire field and to dedicate himself to the problems already established by his contemporaries as the most salient. His personal research into stereoscopic vision and depth perception seems to have begun in the early 1860s, just when the volume sequence of the *Handbuch* dictated. He quickly found himself immersed with his contemporaries in the controversies and uncertainties sketched in the previous chapter.

In turning to the third volume, Helmholtz started with the question of the horopter, a problem to which his mathematical skill naturally inclined him. A brief preliminary treatment, published in 1862, suggests that the horopter problem was then rather new to Helmholtz (*WAH*

2:420–26, no. 75). It analyzed only the simpler special cases, and in terminology and line of attack closely followed previous treatments by Wilhelm Wundt, then Helmholtz's assistant at Heidelberg.

During the next two years, however, the complexity of the problem was brought fully home to Helmholtz (*WAH* 2:427–78, no. 85). Sometime in 1863 he learned of the so-called retinal incongruity, a phenomenon discovered almost simultaneously by Recklinghausen, Meissner, and Volkmann. Imagine the eyes in the primary position, with the left eye closed and the right eye fixated on the midpoint of a physically vertical straight line drawn in the median plane of the body. Curiously, for eyes that show retinal incongruity, that line will not *appear* to be vertical, but instead will seem to be rotated slightly counterclockwise by a degree or so around its midpoint. The same line, viewed with the left eye, will appear rotated slightly clockwise by roughly the same amount. When the line is viewed with both eyes, the monocular effects cancel out, although the extremities of the line may be seen in double images. All this means that the retinal meridians that are physically vertical when the eye is in the primary position are not those on which external lines must image if they are to appear vertical; we must locate corresponding *apparent vertical meridians*, which when stimulated give the appearance of verticality.

Now the retinal incongruity might plausibly be explained as arising from very small, equal, and opposite cyclorotations of the eyes about the lines of sight. In that case, there should be a similar incongruity between the physically horizontal and the apparent horizontal retinal meridians, just as between the vertical ones. Volkmann and Hering, both formidable observers, claimed to have detected precisely this effect. But Helmholtz, on the basis of his own experiments, concluded that retinal incongruity exists only for vertical meridians and dismissed incongruities of the horizontal meridians as a different and secondary effect, induced by eye fatigue and a rolling of the eye in consequence of it. Retinal incongruity, he decided, indicates that the pattern of corresponding retinal points is different from that traditionally assumed. Figure 3.1a is a heuristic representation of the pattern of corresponding meridians that had been traditionally assumed (the figure ignores projective distortions). Helmholtz concluded that the correct pattern of corresponding points must be like Figure 3.1b, where *ab* and *a'b'* constitute the apparent vertical meridians.

This new assumption about the pattern of corresponding points necessitated a new mathematical attack upon the horopter problem, which Helmholtz published in 1864. There he introduced a new coordinate system based upon angles of longitude and latitude, measured from the horizontal and apparent vertical meridians (as defined with the eye in the primary position and subsequently assumed to move with the eyeball) (*WAH* 2:427–77, no. 85). He derived the point-horopter by finding the

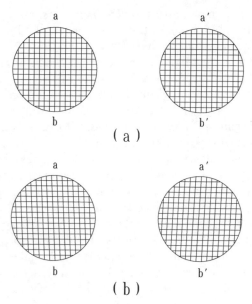

Fig. 3.1 Schematic representation of the
pattern of corresponding retinal meridians,
eyes in the primary position, (a) as
traditionally assumed and as accepted by
Hering, (b) as deduced by Helmholtz from
the retinal incongruity. *Source*: Turner
1993a. Reproduced with permission of the
University of California Press.

locus of points at which, for a given set of the eyes, the latitude and longitude have the same value in each eye. The locus of points for which the
latitudes and longitudes *respectively* have the same value in each eye constitute so-called partial or line-horopters. Here Helmholtz deduced the
most general form of the point-horopter as a curve of fourth degree, but
he devoted most of his analysis to special cases. The 1864 derivation re-
appeared, expanded and slightly corrected, in the *Handbuch* of 1866
(*PO5* 3:421–29, 467–83).

By 1864 Helmholtz had learned that the real pitfalls of the horopter
problem had nothing to do with mathematics. He struggled to purge his
horopter discussion of phraseology that could be taken as asserting
claims about the physiology of the retina. Entities such as retinal horizons, apparent vertical meridians, and corresponding points can be understood as characteristics of external visual fields and need not be understood as characteristics of the retina itself. Hence, he wrote, "it matters
not for visual perception . . . , what distortions the images undergo on the

retina, so long as these distortions remain constant one's entire life through" (*WAH* 2:435, no. 85). But if the horopter had no explicit physiological significance, did it have any significance at all? By now Helmholtz was well aware of contemporary skepticism on this question, and a major object of his 1864 paper was to salvage the horopter problem, which he had so elegantly solved, as a meaningful one in the study of vision.

Helmholtz began, as other writers had, by dismissing several traditional definitions of the horopter. First, it cannot be the locus of points seen single in binocular vision, for small objects near but not on the horopter line are also seen single (p. 452). Second, the horopter cannot usefully be determined through experiment and defined as an empirical locus of single vision. Despite the efforts of Meissner and others, individual differences in the ability to resolve fused images into double images make the experimental approach fruitless. Finally, the horopter cannot be the locus onto which we project monocular half-images, as Nagel had suggested. Half-images are, in fact, seen at the distance of the object that cast them, Helmholtz asserted, and he introduced several experiments to support that claim.

Helmholtz then introduced an entirely new principle on which to define the horopter and illustrated it with the experiment shown in Figure 3.2. Here three needles are placed vertically into a small wooden block, not in a straight line but along a cylindrical surface of large curvature.

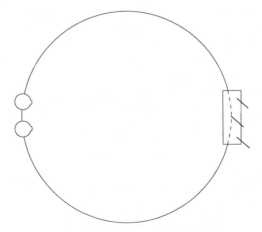

Fig. 3.2 Helmholtz's demonstration of 1863 that the horopter is the region in which perception of relief is most acute (not to scale).
Source: Turner 1993a. Reproduced with permission of the University of California Press.

In Figure 3.2 the eyes are fixated on the center needle; the circle through the eyes and that needle will be part of the mathematical horopter. When the three needles are situated as shown, or anywhere on or near the horopter curve, Helmholtz announced, the eyes show an exquisite ability to judge the three-dimensional relief of the needles. They can, for example, readily judge whether the base is oriented so that the needles present a concave or convex surface. But when the base is displaced even slightly from the horopter locus, the accuracy of judgment falls off rapidly. Therefore the horopter must be understood in a new way, as the locus of points in space around which the perception of relief is most acute.

In describing this experiment in 1864, Helmholtz offered his readers a warning. If the outer needles are spaced too far from the inner one, then what he referred to as a "peculiar visual illusion" spoils the outcome: if the three needles are arranged such that they lie precisely along the horopter curve, then they appear (falsely) to lie in a straight line; if they are arranged in a straight line, the line appears convex, and if objectively convex, more convex than it really is (pp. 448–54). Helmholtz was soon to regret this passing claim about what obviously seemed to him to be a curious but minor phenomenon.

Helmholtz also claimed to have found a further remarkable property of the horopter locus. Consider the special case when the visual plane is horizontal and the eyes are fixated on an infinitely distant point in the median plane. Helmholtz's mathematical derivation showed that the horopter then becomes a plane, parallel to and below the visual plane. Specifically, that horopter plane passes through the point formed by the imagined extensions of the apparent vertical meridians of the two retinas. Now a divergence of 2 degrees, 26 minutes, which Helmholtz measured for his own eyes, put that point of intersection 1660 mm below the level of his eyes, a figure that corresponded closely to Helmholtz's height. The horopter plane, for this special setting of the eyes, corresponds to the plane of the ground.

Helmholtz found great significance in this fact and elaborated it in a long and enthusiastic discussion. He took it as a general rule that an individual's retinal incongruence will be correlated with his or her height, so that with forward-directed, parallel lines of sight the horopter plane will correspond with the ground. This relationship held true, he insisted, for his own children, aged ten and thirteen. The correspondence of the horopter plane and the ground means that when we look at a distant horizon the landscape appears before us with great detail, expanse, and depth. It means that when we walk along with eyes fixed straight ahead, we are maximally equipped to perceive small obstacles or irregularities on the ground ahead of us without glancing at them. When we gaze into the distance with our eyes inverted, as when we look between our legs or invert our head under our arms, the landscape appears flat, constrained, and poor in detail. The same occurs when we view a landscape through inverting prisms, except that low-flying clouds, which then correspond to the horopter plane, are now invested with unexpectedly rich depth and detail. All these claims Helmholtz buttressed with lyrical descriptions of his observations on landscapes and cliffs during walks along the Nekkar and around Heidelberg. His discussion juxtaposed mathematical calculation and theoretical virtuosity with a rich sensitivity to the aesthetic and scientific significance of common visual experience. It also invested the arid and abstract horopter problem with a perceptual significance contemporaries had scarcely suspected it contained. At least temporarily, the horopter problem was saved.

THE DEFENSE OF LISTING

Useful solutions to the horopter problem require assumptions about the degree of torsion present in the eyes for particular angles of elevation and rotation of the lines of sight. Helmholtz therefore tackled the problem of eye movements simultaneously with that of the horopter. He reported his preliminary results to the Naturhistorisch-medizinischer Verein in Heidelberg in 1863 (*WAH* 2:352–59, no. 77), and his major treatment, which was reproduced almost unchanged in the *Handbuch*, appeared in Graefe's *Archiv für Ophthalmologie* the same year (WAH 2:361–419, no. 78). Each treatment shows Helmholtz attempting to synthesize and impose order upon a complex field.

Helmholtz claimed that the current, "rather confused state" of the problem of eye movements resulted from the absence of any widely accepted principle of precisely *how* the eyes move and the lack of clear analysis of the functional principles behind eye movements (p. 360). To meet the former need Helmholtz came forward to champion Listing's rule. That rule, discussed in Chapter Two, held that the eyes move from the primary position as if they had rotated around an axis that is perpendicular to the initial and final positions of the lines of sight. Physiologically complex though kinematically simple, rotations around Listing axes cause the eye to move without undergoing any cyclorotation or true torsional movement around the line of sight.

Helmholtz knew that Listing's hypothesis could be experimentally tested most directly by moving the eye successively from its primary position to various so-called tertiary positions away from the center of the field, mathematically deducing the theoretical angle of torsion predicted by Listing's rule for these tertiary positions, and then comparing these to observations made on the inclination of afterimages. Meissner and

Wundt had followed this involved strategy, however, and had obtained disconfirming results (Meissner 1854; Wundt 1862a, 4:138–41). Helmholtz therefore turned to a new experimental approach, and offered the following ingenious if indirect and heuristic proof.

He sat with his eyes in the primary position, before an orthogonal grid of vertical and horizontal lines mounted on the opposite wall (see Figure 3.3). He stared at two crossed, colored ribbons, so as to imprint the afterimage of a right-angled cross on his retina. When he shifted his gaze vertically or horizontally along the lines of the wall grid, that is, to any so-called secondary position, the arms of the afterimage cross remained horizontal and vertical and right-angled. But when Helmholtz shifted his gaze directly from *P* to a tertiary position in the upper right-hand quadrant of the wall grid (say to point *T* in Figure 3.3), the arms of the afterimage cross were observed no longer to lie at right angles, but rather to have undergone the opposed rotations illustrated in Figure 3.3.

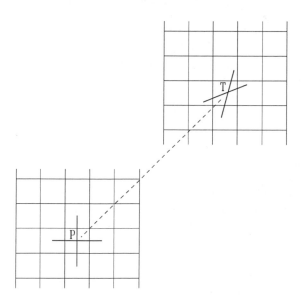

Fig. 3.3 Schematic illustration of Helmholtz's afterimage experiment of 1863 confirming Listing's law of eye movements. *Source*: Turner 1993a. Reproduced with permission of the University of California Press.

Now at least three factors can be thought of as possibly contributing to this result: (1) projective distortions of the grid upon the retina, combined with our subjective tendency to accept the grid lines as horizontal and vertical; (2) changes in the angle of torsion not involving a cyclorotation; and (3) changes in the angle of torsion arising from a possible cyclorotation.[6] The effect is, in fact, quite complicated, and Helmholtz never attempted to analyze the separate contributions directly. He rather negated any contribution of the first factor by rotating the ribbons and the grid pattern on the wall, so that their formerly horizontal components lay parallel to the direction of the line *PT*. Now when the afterimage was imprinted with the gaze at *P*, and the gaze then moved to *T*, the arms of the (oblique) afterimage cross were seen to undergo no distortion at all! The cross remained right-angled, and its two components continued parallel and perpendicular to the lines of the grid. This remarkable behavior of the afterimage is only possible, Helmholtz reasoned, if in both cases the eye has carried out its rotation from *P* to *T* along an axis of rotation perpendicular to the plane that includes the initial and final lines of sight to *P* and to *T* (*WAH* 2:360–419, no. 78; *PO5* 3:44–51). But this is the condition of rotation proposed by Listing, and Helmholtz promptly elevated Listing's proposal to the status of Listing's law.

Helmholtz not only set out to establish Listing's law in 1863, but also to show its significance in light of a functional principle that he introduced and named the principle of easiest orientation. First, he considered the functional significance of Donders' law for vision. Suppose we glance at an object and look away, and then glance back at it and find it has undergone an apparent rotation. If Donders' law were not in effect, then we would be unable to judge whether the rotation were a true rotation of the object or resulted merely from a different torsional setting of our eyes between the first and second glance. Helmholtz argued that the eye's mind, in order to avoid this confusion, learns to control the eye's torsional movements so that particular torsional settings are associated with particular tertiary positions. Similarly it learns through experience what retinal meridian to regard as vertical at each of these positions. The eye therefore *acquires* its obedience to Listing's law, in conformity with the functional principle of easiest orientation.

The principle has an obvious extension. Suppose we move the gaze from point *P* to point *P'* and want to be sure that during the motion other objects seen indirectly in the visual field undergo no subjective rotation or distortion. The condition for this is that all such points in the visual field should seem to move parallel to the line of motion of the point of fixation as it travels from *P* to *P'*. The main kinematic condition for this parallel displacement is that the rotation be carried out about a Listing axis.

Unfortunately, as Helmholtz pointed out, all eye movements cannot be carried out so that they simultaneously preserve parallel displacements *and* obey Donders' law. The gaze can always be moved from any point *A* to any point *B* by rotation around a Listing axis, and this is the rotation that will minimize departures from parallel displacement of image points. It can similarly be moved from any point C to the point B by rotation around a Listing axis. The problem is that if A and C are different points (reflecting different initial orientations of the eyeball), then the two Listing rotations *must* leave the eye with different angles of torsion at point C, and this is not permitted by Donders' law. If Donders' law is to be obeyed, then at least one of these movements must be carried out about a non-Listing axis, and so must be accompanied by some degree of cyclorotation around the line of sight and some subjective distortion in the orientation of objects seen indirectly in the visual field.

Helmholtz then set out to deduce analytically how the eye must move in order that Donders' law be consistently obeyed and departures from Listing rotation minimized, since they cannot be wholly avoided. He expressed analytically the component of the rotation that lies along the line perpendicular to the plane of all possible Listing axes connected with that position—this line will normally be the line of vision—and treated this component as an "error." Using analytic techniques he determined the principles of rotation to which the eye must conform when the squares of the "errors" are minimized. Subject to a series of highly artificial assumptions—which Hering lost no time in pointing out—this formidable mathematical analysis yielded two results. First, the minimization condition guaranteed that from one privileged position at the center of the visual field the eye must make only Listing rotations. Helmholtz defined that position henceforth as the primary position of the eye. Second, the condition specified how the axes are to be defined around which non-Listing rotations from secondary and tertiary positions must be carried out, if Donders' law is to be obeyed and the amount of cyclorotation minimized (*WAH* 2:360–419, no. 77; *POS* 3:62–71, 85–100). Helmholtz had ostensibly deduced Listing's law as well as Donders' law from his principle of easiest orientation.

Helmholtz's analytical deduction of Listing's law did not escape criticism after 1863. Probably few contemporaries fully understood it. Hering, who did understand it, criticized it as artificial and based on questionable premises, and he argued that Listing's law could be deduced more easily from functional principles other than that of easiest orientation (Hering 1864a[25], 245–83). On the other hand, most practitioners readily accepted Helmholtz's experimental demonstration of Listing's law; even Hering called the demonstration elegant and decisive, though lacking in precision (pp. 249–50). Establishment of the law constituted another in the sequence of developments that integrated the formerly incoherent field of vision studies and provided a new basis for its practice; the law played a paradigmatic role in the continuing tradition of research into eye motions during the 1860s and 1870s. Despite the fact that his experimental demonstration was indirect and heuristic, Helmholtz had managed quickly and decisively to quiet the doubts about Listing's law that prevailed among specialists during the 1860s; how he did so reveals much about his particular style of scientific argument.

First, Helmholtz had been at pains to discredit gently the observations by which Wundt and others had cast doubt upon Listing's law. He rejected methods of observing the eye movements by use of the blind spot or double images out of hand as insufficiently accurate. He claimed that even methods based on observing afterimages are subject to serious distortions unless the head is kept absolutely still and unless the primary position of the eyes is precisely identified and used as the origin of every movement. To remedy the first problem, Helmholtz introduced a simple bite-bar device, later a staple item in psychological experimentation. To remedy the second problem, he attached projecting arms to the bite-bar apparatus, so that when the eyes fixated on the distant wall grid, attachments on the arms would be seen in double images. When the eyes were shifted away from the center and then brought back to it, the original orientation of the head with respect to the grid and the center point of the field could be recalled with great accuracy by realigning the two double images with the horizontal line of the grid in the center of the field. Helmholtz cautioned that unless such precautions were observed, fatigue would induce extra torsional effects and invalidate the observations. Helmholtz did not try to prove that the observations of his rivals were faulty; his argumentative strategy merely required casting plausible doubt upon them, in part by introducing instrumental safeguards against error that his rivals had failed to utilize.

Helmholtz's treatment of the primary position was much more subtle. Before Helmholtz the primary position had been defined differently by different observers (as the center of the visual field, as the natural position assumed by the eyes for distant vision straight ahead, as the position at which the ocular muscles are maximally relaxed). Meissner had even assumed the primary position to be slightly convergent. Helmholtz tacitly redefined it as the position (assuming parallel lines of sight) out of which movements to secondary positions (horizontal or vertical movements) will produce no distortion of the afterimage. That position must first be precisely established by every individual observer and fixed by exact adjustment of the bite-bar apparatus and the double images it creates. Only then can the observer proceed to confirm Listing's law for tertiary eye positions. What Helmholtz really demonstrated, therefore, was that there exists one set of the eyes from which eye movements will conform to Listing's law. He then defined that set as the primary position, even if it failed to meet more traditional criteria for the appellation. Helmholtz imposed order upon confusion by fiat and convention as well as by empirical demonstration.

The conventional nature of Helmholtz's achievement shows itself in one further way. Shortly after Helmholtz had established Listing's law, Volkmann showed that raising or lowering the visual plane (with parallel lines of sight), or performing convergent eye movements, produces torsional movements in the eyes radically at variance with Listing's predictions. Volkmann's letters to Helmholtz make clear that he initially regarded these observations as so restricting the generality of Listing's law as to essentially refute it altogether (Volkmann 1856–71, no. 8 [1.10.1864], no. 11 [14.12.1864]). Helmholtz, however, always regarded these movements as secondary effects imposed upon the eye's basic conformity to Listing's law and in no way impugning its validity in what he regarded as the normal case. Indeed, Helmholtz always saw a deep functional importance in Listing's law and was reluctant to admit departures from it. Forced to consider convergent eye positions in the *Handbuch*, Helmholtz and his assistants consistently reported deviations from Listing's law more than nine times smaller than those detected by so reliable an observer as Volkmann (*PO5* 3:37–126, esp. 52). Hering followed Helmholtz in treating Listing's law as the baseline expectation about eye movements from which deviations were to be measured. But he, too, found deviations greater than those Helmholtz could comfortably countenance, and this was to be one more element in the confrontation between them that was already looming in 1863.

CHAPTER FOUR

Hering on Spatial Perception

As A PHYSIOLOGIST Helmholtz awed his contemporaries with his mastery of physical and mathematical techniques, skills nowhere more impressively displayed than in his analytic derivation of Listing's law and the horopter. Hence contemporaries' surprise when in 1863 an unknown young physiologist from Leipzig published a horopter derivation fully as rigorous and general as that of Helmholtz's (Hering 1863a[25], 1864a[25]). Ewald Hering not only independently duplicated Helmholtz's achievement, but also used a new and different mathematical approach (the projective geometry recently developed by Jakob Steiner at Berlin) and had the audacity to criticize Helmholtz and hold his errors up for ridicule (Hering 1865a[25]).

EWALD HERING

Less is known about Ewald Hering than about his more famous rival. Few private papers have survived to supplement the limited biographical information provided in official sources and obituaries by his students.[1] Those sources say that Hering was born in the village of Altgersdorf in Saxony, the son of a rural Lutheran pastor. The family was probably poor, but the financial assistance traditionally available to the sons of clergy would have made it possible for Hering to attend the gymnasium in Zittau and to enter the University of Leipzig in 1853. There, according to reports, he was attracted to zoology and to philosophy and studied medicine as a *Brotstudium*, completing the M.D. degree in 1860. Little is known about his long student years, except that he spent the winter of 1858–59 in Sicily with the elderly Leipzig professor J. V. Carus. There he prepared a dissertation on the genital and excretory organs of *Alciopida*, a genus of ringed worms.

Between 1860 and 1865 Hering practiced as a private physician in Leipzig, serving part of that time as an assistant in a clinic run by internist Ernst Wagner. The obituaries refer to financial hardship during this period, and certainly Hering was scarcely devoting all his time to practice. In 1862 he became privatdozent in physiology at the university, a teaching post that entitled the holder to lecture fees but no salary. In 1863 he married Maria Antonie Lincke (born 1838), and they had a son, Heinrich Ewald Hering (1866–1948). Hering's earliest scientific work dates from this period; he published the five installments of his *Beiträge zur Physiologie*, which dealt with binocular vision and depth perception, between 1861 and 1864; installments three and four contained his horopter derivation. Hering later quipped that he had turned to this line of research "because it was cheap," meaning that it required practically no resources or apparatus (Tschermak-Seysenegg 1934, 1231).

Through the patronage of two prominent ophthalmologists, Hering in 1865 was appointed professor of physiology at the Military Medico-Surgical Academy in Vienna, the so-called Josephinum, a post just abandoned by Carl Ludwig. In the five busy years Hering spent in Vienna, he continued to publish on binocular vision and investigated the comparative anatomy of the mammalian liver. In 1868 he and his student Josef Breuer demonstrated the "self-regulation" of the respiratory function. They showed that artificially inflating the lungs of curarized animals triggered receptors that transmitted a nervous impulse to the respiratory center in the brain via the vagus nerve. These impulses induced expiration, and the emptying of the lungs in turn triggered inspiration as a similar reflex action. In other work Hering showed that inflation of the lungs accelerated the activity of the heart and also stimulated the vasoconstriction centers of the brain, giving rise to the so-called Traube–Hering pressure waves in the blood and explaining their correlation with respiration.

In 1870 the Josephinum was abolished, and Hering was called to be the successor to Jan Evangelista Purkinje at the University of Prague, where he worked for twenty-five years. There he developed and published his opponent process theory of color vision and light perception (1874–76), extended the same explanatory scheme to the temperature sense (1875), and tenaciously defended and further developed his whole theory of visual perception in a long series of papers and polemical exchanges. From the late 1870s to the mid-1880s Hering studied the electrical action of nerves and muscles. In 1884 he claimed to have discovered a positive afterpotential in nerves, an assertion opposed by du Bois-Reymond in a sharp exchange. At Prague Hering operated a very successful institute, which attracted students of physiology and ophthalmology from all over Central Europe, although primarily from the Austro-Hungarian empire and Russia.

The Prague years also saw Hering active as a public figure. In the 1870s the university in Prague became the focus of bitter nationalistic disputes over the language of instruction. The university had traditionally been German, but as lectures were increasingly offered in Czech, the German minority began to fear for the institution's German character. Hering led the public defense, becoming "the most hated by the Czechs of all the

German professors" and, according to one source, was "primarily to thank" for the creation of a new and separate German university in Prague in 1882, a university of which Hering became the first rector (Garten 1918, 510; Koertling 1968, 15–32, 118–19).

In 1895 Hering was called to succeed Karl Ludwig at the University of Leipzig. He had already turned down a call to the new imperial university at Strassburg in 1872, and the Leipzig chair was among the most prestigious in Europe. Already sixty-one when he went there, Hering was less productive during the Leipzig years and trained fewer important students, but he continued to defend and refine his theory of vision. At Leipzig, as he had done at Prague in the 1880s, he developed in popular lectures the philosophy of biology evident in his scientific works from the 1860s. Hering retired in 1915 at the age of eighty and died from tuberculosis in 1918, still busily writing on physiological optics until the end.

Sketchy as are the facts about Hering's career, strong conclusions can still be drawn about the individual behind that career. The harmony, balance, and magisterial calm that marked Helmholtz's writing were opposed on Hering's side by a tortured, vitriolic, argumentative prose, which lost nothing in rhetorical or logical potency for seeming to flow straight from the depths of his personality. His students remembered him as a modest and unpretentious man, solicitous about their well-being and tirelessly involved in their research and its presentation. One also remembered Hering as he appears in his scientific papers: a rigid individual, ready to explode at any offense real or imagined, and implacable in the pursuit of those who had given offense (Garten 1918, 522).

Hering's self-assumed role as the anti-Helmholtz invite comparisons between the two men. Helmholtz's social roots lay in the *Oberlehrerschicht*, a rising element that had harnessed its social identity and ambitions to the lofty ideals of Prussian neohumanism. Hering came from the lesser Lutheran pastorate, the most marginal group among the *Gebildete*, and a group whose upwardly mobile sons had for centuries struggled to reconcile their social aspirations with their sense of religious duty and their desperate inner need for calling (La Vopa 1988, 326–40). This background may explain the stern, implacable sense of righteousness—sometimes leavened by sardonic humor—with which Hering fought his particular wars of truth. So formidable and ready a polemicist was he that he inspired real fear among the scientists of his day, and few who challenged him came out unscarred.

Hering's intellectual formation also invites comparison to that of Helmholtz. Both were influenced by Johannes Müller—Helmholtz as student and protégé, Hering as intellectual disciple. Hering liked to portray his theory of spatial perception as a logical extension of Müller's own approach to the problem. He would later attack Helmholtz and du Bois-

Reymond for perverting Müller's doctrine of specific nerve energies and for abandoning Müller's view of life as an autonomous, holistic, self-regulating process.

If Berlin during the 1840s was one cradle of organic physics and quantitative physiological experimentation, then the University of Leipzig was another. There physiologist E. H. Weber analyzed the mechanics of the blood circulatory system, studied the nature of the pulse wave in the arteries, and discovered the inhibitory action of the vagus nerve upon the heartbeat. In sensory physiology Weber's famous study of the tactile sensation introduced the crucial concepts of the threshold and the just-noticeable-difference and pioneered the techniques of quantitative investigation of perception (Kruta 1976, 199–201). Hering's own research faithfully pushed forward exactly those lines of investigation pursued by his mentor.

No less important to Hering was Leipzig physicist Gustav Theodor Fechner. Fechner created and named the field of "psychophysics," which attempted to study the quantitative relationship between sensation and stimulus intensity. Fechner developed many of the methods that soon became fundamental to experimental psychology, and published the so-called Weber–Fechner law, which sets sensation proportional to the logarithm of the stimulus, the stimulus measured in just-noticeable-differences of intensity (Jaynes 1971; Boring 1942, 34–45; Brozek and Gundlach 1987). By the 1870s Weber and Fechner were reckoned among the founders of experimental psychology, and Fechner's psychophysical law greatly influenced both Helmholtz and Hering. In 1876 Hering argued that Fechner's law should be replaced by a linear formula relating sensation and stimulus, but even in doing so he proudly acknowledged himself a student of Fechner's and claimed that "my conception of the functional relationship between body and soul stands in better agreement with the philosophy of Fechner than his own psychophysical law" (Hering 1876, 310; Turner 1987b, 145–49).

What was that "conception of the functional relationship between body and soul"? Late in his career Hering claimed that his life's work had flowed from a single doctrine: that the sensory and motor processes are products of a long evolutionary development. He had, Hering insisted, read Lamarck and become convinced of the theory of descent long before the doctrine had appeared in its Darwinian form. Far from contradicting one another, Lamarck and Darwin represented the two halves of a stereogram: different from each other, yet capable of being fused into the perception of a third dimension absent from either alone (Hering 1906). To Hering, the parallelism of those doctrines—Darwinism representing the physical and material in biological development, Lamarckism the role of perception and intentionality—reflected the similar parallelism upon which Fechner had erected his doctrine of psychophysics. On the one hand life consists of material changes in the body, on the other the phenomena of consciousness; each realm is a function of the other, but neither can be taken as more real or more directly causal (Hering 1902/1870, 5). In a famous lecture of 1870, Hering set out to blur the line between these parallel realms. He refused to distinguish between the conscious "memory" of daily life, and the phylogenetic "memory" acquired by all organisms through the inheritance of acquired characteristics. "Every organized being of our present time," he wrote, "is the product of the unconscious memory of organized matter" (p. 20).

AGAIN, THE HOROPTER

The first clash between Helmholtz and his nemesis showed few traces of the deep philosophical differences about life and the organism that permeated their later controversies. They published their major treatises on the horopter almost simultaneously in 1864 (Hering 1864a[25]; WAH 2:427–77, no. 85), and although they employed quite different mathematical techniques, neither disputed the overall correctness of the other's results. Helmholtz even called Hering's approach "very elegant, comprehensive, and complete" and the projective geometry especially suitable to the problem (WAH 2:478–81, no. 82). That did not prevent Hering from launching a running critique of Helmholtz's work, which in turn goaded the latter into a reply in 1864 and an aloof review of the whole controversy in the Handbuch two years later (Hering 1865a[25], 1865c[33]; WAH 2:478–81, no. 82; 3:21–25, no. 83; POS 3:484–85).

Jealousy over priority lurked dangerously below the surface of the horopter dispute, but neither participant made that charge explicit. Hering criticized Helmholtz for the excessive complexity of his analytical derivation; for including as part of the real horopter elements of the mathematical locus that lie between or behind the eyes; for errors in verbal descriptions of his mathematical results; and for one real though nonconsequential mathematical error, a charge that wrung an embarrassed admission from Helmholtz (POS 3:484–85). Hering's tone was alternately sycophantic and pugnacious; Helmholtz's grew increasingly exasperated, as it became obvious that neither acknowledgment nor praise would placate Hering. No contemporary seems to have publicly commented on the dispute. Volkmann, however, privately expressed envy of Hering's mathematical achievement and skepticism about whether it was really his own. He wrote to Helmholtz that he had heard from his brother-in-law, Fechner, that Hering had had the mathematical derivations carried out by the young mathematician Hermann Hankel at Leipzig (Volkmann 1856–71, no. 7 [7.8.64]).[2]

While the horopter dispute turned mainly on trivial issues, Hering did raise several substantive objections to Helmholtz's treatment. He attacked Helmholtz's concept of the horopter as the locus at which the perception of three-dimensional, visual relief is most accurate, and charged him with misinterpreting the results of the very experiment done to confirm that attribute. On Hering's view, that definition confused the subjective relationships of visual space with the objective ones of physical or mathematical space and reflected Helmholtz's lingering loyalty to the theory of projection. It also ran counter to the theory of spatial localization Hering was then developing (Hering 1865a[25], 357–58).

Helmholtz in turn criticized Hering's treatment because it did not take retinal incongruity into account. Hering, for his part, could detect no significant retinal incongruity in his own eyes, and he regarded it as one of the many potential eccentricities among individual eyes for which no general horopter derivation should try to account. Hering reached sardonic peaks in arguing that the angle of incongruity varied widely among individuals, that there was little correlation between individual height and the angle of retinal incongruity, and, hence, that the enormous functional significance Helmholtz read into the phenomenon was mostly imaginary. Equally damaging, he could draw upon the published experiments of Volkmann in support of this view (pp. 302–3). Helmholtz refused to retreat from his earlier claims in the face of this criticism, but his ambivalent discussion of the functional significance of retinal incongruity in the *Handbuch* shows that his confidence in them had been shaken (*POS* 3:421–25, 466–82).

The horopter exchanges point out a significant difference between Helmholtz and Hering. A strong (and historically little-noticed) emphasis on functionalism and functional explanation runs through all Helmholtz's work on sensory physiology. He was deeply concerned with the principles that lie behind the form of the horopter, the eye's obedience to Listing's law, the correlation of accommodation and convergence, and other phenomena. Hering also discussed functional principles at length (Hering 1864a[25], 253–83). But he insisted that the choice of functional principles is often arbitrary and that in themselves they do not constitute explanations or confirmations of phenomena. He accused Helmholtz of carrying functional explanation to the point of teleology: of adopting a functional principle and then assuming that the eye, to whose physiology everything is initially possible, has somehow learned to act in conformity with that principle (Hering 1977/1868, 140–45; 1865a[25], 274; 1868a, 102–7).

The disagreement over the size and prevalence of retinal incongruity also points out a methodological problem endemic to physiological optics at this time. The central controversies in the field hinged on difficult subjective experiments that required an exquisite ability to hold rigid fixation of the eyes, observe phenomena in indirect vision, and avoid muscle fatigue. Experimenters differed widely in their conventions about reporting the exact circumstances of experiments, the numbers of experimental trials, and the measured outcomes, if quantification was sought. They frequently substituted detailed, highly personal descriptions of their subjective experiences in order to give verisimilitude and credibility to observations that readers and rivals were likely to find difficult to confirm (cf. Shapin and Schaffer 1985, 22–79). One's reputation as a credible, expert, introspective observer counted for much in scientific disputes. Physiologists tended to dismiss anomalous observations by other scientists as resulting from inattention, inability to hold hard fixation, or individual eccentricities of vision. Experiment served as a loose constraint upon the polemical exchanges and theory making of the period.

HERING AND THE THEORY OF IDENTITY

The five installments of Hering's *Beiträge zur Physiologie* (1861–64) contained much more than his horopter derivation and his exchanges with Helmholtz over them. Hering also presented a disordered, rapid-fire mix of subjective experiments interspersed with attacks on most of the German scientists then writing on depth perception. Except for the exchanges with Helmholtz over the horopter derivation, the *Beiträge* themselves attracted little attention. Fully aware of this, Hering published shorter, calmer, and more cogent accounts of his views in Reichert and du Bois-Reymond's prestigious *Archiv* in 1864 and 1865. In the same years he conducted polemical exchanges with Wundt, Classen, and Volkmann.

In all this work Hering presented himself as a man out to impose order upon the prevailing chaos in the study of binocularity and as one who knew precisely how this could be done. Ignoring the ambiguities and confusions that really prevailed in the field, Hering caricatured the study of depth perception as sharply polarized between the defenders of projection and identity, with the former coming rapidly into ascendancy (Hering 1862[25], iii). He insisted that the reform of physiological optics depended upon squelching the theory of projection and its many alleged defenders and rebuilding the science of visual perception upon a renewed and extended theory of identity.

Hering began characteristically with a devastating attack upon the theory of projection. He insisted that despite its veneer of geometrical plausibility, it fails on all counts as a description of visual experience. First, it cannot explain the basic facts of apparent visual direction. Hering showed that the direction of an object seen in indirect vision varies, according to whether it is being looked at with one or both eyes; the simple theory of projection cannot account for this fact (Hering 1861[25], 30–31). Second, projection cannot explain without ad hoc hypotheses why we see double images at all, and even the ad hoc hypotheses do not correctly predict how double images are localized. Experiment shows that double images of objects in the median plane are normally seen at the distance of the object that cast them, contrary both to the hypothesis of a plane projection surface and to Nagel's ingenious but wholly implausible notion of projection spheres (Hering 1862[25], 132–58). Hering devoted particular critical attention to claims that Wilhelm Wundt had made about the projection of afterimages onto plane surfaces. Hering viciously criticized both Wundt's observations and his mathematical analysis, finding "one as unreliable as the other," and forcing Wundt to retract the mathematical results. Wundt and other advocates of projection surfaces forget, Hering jeered, that these surfaces are themselves retinal images, the projection of which must themselves be explained (Hering 1862[25], 148; 1863b[26]; 1864b[28]).

Piling attack on attack, Hering complained that the projection theory predicts a visual competency in depth perception that the eye simply does not exhibit. Objects are really seen in the binocular field projectively foreshortened and spatially distorted in other minor ways that cannot be deduced from the theory of projection (Hering 1862[25], 132–58). As for Wheatstone's criticism, Hering admitted that the evidence of stereoscopy forces us to acknowledge that images falling on noncorresponding points can be fused and seen single; indeed, this capacity is somehow associated with our ability to see these objects in relief. But Hering insisted that we are not obliged to concede that images on corresponding points may be seen double, and he mounted lengthy criticisms of the stereograms of Wheatstone and Nagel purporting to show this (pp. 81–96).

Worse still, according to Hering, the theory of projection requires that we possess an exquisite subliminal awareness of the tension in our eye muscles, so that we can know the instantaneous orientation of the eyes in our heads and hence of the hypothetical lines of visual projection. Hering admitted that eye movements and changes of convergence play a role in localization and depth perception, but he denied that in the absence of visual cues we can sense the "set" of the eyes in our heads with the accuracy required by the projection theory. Hering gleefully cited experiments done by Wundt himself that showed that accommodation and convergence alone are relatively inaccurate guides in estimating distance (p. 138; Wundt 1862a, 181–99).

Finally, Hering found it inherently implausible that the eye's mind should constantly be recalculating the distance of external objects and projecting their images appropriately. He charged that projection theories merely reify the geometrical abstractions of the physicist and substitute them for real subjective perceptions and their underlying physiological mechanisms. This criticism encapsulated his lifelong hostility to explanations that portrayed the processes of sensory perception as analogous to higher, intellectualistic functions of the mind, rather than as immediate expressions of the life forces in the sense organs themselves (Hering 1864a[25], iii–v).

Hering's contemporaries found his determination to portray the theory of identity as an alternative and rival to the concept of projection characteristically perverse. After all, most writers happily combined both concepts; they regarded projection as an explanation of spatial localization, and retinal identity or correspondence as a theory of single and double vision. Hering almost alone in the early 1860s saw retinal correspondence as directly involved in the determination of visual direction and visual depth.

Early in the first installment of the *Beiträge* Hering described an experimental observation that he self-consciously generalized to "the law of identical visual directions." His classical description runs as follows. Sit at a window with the head still and the right eye tightly shut. Then with the left eye look at some prominent object in the distance (say a tree) that lies somewhere on the right-hand side of the median plane. With the left eye still fixated on the tree and the right eye closed, make a black mark on the place on the glass window pane that lies on the line of sight from the left eye to the tree. Then close the left eye, open the right eye, and notice what distant object lies along the line of sight from the right eye to the mark on the window, so that it is partly obscured by it. Imagine the object to be a distant chimney. Then open both eyes and fixate the black mark with binocular vision, noting at the same time what distant objects appear to lie directly behind the mark and so be partly obscured by it. To the surprise of most observers performing the experiment for the first time, both the tree and the chimney will be seen to lie in a straight line through the black mark on the window; that is, seen binocularly, they will all appear to lie in the same *visual* direction, even though we know they cannot lie in the same *physical* direction. As Hering was later to insist, objects in visual space (*Sehraum*) are not subject to the same laws and relationships as objects in physical space (Hering 1861[25], 28–29; 1864c[29], 38–42).

What has happened here and why is it important? Hering's law (as Hering interpreted it) declared that external objects that image on corresponding retinal points always have the same visual direction in the unified binocular field. That direction will be the same as if the two retinas had been displaced toward the nose, so that their pattern of corresponding points perfectly overlapped, and they formed the retina of an imaginary, "double eye" midway between the two physical eyes. This simple

observation seems to have confirmed Hering's conviction of the phenomenological and physiological existence of retinal correspondence. Identical points not only determine single and double vision; they also
determine the lines of identical visual direction, and so the whole two-
dimensional spatial configuration of the binocular field.

The law of identical visual directions gave the theory of retinal identity
a new claim to sensory significance. Hering also tried to fortify that theory by altering its epistemological status. His earliest and most succinct
statement came in an attack on August Classen, which he launched in
1863 in Virchow's *Archiv* (Hering 1863c[27], 560–72). Like many defenders of the projection theory who attempted to deny retinal identity,
Classen (according to Hering) confused the *fact* of retinal identity with
hypotheses as to why it is true. Hering insisted that the theory of identity,
correctly understood, is not a theory at all, but an indisputable generalization from observations on visual direction. It does not depend on the
assumption of some neural linkage between corresponding retinal points,
nor does it matter to the correctness of the theory whether the correspondence is innate or acquired. Although he opined that the correspondence
probably rests upon a neural linkage between points of the two retinas,
Hering was content to remain agnostic on the anatomical connection
(ibid.; 1865b[32], 80).

Now Hering was soon to learn that the most controversial hypotheses
are those that claim to be self-evidently true, but as a rhetorical strategy
of argumentation this ploy was nevertheless extremely adroit. Most contemporaries thought of retinal identity as a strong theory for which, it
was agreed, there was little direct anatomical support. They regarded
projection as a weaker and less controversial formulation, perhaps little
more than a short way of stating the indisputable fact that we do not
"see" images on our retinas, but in orderly patterns in space outside our
eyes. Hering attempted to invert this popular perception of the two theories. The theory of identity, cut loose from anatomical claims, would take
on an uncontroversial, phenomenological immediacy. Projection would
become a complex, little understood, hypothetical visual capacity, to be
measured against the facts of perception and found consistently wanting.

THE THEORY OF RETINAL SPACE VALUES

Hering's program for the reform of physiological optics required him to
show that the theory of identity could actually do what the theory of
projection only promised to do: explain the principal facts of depth perception. To provide this demonstration, Hering first drew a sharper distinction than any contemporary between absolute depth localization (by

which we estimate the distance from our bodies of the instantaneous point of fixation) and relative depth localization (by which we perceive objects to lie nearer or farther than the point of fixation). Hering conceded that the former depends mostly upon learned, empirical cues, but insisted that the latter depends upon binocular disparity that may be supplemented by empirical cues. Point-objects not lying on the horopter will cast their images onto noncorresponding retinal points, and these pairs of retinal points will be increasingly disparate as the objects lie increasingly behind or in front of the point of fixation. Until the disparity becomes so great that the object begins to appear in double images, it is somehow responsible for our direct awareness of the object's depth vis-à-vis the instantaneous point of fixation (Hering 1865a[25], 287–358; 1865b[32], 79–97, 152–65). This claim was commonplace by 1865; no one doubted that the disparity of retinal images somehow triggers binocular depth perception.

Hering went beyond this commonplace claim, however, in his theory of retinal space values—an ingenious extension of the doctrine of local signs that implied that the retina possessed innate physiological mechanisms for assessing image disparity and converting it to spatial perceptions (Hering 1864a[25], 287–303; 1865b[32]). To an adequate approximation, Hering wrote, we can think of the retina as a flat surface overlaid by an orthogonal grid, the central axes of which are the "middle horizontal section" (Helmholtz's retinal horizon) and the "middle vertical section" (Helmholtz's apparent vertical meridian). Hering hypothesized that every point on the retinal grid is endowed with three separate, spatial-sensory qualities called "space values" (*Raumwerthe*). On analogy with Cartesian coordinates, he associated a particular "height value" (*Hohenwerth*) with each horizontal section, increasingly negative below the middle horizontal section, increasingly positive above it. Corresponding horizontal sections on each retina have identical height values. Hering associated a particular "breadth value" (*Breitenwerth*) with each vertical section, increasingly positive on the temporal side of each middle vertical section and increasingly negative on the nasal side. Each corresponding pair of vertical sections has the same breadth value.

When a point on one retina is stimulated we *immediately* experience the image as lying above or below, to the left or right, of the point of fixation, with the distance from that point determined by the height and breadth value of the particular point that was stimulated. If both eyes are being used, Hering went on, then the visual direction of a point in the binocular field will be the *algebraic mean* of the height and breadth values evoked by the point stimulus on each of the two retinas. A small external object imaging on corresponding retinal points will therefore be seen in the same direction in the binocular field as in either of the monocular fields alone. If it images on noncorresponding retinal points it may be seen in double images; if so, each will lie in slightly different directions in the binocular field. Or the object may be seen single, in which case its visual direction in the binocular field will not correspond to its precise direction in either monocular field. From this scheme, Hering noted, his law of identical visual directions could be fully deduced.

More intriguing and more controversial was the third space value, the "depth value" (*Tiefwerth*), which Hering associated with each retinal point. Unlike the other space values, these are symmetrically distributed across the two retinas: increasingly negative for the vertical sections on the temporal side of the two middle vertical sections, increasingly positive for the vertical sections on the nasal side. All points on every vertical section have the same depth value; corresponding retinal points have depth values of opposite sign and equal absolute values. As with the other space values, the depth value associated with a point-image in the combined binocular field is the algebraic sum of the depth values excited in the two monocular fields.

On this scheme an external point-object imaging on the two foveas will excite monocular depth values of zero, and so will have a combined depth value of zero in the binocular field. This means, Hering explained, that the distance of the object from us cannot be determined by depth values; any assessment of the distance of the point must be made on the basis of other cues. On whatever basis we do localize the point in visual space that excites respective depth values of zero and zero, that point then becomes what Hering called the *Kernpunkt* or "core point" of visual space. He rejected the more traditional term, the "point of fixation," because of its projectionist connotations.

If an external point-object lies in the horopter and images on corresponding retinal points other than the foveas, it will excite equal and opposite depth values and so have a combined depth value in the binocular field of zero. Hence, Hering reasoned, all such external points will be see as lying at the same distance from us as the core point, whose distance we have obtained by guess or by other cues. They must lie in what Hering called the *Kernflache*, the "core surface," which is a frontal plane perpendicular to the line of primary visual direction and passing through the core point. Its perceptual significance is that all external points imaging on corresponding retinal points will *seem* to lie in this plane, even though physically they may not do so at all. Hering readily admitted, however, that when viewing real objects with parallaxes, shadows, and superpositions, empirical cues may override the organic depth values and cause us to localize these objects at distances more correctly corresponding to their physical distance.

Finally, consider external objects imaging on noncorresponding retinal points but still seen single. These objects will have nonzero combined depth values in the binocular field. If that value is negative, Hering specified, then we will see the object as lying nearer to us than the core surface; if positive, as lying beyond the core surface. In this way our rich perception of visual *relief* is built up. Hering insisted that binocular depth perception, insofar as it depends upon organic depth values, is always perception of relief relative to the core surface.

As proof of his theory of the core surface and localization with respect to it, Hering gleefully invoked Helmholtz's own experiment (illustrated in Fig. 3.1) viewing erect needles aligned along the horopter circle (Hering 1865a[25], 298–302). According to Hering, what Helmholtz had dismissed as an "optical illusion" occurring when the needles are spaced too far apart, expressed in fact the essence of the phenomenon: that when aligned along the horopter circle, the needles appear to lie in a frontal plane, namely, Hering's core surface. He claimed that the "illusions" of convexity or concavity that Helmholtz had observed when the needles were not aligned precisely along the horopter circle follow precisely from the retinal depth values excited by the images. That Helmholtz could dismiss this phenomenon as an illusion, Hering charged, reflected his chronic inability to distinguish the subjective nature of visual space from the objective but nonperceptual nature of physical or mathematical space (pp. 357–58). Far from confirming Helmholtz's conception of the horopter as the spatial locus along which our perceptions of relief are most accurate and most acute, the experiment actually proved the opposite. Objects in or near the horopter are perceived in relationship to the subjective core surface, not in their physically correct relationship to the point of fixation.

When Hering sprung this infamous theory of space values upon his contemporaries in 1865, he insisted that the "laws" of depth perception it embodied are "independent of every preconceived theory about identity or non-identity and so forth" (Hering 1865b[32], 80). It has no hypothetical character, he wrote, for it is "merely abstracted from the facts of experience," and hence beyond dissension or controversy. This claim remained a dogma within Hering's school right down to the 1920s, but Hering himself, who was always profoundly sensitive to the theory-laden nature of terminology and description, must have recognized how disingenuous it was. The scheme explicitly extended the theory of identity to render it a theory of depth perception as well as a theory of single and double vision; Hering's terminology made it possible for the first time to discuss depth perception in terms of the retinal correspondence without any reference to projection or direction lines. Hering, no less than Wundt or Lotze (whose influence he acknowledged), was out to place depth perception on the same epistemological and explanatory basis as directional perception. Hering insisted that perceiving an object in relief or at a distance is as immediate and as primitive as perceiving it as "up" or "down" in the visual field or, for that matter, as perceiving it as "green" or "bright." The only difference is that one eye suffices for the spatial perception of direction, whereas the simultaneous action of both eyes is required for the visual perception of depth. These unprecedented claims set the stage for the dispute with Helmholtz that became the nativist-empiricist controversy.

CHAPTER FIVE

The Nativist-Empiricist
Controversy Begins

THE REFORM OF PHYSIOLOGICAL OPTICS

During the early 1860s Helmholtz and Hering pursued different programs intended to impose order upon the chaotic field of binocularity and depth perception. Of the two strategies, Hering's was by far the blunter instrument. Through the 1860s he portrayed the study of spatial perception as polarized between the theories of identity and projection, attacked projectionists wherever he found them, and rallied support for his own extended theory of identity. With at least the first two objectives, he enjoyed considerable success. Volkmann adopted some views about spatial localization so similar to Hering's as to lead Hering in 1864 to hint that Volkmann had borrowed them from him (Hering 1864e). August Classen recanted his former advocacy of projection in the face of attacks by Hering and in 1863 became a supporter of identity (Classen 1863; Hering 1863c). Hering never compelled Wilhelm Wundt to recant his projectionist views, but he forced him onto the defensive, so that Wundt's later discussions of projection and localization were considerably more tentative than those of 1862 (Wundt 1862b, 1863a, 1863b). Best of all for Hering's program, Hermann Aubert concluded in his judicious survey of physiological optics that the projection theory of Panum, Nagel, and Wundt had been so roundly refuted by Classen, Hering, and Volkmann that "I need not go further into it here" (Aubert 1865, 307). This success so cheered Hering that he temporarily abandoned his public persona as the embattled underdog and concluded triumphantly that his "attack upon the theory of direction lines" had been fruitful (Hering 1865b, 79).

Through it all Hering considered the greatest prize to be Helmholtz himself, the "coryphaeus of physiological optics." Hering's program needed Helmholtz, and that need showed in the ambivalent attitude Hering displayed toward the master. His vituperative early criticisms of Helmholtz's horopter derivation are interspersed with passages of surprising deference, written clearly without ironical intent. Helmholtz was always "this researcher whom I value so highly," this "famous physiologist," "the student of whom, if not in a personal sense, [I] gladly call myself" (Hering 1864a[25], i; 1865b[32], 84). The papers written during these years frequently open with a public update on what (in Hering's view) was the current trend in Helmholtz's thought, either toward the projectionist language and explanations of his students Wundt and Nagel, or toward the opposite perspective Hering claimed as his own.

By 1865 Hering's program to win Helmholtz away from the projectionist cause had enjoyed ostensible success. He and Helmholtz had reached quite similar positions on many of the major questions that had racked physiological optics. They had deduced similar forms of the horopter curve, had reached a rough consensus on the nature and purpose of eye movements and the foundational status of Listing's law, and had accepted an approximate retinal correspondence and how it could be empirically determined. More important, Helmholtz in 1864 had repudiated projectionist explanations of the horopter, explicitly citing experiments done by Hering, and he repeated and expanded these arguments in the *Handbuch* (*WAH* 2:450–51; *POS* 3:267–68). He broke with Wundt by (politely) rejecting his assistant's theory that the eyes move in accordance with a "principle of least muscular exertion" and that the particular torsional setting at any tertiary position is dictated by this principle. Similarly, Wundt had argued that the eye estimates distances on the visual globe by the muscular exertion required to move the point of fixation over those distances. Helmholtz rejected this claim, citing with approval Hering's arguments that muscle-related cues are highly inexact unless constantly compared to those available in the visual image (*WAH* 2:352–59, no. 77; 2:360–419, no. 78; *POS* 3:70, 121, 293–30). No less important was their common utilization of a whole series of new experimental techniques to investigate these questions, some invented by Helmholtz or Hering, others borrowed from Volkmann, Meissner, or Wundt. This basic agreement between Helmholtz and Hering on several key issues made up another element in the broad integration and transformation of vision studies that occurred in Europe shortly after midcentury.

THE DISPUTE OVER SPATIAL LOCALIZATION
BEFORE THE *HANDBUCH*

As Helmholtz and Hering were moving toward consensus on some key questions, they were simultaneously moving toward irreconcilable opposition over others. Throughout his career, Helmholtz insisted that the processes that mediate sensory perception are psychological or quasi-inferential in nature, occur high in the central nervous system rather than in the end organs, and depend heavily on learning and experience acquired by the individual during a lifetime. Helmholtz set out these views loosely in his popular lecture of 1855 and drew on them to explain various phenomena in visual and auditory perception between 1855 and 1865, but he did not formulate them definitively for spatial perception until 1866.

Hering also acknowledged the importance of empirical elements in conditioning human perception, but he insisted on a primitive residue of spatial perception that is largely fixed by inherited organic structures and so prior to all learning and experience. This view is implicit in Hering's earliest writings, but its first explicit statement occurs in 1864 in the fifth *Beiträge*, where he distinguished between our "acquired capacity for seeing in depth" and our "inborn sensory energy for visual depth, which is fully independent of all experience." Empirical cues readily override localizations based upon the innate spatial sense, Hering went on, but experiments designed to eliminate empirical depth cues allow us to isolate and study the innate spatial sense as it is given directly by the retinal depth values (Hering 1865a[25], 287–89).

These two, opposed orientations to the problem of spatial perception run through the entire history of the Helmholtz–Hering dispute. They were soon to be amplified into the nativist-empiricist controversy; they can be traced far back into the history of philosophical speculation about spatiality and the mind; and in different guises they persist, as formative and influential as ever, in vision research today. These facts make it tempting to present the Helmholtz–Hering dispute as a natural consequence of the fundamentally opposed positions the protagonists adopted, and to interpret the dispute as a particular recurrence of an almost transhistorical confrontation of nativist and empiricist positions. Helmholtz himself urged this view and invested it with his authority. Much evidence, however, supports a rather different and unexpected account of the dispute. In adopting the positions they did, Helmholtz and Hering did not simply choose sides in an established and preexisting controversy, did not come to the study of depth perception with fully developed positions, and did not insist from the beginning on the fundamentally antagonistic nature of their approaches. On that alternate telling, the nativist-empiricist controversy in its modern guise emerges as a consequence of the Helmholtz–Hering dispute, as much or more than as its cause.

In support of that alternate interpretation, Chapter Two stressed that in the context of the early 1860s, the question of whether visual capacities are acquired and inferential or innate and physiological existed as one contentious issue among many in the confused debates over spatial perception. Neither Helmholtz and Hering nor their contemporaries regarded this question as the central axis of controversy in the field during the early 1860s. Hering regarded identity versus projection, not physiology versus psychology, as the central question facing the field, and he happily made common cause with the infamous psychologizer Volkmann when doing so seemed to strengthen the case for identity. When Hering did attack the advocates of psychology during this period, he did not identify Helmholtz as a particular offender. In 1864 Hering momentarily interrupted his running attack on projection in order to criticize Volkmann and Wundt for their psychological explanations of fusion and other perceptual phenomena. He objected that through these explanations they made physiology the "stepdaughter" of psychology, and he went on to criticize any appeal to "unconscious inferences" to explain perceptual processes. Hering traced this line of psychological explanation back to Kant and philosopher J. F. Herbart, and among contemporaries he identified Wundt as its principal defender (Hering 1865a[25], iii–v). Hering did not then include Helmholtz among the advocates of unconscious inference, even though he must have known that Helmholtz had already made wide use of this concept to explain stereoscopic luster, simultaneous contrast, and elements of auditory perception.

As for Helmholtz, the language of learning and inference runs all through his classic papers on the horopter and eye movements, but there is little self-conscious discussion there of empiricism as a methodology, and almost no explicit recognition of a nativist alternative. Helmholtz had offered a classic empiricist interpretation of stereoscopic luster as early as 1855 and had used it to reject claims for an innate neural connection between corresponding retinal points. This was not, however, a position that Hering defended or considered essential to the nativist case. In a popular lecture the same year, Helmholtz held up to ridicule "those who do not want to bring themselves to acknowledge a role for thought and inference in sensory perception," but the only offenders he could muster were ancient emissionists, Plato, and animal magnetists (*VuR* 1:112). Later Helmholtz would criticize the teachings of Kant and Johannes Müller as nativistic in orientation and therefore as offending against this principle; if he held that view in 1855, however, he carefully refrained from stating it, and he praised both men in the lecture.

During the mid-1860s a series of very specific empirical problems and the local disputes they occasioned polarized the positions of Helmholtz and Hering and led them to develop and harden their broad methodological commitments to the study of spatiality. Several specific issues of contention arose from Hering's claims concerning retinal space values. Helmholtz was prepared to accept that scheme as a mere restatement of what was known about the role of binocular disparity in stereopsis, but he would not accept the implication that spatial awareness emerged directly from innate, sensory-physiological capacities of retinal points. What rankled Helmholtz most was that Hering should base his hypothesis of the core surface on Helmholtz's own experiments with the vertical needles. He was forced into the embarrassment of repeating his original experiments, this time using suspended black threads that could be aligned along the horopter circle. In a major reply to Hering of 1865 and again in the *Handbuch*, he reported that when the set of hanging threads lies on the horopter circle it is usually *not* perceived as plane. This new result violated his own earlier, erroneous reports, but it also ran contrary to the predictions of Hering's theory of depth values. Helmholtz was also forced to concede that hanging threads arranged along the horopter circle usually are not seen correctly as lying in a circular arc, but appear to lie in some other, more convex or concave configuration (*WAH* 2:492–96, no. 88; *POS* 3:318–22, and cf. 488–90).

Other issues saw Helmholtz on the offensive. Hering's scheme of depth values predicted that only horizontal retinal disparities, not vertical ones, provide cues to depth perception. Helmholtz attached small beads to the suspended threads, so creating a vertical disparity between retinal points, and showed that the eye can then immediately and accurately judge the true configuration of the set of hanging threads. In the *Handbuch* he provided a series of stereograms designed to prove that vertical disparities could generate the perception of stereoscopic relief as readily as horizontal ones (*WAH* 2:492–96; *POS* 3:318–22, Plate I).

Helmholtz and Hering also clashed over the status of Hering's law of identical visual directions. Helmholtz fully accepted the law's correctness and its damaging implication for the theory of projection, but not its role as a central principle of space perception. That we refer all visual directions to an imaginary central eye, even in monocular vision, merely reflects the fact that we *normally* look at objects with both eyes, Helmholtz argued. We have therefore learned to refer visual direction to a point midway between the two real eyes, and now persist in doing so even when one eye is closed, or when experiments show us that this habit produces curious anomalies in the apparent directions of objects outside the point of fixation (*WAH* 2:492–96; *POS* 3:258–59).

Most contentious among the specific issues that divided Helmholtz and Hering was Helmholtz's conviction that the eyes are separate organs that in principle may be moved wholly independently of each other. In 1863 and again in London in his Croonian Lecture of 1865, Helmholtz expressed his belief that adherence to the laws of Donders and Listing is a habit acquired by an individual during early life in order to facilitate clear and easy visual orientation. Once acquired and ingrained, however, the facility cannot be overridden by acts of the will. Accordingly, some eye movements are impossible for adults to make voluntarily—notably, cyclorotations, vertical divergences, and horizontal divergences beyond parallel lines of sight. But these movements are not *anatomically* impossible, Helmholtz insisted, for through the use of prism glasses, which produce a constant, abnormal angular separation of the visual rays entering the eye, we can induce the eyes to perform fusional cyclorotations as well as vertical and absolute divergences in order to bring the distorted images onto corresponding retinal places in the interests of clear vision (*WAH* 3:25–43, no. 80; 2:360–95, no. 78; 3:44–48, no. 89).

Hering did not immediately contest Helmholtz's experimental support for these claims, but he reasserted his conviction that the harmony and expediency of eye movements suggest that "they are prescribed in their essential elements through innate mechanisms" (Hering 1865a[25], 320). He did heap sarcasm upon Helmholtz's report that, while drowsing over a book late in the evening, his eyes had seemed to perform independent and opposite cyclorotations (movements that cannot be voluntarily induced) as a result of this involuntary relaxation of the will. Much more likely, Hering contemptuously observed, the great Helmholtz in his dozing state had simply allowed his head to nod involuntarily to one side and been misled by the resulting appearances (Hering 1864a[25], 274)! Stung by this exchange, Helmholtz seems to have concluded that henceforth any concession on the principle would expose him not merely to charges of inconsistency but to ridicule as well. In the *Handbuch* he defiantly repeated and strengthened these claims, including his view "that the rotation of the eye round the visual axis cannot be effected by our will, because we have not learnt by which exertion of our will we are to effect it, and that the inability does not depend on any anatomical structure either of our nerves or of our muscles which limits the combination of movements" (*WAH* 3:34–35, no. 80; *POS* 3:54–62 and *passim*).

THE DISPUTE OVER SPATIAL LOCALIZATION
IN THE *HANDBUCH*

Down to 1866 the exchanges between Helmholtz and Hering had hinged mostly on specific issues, not on abstract principles. The tone of these exchanges had been pointed, but nevertheless mild in comparison to Hering's concurrent polemics with Wundt, Classen, and others. On many of the specific issues of the field, Helmholtz and Hering remained in close agreement. Yet the exchanges had made their mark on Helmholtz, forcing him repeatedly onto the defensive, exposing him to public embarrassment, and blocking his routes of retreat.

As Helmholtz labored over the final volume of the *Handbuch*, he had no reason to expect that Hering would mitigate his future attacks. Perhaps for this reason, he allowed the project, once scheduled for completion in 1864, to drag on and on. Helmholtz's correspondence with du Bois-Reymond from this period abounds with melancholic, agonized passages in which he described his work on binocular space perception as "disheartening," a "hopeless enterprise" and an "abominable ordeal."

He bemoaned the confused state of the phenomena, the many disputes arising merely from individual particularities, and the prevalence of "theoretical prejudices" among researchers; and he expressed fear of damage to his own eyes from the constant experimentation. Concern with rhetoric and persuasion figured large in Helmholtz's letters. On one occasion he complained that the work had drawn him into what he disparagingly referred to as "philosophical questions" about which it was impossible to "persuade people" of any definitive answer. On another he wrote of spatial perception as the "most confused chapter" in physiological optics, where the omnipresence of psychological influences on perception made it difficult "to persuade people" even with the "most superior arguments" (Kirsten 1986, 207–21, nos. 90, 91, 96, 97, 101).

Ewald Hering also occupied Helmholtz's thoughts. Helmholtz did not always speak freely to du Bois-Reymond on this sore subject, but in February 1865 he wrote to his friend with uncharacteristic smugness. He had so far refrained from "putting Hering in his place," partly out of respect for the intelligent and consequent nature of Hering's writings, and partly because of rumors that he had earlier been mentally disturbed. But, he went on, "Hering has annoyed me with his insolent way of condemning other people's work, when for the most part he hasn't even made the effort to really understand it" (Kirsten 1986, 215–19, no. 97). Hering, as Helmholtz knew much better than his words suggest, was the obnoxious and potentially dangerous specter who hung over his program for the reformation of sensory physiology. Helmholtz already knew that in the final volume of the *Handbuch*, that specter would have to be laid to rest.

The final volume, which appeared in 1866, extended and recapitulated Helmholtz's earlier results. Yet it presented those results in a new framework. The third volume of the *Handbuch* grounded those results in a deep theory of epistemological and perceptual processes, presented and interpreted them as explicit consequences of empiricist methodology, and reinterpreted the whole field of visual perception as polarized around as the competing methodologies of nativism and empiricism.

Helmholtz set the stage by opening volume three with one of his most famous epistemological discussions, "Concerning the Perceptions in General" (*PO5* 3:1–36). There he restated his conviction that our perceptions of objects localized in space reach consciousness already psychologically "processed" by factors of expectation, habit, and memory acquired through past visual and tactile experience. He again described the psychological operations through which primitive sensation is processed to conscious spatial perception as "unconscious inferences." Of course, formulations like this were not uncommon; Wilhelm Wundt, especially, had published very similar ideas between 1858 and 1862 (cf. Hatfield 1990, 199–208). But Helmholtz elaborated for the first time his more unusual conviction that these unconscious inferences are inductive and syllogistic in nature, and differ from logical inferences only in being imagistic rather than linguistic in nature.[1]

Helmholtz quickly moved from epistemology to methodology. The perceptual task of the eye's mind, Helmholtz argued, is wholly pragmatic and utilitarian: to localize and to identify external objects sufficiently for the purposes of life. This implies, however, that the unconscious inferences that mediate perception are susceptible to a functional analysis. Helmholtz deduced three methodological tenets for the study of perception which, in his view, followed immediately from the empiricist theory.

The first of these methodological tenets is that a perception is "explained" when we can plausibly show that perceptions of that kind normally yield correct or useful information about external objects. Contemporaries familiar with the literature would readily have recognized how this methodological tenet positioned Helmholtz to resist Hering's key claims. It implies, for example, that introspective analysis offers a poor guide to understanding our perceptual processes. In the radical pragmatism of perceptual experience, unconscious inference routinely ignores or suppresses sensations that do not give us useful information about external objects. We do not, for example, "see" the retinal blindspot, since awareness of it would provide no useful information about the external world. We are interested in our complex perceptions only as they are "signs" of external objects, and so we normally cannot decompose perceptual compounds into their uninterpreted sensory elements (POS 3:6). The phenomenological immediacy of a perceptual experience, including our awareness of space, therefore permits no inference to its primitive and uncompounded nature. This methodological tenet distanced Helmholtz's approach from Hering's phenomenological orientation.

Helmholtz's second methodological tenet proclaimed that what we call an "illusion of the senses" is really an "illusion in the judgement of the material presented to the senses, resulting in a false idea of it" (p. 4). What distinguished Helmholtz's assertion of this commonplace claim was his rigorous insistence that every perceptual illusion arises out of the inappropriate application of some inferential procedure, which under ostensibly similar stimulus conditions is known to yield correct information about objects. A methodologically legitimate explanation of a visual illusion must specify the normal inference involved and also show how unusual patterns of stimuli "tricked" the perceptual processes into an inappropriate application of it. This tenet, too, strategically anticipated the objections of Hering and Panum, already directed against Volkmann and Wundt, that appeals to "psychological" explanations of perceptual regularities must be arbitrary and hypothetical (ibid.).

Helmholtz's third tenet defied Hering much more directly. Helmholtz postulated that in any situation in which practice, concentration, or external aids can cause a familiar pattern of stimuli to be perceived differently, we may conclude that the original perception was itself an interpreted experience somehow conditioned by expectation and prior learning. This tenet therefore yielded a sufficient (but not necessary) criterion for detecting the role of learning and experience in the formation of our perceptions (p. 13). Hering, however, had already considered and rejected the claim in 1865 (Hering 1865b[32], 164).

This discussion also set out for the first time Helmholtz's conception of a physiological optics starkly polarized between the methodologies of nativism and empiricism. Helmholtz claimed that the central problem of a theory of human visual perception is to determine how much of perception is due directly to sensation and how much is due to experience and training. This dictum in itself merely echoed many previous writers; Helmholtz, however, went on to portray the problem as the central cleavage of the field. The methodological predisposition to "concede to the influence of experience as much scope as possible, and to derive from it especially all notions of space," is the "empirical (*empiristisch*) theory" of perception. On the other hand, researchers who "believe it is necessary to assume a system of innate apperceptions that are not based on experience, especially with respect to space-relations," may be said to adhere to the "intuition theory" (*nativistische Theorie*) of the sense perceptions (*POS* 3:10).[2]

Nativists, Helmholtz went on, try to explain the relative constancy of an individual's perceptual experience (which really arises from "fixed and inevitable associations of ideas") by seeking "some mechanical mode of origin for this connection [between the sensation and the conception of the object] through the agency of imaginary organic structures." As he had pointedly not done in 1855, Helmholtz in 1866 explicitly attributed this approach to Kant and Johannes Müller, as well as to contemporaries Panum and Hering. Nativist doctrines like theirs, he wrote, do not *explain* our perceptual images of space; they merely postulate innate mechanisms, which in the presence of proper neural stimulation give rise to these perceptions (pp. 17–18).

The substantive chapters of the *Handbuch* laid out Helmholtz's findings on the nature of perception in such a way as to massively confirm the empiricist theory and to portray those findings as direct consequences of his three methodological tenets. Helmholtz's long discussion of geometrical and other illusions, for example, attributed most of these effects to eye movements, or to the principle of psychological contrast—the mind's tendency to perceive clearly demarcated divisions or differences to be larger than those more vaguely demarcated or not demarcated at all. This discussion included a blistering refutation of an unfortunate early suggestion by Hering that certain geometrical illusions arise because the eye estimates distances on the retina by the chord of the arc subtended rather than by the arc itself. Helmholtz branded that suggestion as epitomizing a dangerous nativist tendency, derived from Müller, to endow the retina with direct awareness of its spatial attributes (p. 192).

In his discussion of the monocular visual field, Helmholtz followed Lotze and Wundt in arguing that our knowledge of distance and direction on that field is gradually acquired from intrinsically nonspatial cues. His explanation differed from Wundt's mainly in attributing a minimal role to muscle kinesthesia and in denying that the local signs are known through qualitative variation in sensation. Here as elsewhere in his writings, Helmholtz drew no distinction between spatial awareness per se and the visual assessment of the distance and direction of points in that space. He most frequently treated the former as if it were given in the sense of touch and were merely assimilated to the visual sense (pp. 154–232).

Like others before him, Helmholtz found support for empiricism in various reports of blind persons who had sight surgically restored in one eye. One of these was the celebrated Cheselden case of 1728, in which the recovering patient was supposedly incapable at first of all visual perception of distance, and to have reported that all objects seen "touched his eyes (as he expressed it) as what he felt did his skin." The inability of the patient in a second case immediately to identify visually such familiar objects as a ring or a key—well-known through the sense of touch— spoke, according to Helmholtz, against the existence of "an innate power in the retina of recognizing the form of images there," since "the surface of the key, with its ring and tag, must have been represented on the retina in the same form as it feels to the touch" (pp. 220, 226).

Ironically, this same evidence compelled Helmholtz to make a major concession to nativism. The newly sighted acquire monocular spatial vision so quickly, Helmholtz admitted, that the local signs that make that learning possible cannot be "disconnected and unsystematic signs, whose connection with the adjacent retinal points can only be acquired by experience." The local signs must vary continuously across the retina, so that, prior to all experience, adjacent retinal points must be recognized in the sensation as adjacent (p. 227). That passing statement brought Helmholtz perilously close to conceding the innate spatiality of the two-dimensional retinal image and rendering his position on directional localization almost indistinguishable from Hering's own.

In discussing the perception of visual direction, Helmholtz presented an ingenious new demonstration that our sensation of a change in visual direction is cued by the effort of the will in moving the eyes, not by the resulting tension in the muscles, or by any change in the visual sensation or any kinesthetic awareness in the eye muscles that might result from the actual movement (pp. 242–70, esp. p. 243). That demonstration supported empiricism no more than nativism; but in the course of the discussion, Helmholtz reasserted his belief that visual depth perception is constantly adjusted by, and so is dependent on, the more reliable evidence of touch. Nativists, Helmholtz countered, insist that primitive visual perceptions of space are independent of tactile experience, and for this reason they must assume a "pre-established harmony" between visual and tactile localization in order to explain the coordination of the two. Such an approach, he cautioned, opens the way to the "wildest speculations" (p. 252).

In his discussion of binocular double vision, Helmholtz offered his own genetic account of retinal correspondence and how it is acquired by every individual. The infant, Helmholtz implied, is simultaneously conscious of both monocular fields. In order to perceive the external world more clearly, it learns to focus both eyes on a single object so that the object images on the two foveas; through the sense of touch, it comes to identify these foveal images as signs of a single object at a particular distance before it in space. The infant then superimposes the two monocular fields onto one another so that the two foveal images correspond and are seen single. Through a similar process all individuals have learned to see lines imaging on the retinal horizons and apparent vertical meridians single, and so they build up an entire pattern of correspondence. We "construct" this correspondence in order to exploit the retinal disparities in the binocular field as useful cues to the distance of objects with respect to the point of fixation (pp. 400–488 and *passim*).

As proof of the acquired nature of retinal correspondence, Helmholtz introduced ophthalmological evidence drawn from patients who suffered from fixed-angle strabismus, or squint. These people cannot fixate, that is, when they bring the image of an external object onto one fovea it will not image on the fovea of the other eye, so that external objects can never be imaged on corresponding points. Most of these individuals simply suppress the image from one eye and see the world monocularly. A few, however, continue to see the world with both eyes simultaneously. They ought to see everything in double images, yet they do not. This suggests, Helmholtz argued, that in response to their handicap they acquire an anomalous retinal correspondence, different from the correspondence of normal individuals (pp. 405–7).

In 1838 the first operation to correct for fixed-angle strabismus had been performed in Berlin. This allowed the patient to converge his lines of sight and image an external object upon both foveas simultaneously. As the operation became more common through the 1850s with use of anaesthesia, it was frequently reported that following such an operation the patient saw double. Within weeks, however, single vision gradually returned, suggesting that the patient had not only developed an anomalous correspondence to correct the handicap, but that after the operation had reacquired a normal correspondence in the interests of clear vision. Helmholtz cited these cases as "of fundamental importance for the theory of binocular vision," and as prime support for the empiricist theory (pp. 405–7).

As further evidence that retinal correspondence is acquired, Helmholtz argued that it may be overridden by empirical factors. He conceded that critics had successfully discredited Wheatstone's famous experiment, but he maintained that the conclusion that Wheatstone drew from it "cannot be well contradicted." Helmholtz put forward stereograms of his own purporting to show that points imaging on corresponding retinal points could be seen at different places in the binocular field. He agreed with Volkmann that binocular fusion was a psychological act arising from the unconscious conclusion that the eyes are viewing a familiar object or image in binocular perspective (p. 222).

Helmholtz concluded his case by examining the phenomenon of retinal rivalry, the condition that arises when the separate monocular fields "cannot plausibly be combined into the image of a single object" (pp. 493–528, on p. 494). This phenomenon did not give unequivocal support to the empiricist position, as Helmholtz knew. Numerous observers reported that uniform monocular fields of different colors could often be combined into a binocular field showing the same mixed color that would have arisen from monocular mixing. Panum and Hering had argued from this and other phenomena to the existence of an innate mechanism at work in combining the two fields. Helmholtz could only reply that he and others had been consistently unable to achieve this binocular color mixing; to him the binocular field showed an active rivalry of the two colors but never a mix of the two. He interpreted this struggle for dominance between the two fields as a psychological wavering of the concentration in the absence of other cues as to how to interpret the fields.

One kind of rivalry offered what Helmholtz regarded as the single strongest support of the empiricist interpretation: stereoscopic luster. Look at a stereogram that shows the outlines of an object or area, with one-half of the stereogram showing the object or area darkly colored and the other half the same scene lightly colored. The binocular perception is not that of an intermediate gray; rather, the object or area will seem to shine with a metallic luster. Now the circumstances under which a real object appears lustrous, Helmholtz explained, are those in which the object has the property of a mirror, reflecting light regularly off its surface rather than diffusely. Under such circumstances, it frequently occurs that more light from the object will fall onto one eye than onto the other, so that one of the two monocular fields appears much brighter than the other. When this occurs artificially, as in viewing a specially prepared stereogram, the judgment infers from past experience that it is looking at an object that is lustrous, and so the binocular apperception is of a lustrous object, not of an object of brightness intermediate between the two fields (pp. 512–13).

Helmholtz always regarded binocular luster as a crucial observation supporting the empiricist position. It and other phenomena associated with rivalry proved "that the content of each separate field comes to consciousness without being fused with that of the other field by means of organic mechanisms; and that therefore, the fusion of the two fields in one common image, when it does occur, is a psychic act" (pp. 499, 512–13). Above all, stereoscopic luster ostensibly proved that binocular perception depends heavily upon our prior experience of viewing real objects under normal viewing conditions. Here, as throughout the *Handbuch*, Helmholtz wove into his presentation of the material a skillful utilization and defense of his empiricist methodology and did so even when he chose not to invoke empiricist principles explicitly.

THE REFUTATION OF HERING

The third volume of the *Handbuch* bore a double burden as a work of scientific argumentation and persuasion. It had to persuade contemporaries to accept Helmholtz's portrayal of physiological optics as polarized around the two great methodological alternatives of nativism and empiricism, and also leave them in no doubt of the superiority of the latter. The thematic structure of the book made it particularly effective in achieving these rhetorical ends. The volume opens with the famous introductory chapter, "Concerning the Perceptions in General," in which Helmholtz defined the nativist and empiricist positions and introduced the first of his two themes. His following chapters survey the particular topics of visual perception, progressing from the movement of the eyes and the monocular field of vision to the perception of depth to binocular double vision. As was shown in the previous section, these chapters offer interpretations of these phenomena that either presuppose the empiricist theory or that serve to amplify and defend it. Sometimes those interpretations are implicit, sometimes explicit, but always they serve to bind Helmholtz's methodology tightly to the empirical claims he advances. This strategy, in addition to advancing the argument for empiricism, allowed Helmholtz to impose a degree of thematic unity upon the material that was rare in the *Handbuch*-genre of the day.

Helmholtz mentioned Hering only occasionally in the very early chapters and offered few direct attacks on his views, but he kept the dramatic juxtaposition of empiricism and nativism before the readers' eyes. In successive chapters, however, the refutation of nativism becomes ever more prominent as a subtheme. That theme becomes particularly insistent as the work moves toward considerations of binocular depth perception and then to retinal rivalry, the penultimate chapter and Helmholtz's most powerful empirical argument. The stark juxtaposition of nativism and empiricism—the leitmotif of the whole book—imposes on the work a narrative tension that leads on from chapter to chapter, tightening and intensifying at every turn, toward its final confrontation and resolution. The work achieves that culmination in the final chapter, Helmholtz's "Review of the Theories." There the attack on nativism is finally brought center stage. Nativism, portrayed earlier mostly as a methodological abstraction, appears incarnated there as Ewald Hering and his theory of depth values. In that incarnation, Helmholtz subjects nativism to one final, massive critique. The entire argument of the *Handbuch* lost nothing in passion or effectiveness for being presented in a judicious, understated tone of scrupulous fairness.

The rhetorical strategy of Helmholtz's critique invoked many of the classical topoi of scientific argument. From the start he judiciously positioned his own empiricist perspective on the inductivist high ground, from which he could assail his nativist opponents with charges of philosophical idealism, theoretical dogmatism, and disregard of Ockham's razor. Historical precedents figured large in Helmholtz's presentation. He traced the empiricist tradition to the British "sensationalists" of the eighteenth century by way of Herbart and Lotze, also including in it his contemporaries Wundt, Nagel, and Classen. Nativism, too, Helmholtz provided with a lineage. He identified Hering as the latest and most distinguished member of a nativist tradition reaching back to Kant and Johannes Müller and also including Panum. By associating Kant and Müller with those who denied "a role for thought and inference in sensory perception," as he had declined to do in 1855, Helmholtz strengthened his interpretation of nativism and empiricism as methodological alternatives deeply rooted in the history of the field (*VuR* 1:112). That step also associated nativism with Kantianism, which was regarded with growing suspicion by young scientists in the 1860s, and with Müller, who had died in 1858 and whose approach was regarded by the younger generation of physiologists as passé.

Turning to an empirical attack, Helmholtz zeroed in unerringly on the weakest element of Hering's position, the theory of retinal depth values. Two of his arguments suffice to capture the tenor of that attack. In developing his theory, Hering had left the role of the innate depth values in *monocular* depth perception rather ambiguous. On Hering's theory, when we look at a scene with both eyes, the apparent distance of any object in front of or behind the core surface will be (in the absence of all other cues) the algebraic sum of the depth values from the two retinas.

Suppose we now close one eye. Does the depth value from the one retina still being stimulated influence our estimate of depth in the monocular image? If the answer is no, then depth values function in a way that makes them scarcely distinguishable in practice from a retinal disparity cue. If the answer is yes, then retinal depth values function quite differently and form the basis of a much stronger theory of perception.

While avoiding explicit discussions of this question, Hering had nevertheless maintained that monocular depth values do contribute to depth perception, but that they are even more regularly overridden by empirical cues than is the case in binocular vision. Hering discussed the case illustrated in Figure 5.1. If we look at a frontal plane (for example, the wall of a room) with one eye closed, and if monocular depth values determine perception, then the wall ought to appear rotated clockwise about a vertical line through the core point of visual space P_f. This is because our perception of the wall's relief will be governed only by the depth values of one retina. Points on the right-hand side of the wall will image on the nasal half of the retina and so evoke positive depth values; those points should appear farther than the fixation point. Points on the left-hand side of the wall will image on the temporal half of the retina, will evoke negative depth values, and should seem closer than the fixation point. Under real viewing conditions, of course, frontal planes show no such distortion. Hering conceded that in these cases the monocular depth values are overridden by experiential factors, which cause us to "reorient our visual space" and rotate the core surface so as to preserve its perpendicularity to the visual axis (Hering 1865a[25], 346).

Helmholtz in his critique responded with the clever experiment illustrated in Figure 5.2 (cf. Hochberg 1962, 286). Here we look at the wall with two eyes, but with a strip of black paper cut the same width as the interpupillary distance held before the eyes. Thus, each eye has the inner half of its normal visual field cut off. Points from the visible left-hand side of the wall ba will image only on the nasal side of the left retina. There they excite positive depth values that begin at zero at the fovea and become increasingly positive with the eccentricity of the retinal point. If those monocular depth values determine the perception of relief in the binocular field, then points along ba will all appear farther than the core point p of visual space, and specifically should appear to lie along an apparent locus like pp'. The same reasoning suggests that the visible right-hand segment of the wall $b'a'$ should appear to lie along pp''; the visible portions of the wall should seem inclined to one another. Yet they do not. Experiential factors again seem to override the primitive monocular space values, and this time in a more complicated way than by simply rotating the core surface (POS 3:545–55).

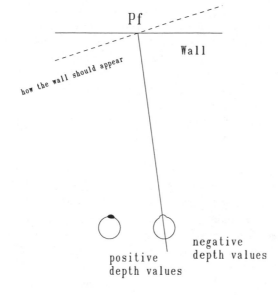

Fig. 5.1 On Hering's theory of retinal depth values, viewing a frontal plane with the left eye closed should induce an apparent rotation of the plane around the core point of visual space. *Source*: Turner 1993a. Reproduced with permission of the University of California Press.

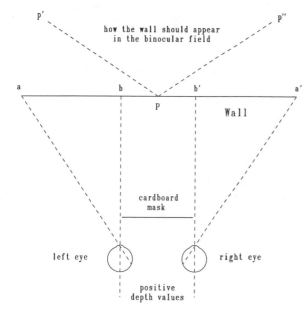

Fig. 5.2 Helmholtz's experimental elaboration of the situation illustrated in Figure 5.1. On the hypothesis of monocular retinal depth values, a cardboard mask held before the eyes as illustrated should induce the indicated distortion of the visual image of a wall or other frontal plane.

On the basis of these and similar observations Helmholtz attacked the theory of depth values for its lack of simplicity and predictive power. Whenever the depth values conflict with experiential factors, he claimed, they seem to cease entirely and are totally overridden by the latter. "Are we not then forced to conclude," he inquired rhetorically, "that those depth-feelings, if they exist at all, are at least so weak and so vague that their influence is negligible in comparison with the factors derived from experience? And therefore, that the apperception of depth might arise just as well *without* them as *with* them, as is supposed to happen on Hering's assumptions?" (p. 556).

By insisting on the efficacy of depth values in monocular vision, Hering had opened his theory to serious objections. Nevertheless, Hering had a strong reason for doing so: his need to explain the localization of half-images in the binocular field. Remember that Hering's empirical case against the theories of projection hinged on two arguments: first, that these theories could not readily explain perceived visual direction, and second, that they could not explain why we localize half-images in space as we do. Consider the simple observational situation shown in Figure 5.3, where *Pf* is the point of fixation. In the binocular visual field (corresponding to the central double-eye) the small object *A* will be seen in double images, the half-image *A″* on the right of the median plane coming from the left retina, the half-image *A′* on the left coming from the right retina. Hering and Helmholtz both agreed that these half-images seem to lie on the near side of the point of fixation, at the approximate distance of the object *A* that cast them, and that this result is not in accord with projectionist concepts. In this situation Hering's theory of monocular depth values correctly predicts the observed outcome, since the object stimulates equal, negative depth values on both retinas.

Monocular depth values also offered Hering the crucial experiment in defense of his theory illustrated in Figure 5.4 (cf. Hochberg 1962, 285). There a vertical wire is positioned slightly to the left of a pin or needle and somewhat nearer the eyes. When the pin is fixated, the wire will image on point *ii* of the right retina, where it will excite negative depth values, and on the point *i* on the left retina, where it will excite positive ones. In the binocular field the wire will be seen in double images, the directions of which will be given by lines from *i′* and *ii′* through the entrance pupil of the imaginary double eye. If its relief is determined by the depth values it excited at *i* and *ii*, then the half-image associated with *i′* (from the left eye) should seem to lie somewhere beyond the core plane of visual space passing through the pin. That associated with *ii′* (from the right eye) should seem to lie nearer than the core plane. Readers can readily confirm that it is, in fact, extremely difficult to form any clear idea of the relative positions of the double images. Most observers are simply unable to maintain

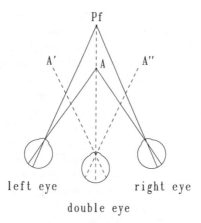

Pf

A′   A   A″

left eye   right eye

double eye

Fig. 5.3 The localization of the half-images of an object A, lying in the median plane. The hypothesis of monocular depth values predicts that the half-images will appear to lie at the same distance and nearer than the point of fixation P_f.

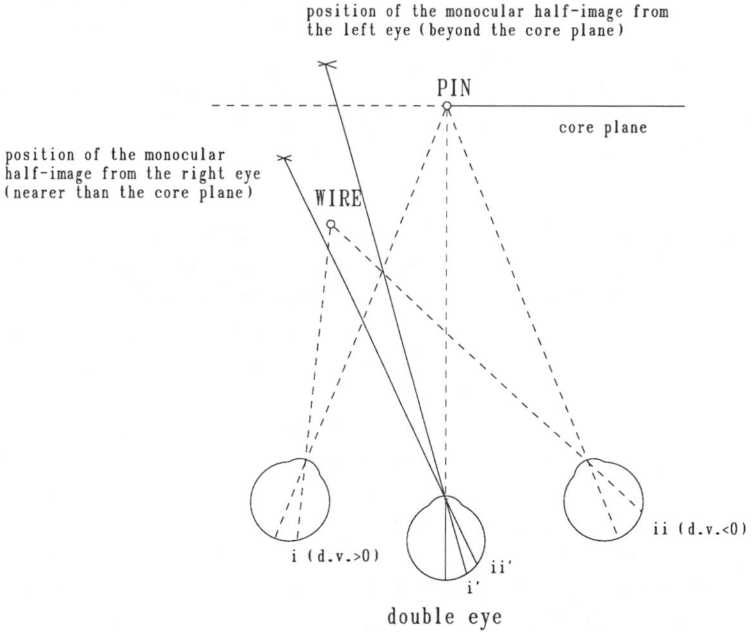

position of the monocular half-image from the left eye (beyond the core plane)

PIN

core plane

position of the monocular half-image from the right eye (nearer than the core plane)

WIRE

i (d.v.>0)

ii (d.v.<0)

ii′

i′

double eye

Fig. 5.4 Hering's crucial experiment to support his theory of retinal depth values. With the eyes fixated on the pin, monocular depth values should make the two half-images of the wire appear to lie at different distances, and on opposite sides of the frontal plane through the pin.

rigid fixation on the needle while directing attention to the apparent distances of the two half-images. Hering nevertheless claimed that after long fixation and rigid attention to the phenomenon, he had observed the half-images at the different distances predicted by his theory (Hering 1865a[25], 340–41). "That with firm fixation the . . . double images really appear as is demanded by the theory," he wrote, "is of the highest interest and was for me an overwhelming proof of the correctness of . . . [my] theory" (p. 340). Out of the chaotic background that attends all such experiments, Hering believed that he had momentarily isolated the fleeting stability that could decide the theoretical point in question.

In his own "Review of the Theories" Helmholtz cited this passage from Hering, described his own attempts to confirm the observation, and concluded with a simple rejection:

> I have gazed at the pin so long and so fixedly that at last everything was extinguished by the negative afterimages. There is a stage when all that can be seen are the nebulous individual parts of the double images of the wire emerging now and then in the course of the conflict with the ground on which they lie and with the afterimages; and then I have noticed that these parts appear sometimes to be far and sometimes to be near, one just as often as the other and just as energetically. But I have never been able to persuade myself that this phenomenon occurred in the main as it ought to occur according to the Hering theory; and I never should have ventured to lay the foundation of a new theory of vision on an observation made with images that are half-extinguished in this fashion. However, I admit that I may have been unskillful. Only, Mr. Hering will have to forgive me for not being able to say that I have been convinced by this 'overwhelming' proof of the correctness of the theory, as he himself puts it. (POS 3:554)

Flat disagreement between interested parties about the outcome of one difficult and subjective experiment can scarcely decide the outcome of a long and complex scientific controversy, and this one did not, in fact, do so. Nevertheless, in the context of the period it proved extremely damaging to Hering. Neither he nor any of his students ever again defended the hypothesis of monocular depth values following Helmholtz's attack of 1866; the issue of where half-images are localized, so pivotal through the early 1860s, largely vanishes from the literature after 1866. Depth values, if they existed, could no longer be distinguished in their effects from retinal disparity cues. In the course of analyzing this one experiment, Helmholtz had called into serious question Hering's experimental and observational competence as well as his objectivity. These powerful topoi of scientific argumentation had special significance for physiological optics at the period. Reputation and credibility counted for much, and by impugning Hering's competence and veracity as an expert observer, Helmholtz had delivered the field's ultimate personal attack.

Helmholtz brought the *Handbuch* to culmination in his ultimate argument. Admitting that "these questions of discussion are not yet altogether ready for final decision," he noted that his preference for the empiricist position followed from the highest principles of scientific method. "I think it is always advisable to explain natural processes on the *least* possible number of hypotheses and on those which are as *definitely formulated* as possible" (p. 558). Having spent a large part of his life in subjective visual experimentation, Helmholtz claimed to have acquired ever greater control over the movements of his eyes and the focusing of his attention. For him, unexpected realms of perceptual experience had been brought under rational control and to scientific understanding by discipline, practice, and the reasoned exercise of the will. With this greater control had come the conviction that "the essential phenomena in this region could not be explained by any innate nervous mechanism" (ibid.). Implicit in this brief passage was a rhetorical appeal to faith in the possibility of the rational mastery of self and experience. In concluding with that implicit appeal, Helmholtz tacitly extended his defense of empiricism beyond physiology and psychology per se, to the ethical realm of the autonomous and responsible ego.

THE RHETORICAL ACHIEVEMENT OF THE *HANDBUCH*

Lawrence Prelli contends that there exists a "rhetorical logic in science" that rationally governs the form of scientific presentations and the reactions of audiences to them (Prelli 1989, 265). If so—and that claim is open to a number of objections—then the *Handbuch* presents a masterful example of that logic in action. Helmholtz's concluding experimental critique of Hering, for example, dealt almost exclusively with the hypothesis of monocular depth values. Impugning that application did not strictly imply that the broader thesis of binocular depth values had been similarly undermined, much less Hering's nativism as a set of claims about organic development. By a looser standard of contextual logic, however, Helmholtz had clearly and legitimately damaged the nativist position in his effective attack upon one of its exposed flanks.

Helmholtz applied this contextual logic to good effect elsewhere. Without strictly misrepresenting Hering's teachings, Helmholtz managed to cast them in a perspective that most contemporaries would find suspicious. He never directly linked Hering's name to those of Hegel or the *Naturphilosophen* (the common whipping boys of scientific polemic in Germany), but he did accuse nativist doctrines of "being connected" with idealist teachings that held that "there was an *identity* of nature and mind, by regarding nature as the product of the activity of a general mind" (*PO5* 3:18). Helmholtz charged that nativism required assumption of a preestablished harmony to explain the correspondence of our perceptions with real things.

At one point contextual logic did shade off into misrepresentation. In linking Hering's doctrine to the teachings of Johannes Müller, Helmholtz was merely pointing out an intellectual debt that Hering readily and frequently acknowledged. But in linking Hering at one remove to Kant, Helmholtz misled readers about Hering's intellectual antecedents. Hering never acknowledged Kantian influence and rarely commented upon Kant's philosophy; indeed, the phenomenological and organicistic tenor of Hering's thought was far removed in substance and sympathy from Kant's. This relative absence of Kantian influence explains in part why Hering, in comparison to Helmholtz, showed so little concern about the epistemological status of "real" or objective space. That unconcern with Kantian problems allowed Hering to maintain a sharper distinction between real space and perceived visual space than Helmholtz ever did, and it left him largely indifferent to how visual and tactile spatial impressions become coordinated. In Helmholtz's skillful hands, that aspect of Hering's thought was made to lend plausibility to the charges of idealism and subjectivism.

The major rhetorical achievement of the *Handbuch* lay in successfully redefining the very issue in dispute. Although earlier thinkers anticipated the positions adopted by Helmholtz and Hering, neither "nativism" nor "empiricism" as doctrines about spatial perception had existed before 1866 in the form that Helmholtz gave them in the *Handbuch*. Although empiricist accounts per se were old in 1866, Helmholtz reinterpreted that position as a predominantly *methodological* one. Empiricism in the *Handbuch* became a methodological prescription for generating preferred scientific explanations of perceptual regularities, rather than a naked assertion about the nature and genesis of those regularities. That rhetorical shift was to prove extremely important in the future controversies.

In nativism, Helmholtz defined a methodological position that perhaps no one before him had seen as a stark alternative to empiricist approaches, and he endowed it with a historically questionable pedigree. Modern scholarship rejects the traditional claim, derived largely from Helmholtz, that Kant was a nativist in any useful sense, and some contemporaries of Helmholtz knew this perfectly well (Hatfield 1990, 101–7, 222–24; Falkenstein 1990). August Classen, himself a militant Neo-Kantian, wrote in 1876 that Johannes Müller, and after him Hering, had substituted innate sensory energies for Kant's transcendental apperceptions, and thus "directly contradicted" Kantian doctrine (Classen 1876, xv; 1865–67, no. 2 [10.5.1867]). Classen declared empiricists like Wundt and Helmholtz to be marginally closer to Kant's true teachings than the nativists.

Similar claims can be made for Johannes Müller's undeniable influence on Hering and his school. Müller had accepted directional localization as an innate power of the retina, but he had regarded depth perception as an acquired capacity; at best Müller was a two-dimensional nativist only. Indeed, until Hering "extended" the theory of identity in 1864, no theorist seems to have asserted the claim that became the central issue of the later dispute, namely, that the retina possesses innate neural mechanisms that compel us to see objects in three-dimensional relief in the absence of all other cues, including kinesthetic ones.[3] Postulating an extended nativist tradition and assimilating Hering to it delivered Helmholtz from acknowledging and confronting the radical nature of Hering's claims and dictated many of the rhetorical strategies he pursued in the *Handbuch*.

HERING AND *DIE LEHRE VOM BINOCULAREN SEHEN* (1868)

In a sense Hering's entire career constituted his inevitable rejoinder to Helmholtz's powerful critique. His first specific reply, however, came in 1868 in his brief treatise on eye movements, *The Theory of Binocular Vision* (Hering 1868a, 1977/1868). There Hering refused to accept the terms of the controversy as Helmholtz had defined them. "In my earlier publications on binocular vision," he protested,

> I have indicated here and there that certain functions of the sense of sight find their basis in inborn arrangements. On this basis my opinion has been caricatured as though I let the child into the light of the world already completely educated as a virtual virtuoso, and as though the images of external objects were shoved from the eyes onto the stage of consciousness fully complete in form and color like sets from the wings of a theater. (Hering 1977/ 1868, 177–78)

In fact, Hering claimed, he had never wavered from believing that "the entire motor system of our body is apparently modifiable by experience in large degree, as much in its nervous as in its muscular part" (p. 178). What must be discovered are the *limits* of that capacity for modification. Indeed, Hering still saw the dispute between projection and identity as the central theoretical fissure, and he viewed the nativist-empiricist issue, as Helmholtz called it, as a relatively insignificant spinoff from it (p. 22).

The *Theory of Binocular Vision* advanced a thesis that itself constituted a direct rejoinder to Helmholtz. The work hinged on Hering's famous claim that "the two eyes should not ordinarily be seen as two separate organs steered by the same commands, but so to say as two halves of a *single* organ" (p. 16). He went on to assert "Hering's law," that all normal eye movements are paired movements induced by a single innervation that is shared equally by both eyes. This claim is, as Hering noted, counterintuitive. When the eyes move their fixation from point P to point P' in Figure 5.5, the left eye obviously turns through a larger angle than the right eye; it appears that each eye must receive a different innervation if they are to arrive separately at P'. But Hering pointed out a common innervation (controlled by visual feedback) must induce both eyes to equal inward convergence movements (l and r, in Figure 5.5) and equal right-versional movements (l' and r'). For the right eye, the impulse to inward convergence will partly cancel the impulse to a right turning, resulting in less net right turning than that carried out by the left eye ($r' - r$, as opposed to $l + l'$). A common innervation does suffice to cause the motion. Hering offered many proofs that this pattern of innervation is what really occurs in such movements, one of the key proofs being (in the case shown in Fig. 5.5) the twitching observed in the right eye as a result of the antagonistic muscle forces at work upon it.

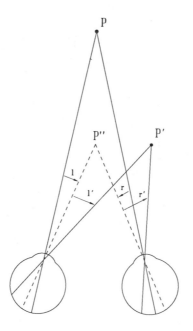

left eye   right eye

Fig. 5.5 Hering's law of equal innervations. Moving the point of fixation
from P to P' can be achieved by a
common innervation to both eyes, a
right turning combined with an
inward convergence.

Hering drew several important "corollaries" from this "law." One is that, contrary to the assertions of Helmholtz, neither adults nor new-borns can move one eye without the other. Donders' law must also be amended, since (as Hering showed in the so-called phenomenon of asymmetrical convergence) the torsion present in one eye will be a function of the position of the other eye as well as of the eye's own line of sight (pp. 83–84). It also follows that one unique innervation suffices to move the point of fixation in any given direction regardless of where the fixation point lay at the start of the motion. We may learn as newborns how to move the eye in a given direction, but we do not have to learn a different innervation for every starting point of an eye movement. Hering supported this claim with a detailed analysis of the ocular muscles and their dynamic relationships in moving the eye. While this analysis was largely derivative, Hering drew from it the highly original deduction that the eye's general adherence to Donders' and Listing's laws is a result of the inborn structure of the musculature (pp. 177–78).

Hering regarded this claim as a direct challenge to empiricism. Two pairs of eye muscles suffice to rotate the eye around any axis. The fact that the eye possesses three such pairs, Hering claimed, had led physiologists and ophthalmologists to believe that rotation around a given axis could be carried out in many different ways by many different innervations. The newborn must therefore *choose* some preferred form of rotation that optimizes vision in accordance with one of several imaginable principles. Hering's analysis showed that the dynamical interrelationships of the ocular muscle pairs ensured that a given rotation could be carried out only by one combination of muscles. The newborn need not, and cannot, *choose* how to carry out a rotation in an optimal manner. But the fit of the muscular apparatus to the needs of vision can still be thought of as optimized, in "that they have developed with one another and through one another in naturally necessary ways through the animal series" (p. 140).

Hering's tone in 1868 was less polemical, abrasive, and ebullient than in his earlier treatises; after all, he was now a recognized physiologist with a secure position in the Josephs-Akademie. But he pointedly criticized Helmholtz's experimental investigations on eye movements as imprecise and insufficiently attuned to departures from Listing's law (pp. 104–30). He also systematically criticized Helmholtz's empiricist assumptions about eye motions. Lowering the visual plane causes the eyes to converge. Helmholtz had argued that this is an acquired association, since we normally look at objects in near vision with a depressed visual plane. In fact, Hering replied, this association can be shown to follow from the musculature; if Helmholtz were correct, then lowering the visual plane should also automatically induce accommodation for near vision, which does not occur (p. 61).

Hering systematically attacked other evidence that Helmholtz had invoked in defense of empiricism. It was known that converging the eyes triggers accommodation for near-vision. Helmholtz had argued that this reflex-like relationship was acquired as a habit. Hering countered with an observation of Donders that certain squinters persist in accommodating their eyes in accordance with the anomalous degrees of convergence produced by their strabismus, even when this made clear vision almost impossible (pp. 187–98). Finally, had Helmholtz paid more attention to newborns, Hering chided, he would have recognized the innate nature of eye movements. While newborns perform primarily symmetrical movements of their limbs (clapping, kicking both feet simultaneously), their eyes show conjugate motions (turning both eyes to the right or the left together), suggesting that the eyes are being moved by a single innervation (pp. 36–39).

Hering addressed the vexed question of the extent to which the compulsion to equal innervations may be overridden. He accepted Helmholtz's demonstration that under experimental conditions we can, for example, deviate the line of sight from one eye upward or downward from that of the other by up to eight degrees, if doing so will eliminate disturbing double images in the visual field. But Hering strongly opposed Helmholtz's further claim that one eye can be induced to perform a cyclo-rotation in the interests of binocular fusion (p. 84). He subjected Helmholtz's central experiment in support of these "cyclofusional movements" to a devastating critique that Helmholtz must have found intensely embarrassing (WAH 3:44–48, no. 89; PO5 3:60–62; Hering 1977/1868, 87–91). Hering was not the only critic of this experimental claim, for Volkmann had also expressed his misgivings to Helmholtz in private correspondence (Volkmann 1856–71, no. 12 [31.03.1865]).

Hering's *Theory of Binocular Vision* invites rhetorical analysis no less than the *Handbuch*. It lacked the cool rhetorical brilliance of Helmholtz's work, but was still a very effective rejoinder. Just as Helmholtz had attacked the theory of depth values as Hering's most vulnerable quarter, so Hering chose in 1868 to attack Helmholtz's vulnerable claims about eye movements. Although he made no attempt to answer Helmholtz's philosophical and methodological charges against his position, the limited aims of the book and its restrained, empirical tone served perfectly in the task of impugning Helmholtz's experimental acumen, exposing the weakness of some of his key claims, and consequently making parts of the *Handbuch* appear inflated and dogmatic.

Also like the *Handbuch*, the *Theory of Binocular Vision* shows how the thought of its author had been actively molded by the controversy. None of Hering's claims in 1868 were inconsistent with his earlier writings, and most of his key results had been anticipated in his previous work. But the treatise of 1868 lacks the phenomenological emphasis of Hering's earlier scientific papers as well as their speculative flights. The *Theory of Binocular Vision* brings center stage an issue Hering had naively taken for granted in 1864, namely, that innate mechanisms (in this case the ocular musculature) determine perception. Despite its lack of methodological discussions, the work is more physiological, more organicist, and more conscious of these positions than Hering's earlier writings on perception had been. In short, Hering by 1868 was more of a nativist than he had been in 1864. Although he continued to disavow that label as Helmholtz's caricature of his real meaning, Hering had been deeply influenced by his opponent's portrayal of the field and by his own teachings seen reflected in Helmholtz's critique.

CONCLUSION

The large scholarly literature on scientific controversy has often ignored to what extent controversy should be considered *constitutive* of scientific change. Do the symptoms of controversy inevitably accompany significant cognitive change in science? Is the role of controversy primarily that of selecting some variants and eliminating others, or does the process actively shape the theoretical and programmatic alternatives defended by rivals? Historian Martin Rudwick has urged the latter view. He argues that the polemical posturing and rhetorical exchanges that occur in scientific controversies constitute a complex and usually tacit negotiation among the parties. The consensual scientific knowledge that emerges with resolution of the controversy (if it is resolved) is neither "discovered" nor "constructed," but is "shaped" by this complex negotiation, and in this sense controversy is deeply constitutive of scientific change (Rudwick 1985, 450–54).

The German disputes over spatial perception between 1861 and 1868 show vividly how controversy molded the views of the major protagonists and drove them to represent the field and its problems in radically new ways. The dispute that flared between Helmholtz and Hering during these years did not so much display the scientific differences between the two men as fundamentally shape them. This applied especially to Helmholtz. Between 1863 and 1866 he struggled toward his great synthesis on spatial perception in the face of cogent, continual criticism by Hering. Before that criticism he tenaciously defended some positions, quietly altered others, and vacillated on still other questions. His thought leading up to the publication of the third volume of the *Handbuch* reflected what Robert Westman once called "the local rationality of the battle field" (Westman 1978, 44). This included the pressing need to consolidate and fortify positions against the attacks of a skilled and implacable critic, and simultaneously to shift the dispute onto some new and more favorable terrain.

This Helmholtz achieved in the third volume of the *Handbuch*. There he not only offered readers a brilliant theoretical synthesis of current research on the problems of spatial perception; he also defined for the first time two philosophical and methodological positions that he called "nativism" and "empiricism" and portrayed them as polar alternatives transfusing the history and logical structure of the field. Now this portrayal of the field was neither historically accurate nor conceptually inevitable, but it was brilliant and highly effective rhetoric. It tacitly rewrote both the history and the future of the field. Despite the protests of Hering, Helmholtz successfully imposed his own version of the nativist-empiricist polarity both upon the psychologists and physiologists who came after him and upon the historians who have studied and evaluated his own philosophical and scientific contributions. The respective positions of nativism and empiricism had very real and very deep historical roots that predated Helmholtz and Hering. But the form that those positions took in the late nineteenth century was in the beginning a rhetorical artifact, created by Hermann von Helmholtz as a weapon in his controversy with Ewald Hering. That artifact constituted one further element in their "negotiation" of a contested field. This angry negotiation would be continued by at least another generation of German scientists.

CHAPTER SIX

Helmholtz on Light and Color

THE PUBLICATION OF THE FINAL VOLUME of the *Handbuch* and the diffi-cult months that preceded it marked a turning point in Helmholtz's life. After 1866 he grew increasingly indifferent to physiology as a research field (Kirsten 1986, 237–38, no. 115). With his interests already turning more and more to hydro- and electrodynamics, he agreed in 1871 to come to Berlin as professor of experimental physics. There he continued to accept physiologists and psychologists into his institute, to revise past work, and to reiterate his basic epistemological position, but until shortly before his death he published little new research on sensory problems.

Hering, on the other hand, found his interest in sensory perception renewed and strengthened in the early 1870s. Buoyed by the reception of his work on eye movements, he resumed his attack upon the Helm-holtzian orthodoxy. Between 1872 and 1875 he published the six install-ments of his famous work, *Zur Lehre vom Lichtsinne (On the Theory of the Light Sense)*. There he challenged the theory of vision that Helmholtz had laid out in 1860 in the second volume of the *Handbuch* and pre-sented his own alternative, the opponent process theory. That story, how-ever, requires the following prelude, which is set in the 1850s and devoted to the small revolution in the study of light perception that occurred in that decade.

HELMHOLTZ ON COLOR MIXING, 1852–55

Helmholtz took his tentative first step into the confused field of color vision and light perception in 1852, when he publicly criticized Brewster's anti-Newtonian, triple-spectrum theory of light (Kirsten 1986, 123–27, no. 30; Sherman 1981, 33–41). Helmholtz brought no new charges against the absorption experiments by which Brewster supported that theory, but he reiterated many made by previous critics and argued that the experiments had been vitiated by various distorting factors. He argued strongly that once those distortions had been eliminated, the re-sults of the experiments conformed entirely to Newton's theory (*WAH* 2:24–44, no. 24; Kremer 1993a; Sherman 1981, 45–59).

Simultaneously with his critique of Brewster, Helmholtz published a short paper on color mixing in which he explored the various senses of the term "primary colors" or *Grundfarben* (*WAH* 2:3–23, no. 23; Kremer 1993a; Sherman 1981, 81–92). He pointed out that "primary colors" can mean the colors from which all others can be compounded, as in the artistic and craft tradition of pigment mixing; or colors corresponding to objective forms of light, as in Brewster's theory; or colors corresponding to particular states of activation in the retinal nerve fibers, as on Thomas Young's. It was therefore possible to distinguish empirical, physical, and physiological senses of the term.

To explore these meanings further, Helmholtz described experiments in which he had allowed sunlight to pass through a V-shaped slit and then through a flint glass prism, producing in the image an area of overlapping spectra in which all possible binary combinations of spectral colors were displayed. Examining these binary combinations, Helmholtz noted that the combination of yellow and indigo-blue (and that combination alone) produced white. That observation, however, clashed with the well-established fact that mixtures of yellow and blue pigments yield green. This conflict led Helmholtz to enunciate the fundamental distinction between additive and subtractive color mixtures and so to clarify the divergent results obtained from mixing pigments and mixing spectral lights. In one stroke the paper reconciled the experience of color derived from the craft and Newtonian optical traditions and clarified the relationship between Newton's color circle and the various pigment color triangles.

In these experiments Helmholtz could find only one binary pair of spectral colors that together yielded white, although in slightly more elaborate experiments he found various three-component mixtures that would do so. He also found himself generally unable to make compounds that would match the various spectral colors by using spectral red, green, and violet as primaries. Using these three spectral primaries he could match the hue of any spectral color, but the compounds—especially those of yellow mixed from spectral red and green and those of blue mixed from spectral violet and green—were always whitish and desaturated in comparison to their spectral, monochromatic equivalents.

Helmholtz interpreted this experimental outcome to mean that Young's theory of retinal action must be false. In his own words,

> If the sensation of yellow excited by the yellow rays of the spectrum were only due to the fact that [these rays] simultaneously excite the sensations of red and green and both together gave yellow, then exactly the same sensation [of yellow] would have to be excited by a simultaneous action of red and green rays. However, the latter never generate so bright and vivid a yellow, as the yellow rays do. (*WAH* 2:22, no. 23)

These remarks embody an assumption about Young's theory, namely, that each retinal receptor type is so highly tuned to a particular light frequency, that light at any one of those three precise frequencies affects that receptor type alone. The remark also assumes tacitly that the sensation corresponding to light of any one of those three primary frequencies is a color of spectral hue and saturation.[1] On those assumptions Young's theory could still explain how all possible hues can be mixed from three properly chosen physiological primaries. It could not, however, account for Helmholtz's demonstration that at least some mixtures of spectral lights lack the degree of saturation possessed by their monochromatic equivalents in the spectrum, or explain how we are able to see those monochromatic equivalents at full spectral saturation.

Helmholtz had feared attack for his critique of Brewster; instead, it was his paper on compound colors that drew criticism, partly due to his exaggerated claims for the originality of his experimental methods and his results. The most important critique, however, came from an unknown mathematics teacher in Stettin, Hermann Günther Grassmann, who claimed that Helmholtz's results were inconsistent with the principles of Newton's color circle (Grassmann 1853). Grassmann argued that any color sensation is fully specified by the three variables of hue, brightness, and saturation. He correlated these sensory variables to the physical ones of wavelength or frequency (for monochromatic lights), amount or intensity of light, and the intensity of the intermixed white. He clarified the relationship of these variables to the geometrical relationships on Newton's color circle and developed a rigorous mathematical interpretation of the barycentric weighting procedures that can be applied to the circle to predict the outcome of color mixing. Grassmann also produced a quasi-mathematical demonstration to show that every spectral light represented on Newton's color circle must have a spectral complementary, that is, another monochromatic light which when mixed with it produces white. He accused Helmholtz of somehow erring in his results of 1852, which detected only one pair of spectral complementaries (Kremer 1993a; Sherman 1981, 93–116).

Stung by this criticism, Helmholtz altered his experimental approach (borrowing techniques first used by Leon Foucault), and announced in a new paper of 1855 that he had indeed been able to find seven complementary color pairs in the spectrum and (by observing Fraunhofer lines) measure their wavelengths (WAH 2:45–70, no. 35). In revising his former result, Helmholtz introduced two conventions that were to be the basis of all subsequent colorimetry.

First, he noted that greens have purples for their complementary colors, and he broke with Grassmann and a long tradition of Newtonian optics by denying that true purples appear in the spectrum at all. Purples are always mixed colors, composed of extreme red and violet. If every prismatic color is to have a complementary as Grassmann required, and if all those colors and their complementaries must form a circle or any other closed curve as traditionally assumed since Newton, then the purple sequence must be inserted by fiat between the reds and violets.

Helmholtz's second innovation was still more radical. The spectral colors in sunlight are the most vivid and highly saturated ones we see; this is to be expected, since as monochromatic lights they contain no intermixed physical white light at all. Since distance from the white center point on Newton's color circle measures the saturation of any color, the prismatic colors had traditionally been represented as equidistant from the center and arrayed along a circumference. The barycentric mixing property then implies that for any complementary pair, equal amounts of the components are required to produce white. But Helmholtz's experiments showed this not to be the case. By varying the width of the slits that admitted light to his experimental apparatus, he was able to measure roughly the relative intensities of each component in each pair of complementary lights. He found the intensity ratios to vary widely and rarely to be equal to one (p. 61).

This surprising result presented Helmholtz with a dilemma: preserve Newton's convention of barycentric mixing, or preserve the circularity of the spectral locus on the color circle (pp. 64–65). He unhesitatingly chose barycentricity. The curve of spectral colors then cannot be a circle, but its exact form can be roughly deduced from the proportions of the components in the complementary mixes. Helmholtz suggested a sketch like Figure 6.1, in which the purples have been inserted as a straight line joining the extremes of the visible spectrum. Helmholtz pointed out that because the points along the spectral locus are not equidistant from white, they should not appear equally saturated, and in fact they do not. Spectral greens, yellows, and oranges appear much more whitish than violets and most blues (pp. 63–64). But nothing in contemporary theory could explain these paradoxical differences in saturation arising from monochromatic spectral lights of equal physical purity. Helmholtz had stumbled upon a major obstacle to mapping physical properties of the light stimulus onto sensory response.

Helmholtz concluded his 1855 paper with a brief, searching analysis of a central problem that Grassmann's treatment had ignored: the question of how the subjective brightness of a color sensation could be defined and measured (WAH 2:66–70, no. 36). If the sensation arises from a mixed light, Helmholtz noted, then one way of proceeding would be to assign arbitrary measures to the brightness of each component in the mix (the units and measures of their *physical* intensities will do). We might then adopt as a convention a tacit assumption made by Grassmann, namely,

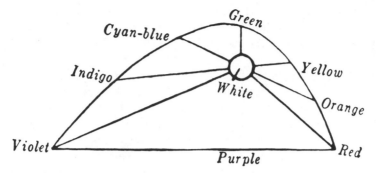

Fig. 6.1 The spectral locus, with interpolated purples, as sketched by Helmholtz in 1855. *Source: POS* 2:139. Reproduced with permission of Dover Publications, Inc.

that the brightness of a light mixture is the sum of the brightnesses of its components. In a far-reaching discussion Helmholtz demonstrated what followed from this convention of measurement. If we postulate positions on the plane of Newton's color circle for any three, noncollinear points (colors), and if we measure their respective brightnesses in any way we like (we may assign unit brightnesses to each), then that information, plus the convention of barycentric mixing, allows us to determine the position on the plane of any other color mixed in known proportions from these three. Conversely, the position of any color point may be expressed in terms of the three initial points; that includes colors that can actually be mixed from the three initial colors (and so lie inside the triangle they form) and those that cannot be so mixed (and hence lie outside the triangle). Helmholtz did not speculate about how this severe mathematical procedure might be realized in experimental practice.

CLERK MAXWELL AND THE ORIGINS OF COLORIMETRY

Another researcher quickly upstaged the important contributions that Helmholtz had made to the study of color vision in 1852 and 1855. Clerk Maxwell was only twenty-four years old in 1855, but he had been conducting experiments on color vision since 1849. He had also read Helmholtz's paper of 1852 and Grassmann's critique of it, and he had reached many of the same insights. In 1855 he published in the *Transactions* of the Royal Society of Edinburgh a paper that went far beyond Helmholtz in demonstrating actual experimental techniques for mixing and matching primary colors and determining the position of mixed colors on the color plane (Maxwell 1855).

So fundamental were Maxwell's procedures to all subsequent colorimetry that we need to follow at least one of his experiments in some detail.[2] Maxwell first chose three colors as primaries. In his initial experiment those were represented by three colored papers that he described as emerald green (*EG*), vermilion (*V*), and ultramarine (*U*). To mix these primaries, Maxwell used the familiar color wheel, a disk such as that illustrated in Figure 6.2 that could be rapidly rotated. The inner circle contained two paper cutouts, one black and one white, made to slide over one another so that the experimenter could adjust the relative amounts of black and white displayed. The outer circle similarly displayed the three colored papers chosen as primaries in three sectors around the circumference. The experimenter could adjust the relative sizes of the sectors by sliding the paper sectors over one another. When the disk was spun very rapidly, the colors of the paper sectors blended into a mixed sensation, the inner circle appearing gray, approaching white as the surface of the white sector was increased at the expense of the black. When the observer looked at the rapidly spinning outer circle, light from the primary colored papers produced in the eye a mixed color. Maxwell reasoned that the contribution of each primary color to the intensity of the mixed color must be in proportion to the area of that primary displayed on the disk.

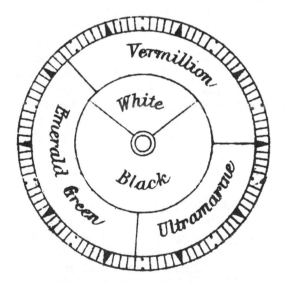

Fig. 6.2 Maxwell's schematic drawing of his rotating color wheel, showing the inner and outer rings with adjustable colored sectors and the outer scale on the perimeter. *Source*: Maxwell 1855, Figure 5 (facing p. 155). Reproduced with permission of Dover Publications, Inc.

Maxwell experimentally adjusted the proportions of the three primary colors displayed on the disk until, upon being spun, they combined to produce a white (or gray) exactly equivalent to the white displayed in the inner circle. Once the match was achieved, Maxwell read the proportion of the inner and outer circles occupied by each colored paper off a perimeter scale, and expressed them in hundredths of a full circle. This yielded a "color equation," which he wrote for the particular papers in question as

$$0.37 \ V + 0.27 \ U + 0.36 \ EG = 0.28 \ W + 0.72 \ Bk$$

If we imagine the three primaries to occupy the three vertices of a triangle, then the color equation allows us to use the barycentric properties of the color plane to locate the point corresponding to the mixed white. We use the color coefficients of the primaries (the contribution of each to the total intensity) as barycentric weightings applied to each of the vertices. Along the triangle-side UV we locate the point a such that $aV/aU = 0.27/0.37$. Then along the line aEG we find the point W such that $aW/WEG = 0.36/(0.37 + 0.27)$. The point W corresponds to the mixed white on the color plane defined by the three primaries.[3]

In principle, similar procedures allow any color C to be expressed in terms of any three primaries. Paper of the color C is substituted for the black and white sectors of the inner circle, and the primary color sectors in the outer circle are adjusted until a match is made; usually black or white must also be added to one side. In practice Maxwell rarely matched chromatic colors in this direct fashion, but rather manipulated the color equations so that the subject always adjusted a mixed gray field, one component of which was the color C, to a given gray (Maxwell 1860, 420). Maxwell found that that procedure often gave rise to negative color coefficients, which suggested negative brightness. Undeterred by the paradox of this concept, he simply declared a negative color coefficient on one side of an equation operationally equivalent to adding that much color to the lights on the other side (ibid. 416–18). Negative color coefficients allow colors that cannot physically be mixed from the primaries nevertheless to be located on the color plane, as Helmholtz had also demonstrated.

In his classic paper of 1855 Maxwell announced his allegiance to Thomas Young's "theory of three distinct modes of sensation in the retina, each . . . produced in different degrees by the different rays" (Maxwell 1855, 136). In principle this was the same theory Helmholtz had considered and rejected in 1852, a fact that the young Maxwell, who stood in some awe of Helmholtz, tactfully failed to mention (e.g., Maxwell 1990, 492). In practice, however, Maxwell understood Young's theory rather differently than Helmholtz originally did. Maxwell assumed Young to mean that every monochromatic light stimulates all three "modes of sensation," even though one or two color responses will predominate in the resulting mixed color (Maxwell 1855, 136). Because the three fundamental sensations together yield white, it follows that every monochromatic light stimulates some white response; all spectral lights appear to us somewhat desaturated. It also follows that the fundamental sensations cannot be spectral colors. If it were possible to stimulate one of Young's modes of sensation without simultaneously stimulating the others, the resulting color sensation would be a hue of greater-than-spectral saturation. Maxwell doubted that these primary sensations could ever be obtained as pure sensations (ibid. 151).

Maxwell's version of Young's theory, which he attributed directly to Young without further comment, obviously avoids the difficulty that had caused Helmholtz in 1852 to reject the theory as he then understood it. Because the fundamental sensations are themselves of greater-than-spectral saturation, they can readily be mixed to yield all the prismatic colors at their observed degree of saturation. This can best be envisioned, as Maxwell carefully explained, in terms of the color plane and the spectrum locus (see Figure 6.3). Maxwell represented the spectral locus as the conventional circle $VGYR$ with white at the center (the argument is unchanged if the locus is not a circle, or if the purples are inserted). The colors corresponding to Young's fundamental sensations (which Maxwell regarded as most likely being species of red, green, and violet) will form the vertices of triangle vrg, which entirely encloses the spectral locus (Maxwell 1856). Mixtures of the three fundamental sensations v, r, and g involve only positive color coefficients, and in practice all those mixtures lie on or inside the spectral locus. Color points outside the triangle are impossible to stimulate physiologically or realize as sensations; points outside the spectral locus but on or inside the triangle could represent real sensations if it were somehow possible to eliminate or reduce one of the primary responses.

Maxwell was still not through. Because we cannot obtain the fundamental sensations in pure form, we cannot empirically derive color equations for them and so locate them on the color plane. Strictly speaking we cannot even know to what spectral hues they correspond, although they are most likely a green, an extreme red, and violet or perhaps blue. Nevertheless, Maxwell was convinced that the visual experience of the color blind allows us to determine the position of one fundamental sensation (Maxwell 1855, 137–42).

Maxwell accepted the hypothesis of George Wilson that color blindness arises from the absence of the red sensory response in individuals so afflicted. In 1854 or 1855 Maxwell conducted color-matching experiments with two color blind individuals at Cambridge, and confirmed that their vision was, in his phrase, "dichromatic." While normal individuals must mix three primary colors if they are to match some arbitrarily cho-

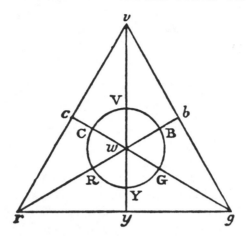

Fig. 6.3 Maxwell's sketch of the spectral
locus, represented as a circle, inside the triangle formed by the color points of Young's
three fundamental sensations. *Source*:
Maxwell 1855, 121. Reproduced with permission of Dover Publications, Inc.

sen color, dichromatic individuals need only two. These results confirmed
Maxwell's conviction that the vision of dichromats is exactly like that of
trichromats who have been deprived of the set of Young's retinal receptors that produce the red response (ibid. 140).

From one of his dichromats Maxwell obtained the equation

$$.19\ G + .05\ B + .76\ Bk = 1.00\ R$$

This individual found 0.24 units of the dark blue-green color located at
the barycentric position b in Figure 6.4 to be equivalent in hue and in
brightness to a full unit of the red primary at R. Maxwell reasoned that
all colors that lie on the line bR must be equivalent in hue for the dichromat and must decrease steadily in unit brightness from b through R. Indeed, there must be some point D on the extension of bR for which the
unit brightness is zero. Assuming the linearity that follows from Grassmann's laws, that point is readily found: $RD/Rb = 24/(100 - 24)$. The
point D, Maxwell argued, "represents the pure sensation which is unknown to the colour-blind, and the addition of this sensation to any others cannot alter it in their estimation. It is for them equivalent to black"
(p. 139).

The point D, Maxwell went on, represents one of the three fundamental sensations (specifically, a sensation of extreme red hue and extraspectral saturation) which is present in normal individuals but absent in the

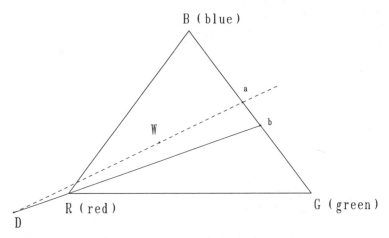

Fig. 6.4 Maxwell's color triangle of 1855, with experimental primary colors *B*, *R*, and *G* at the vertices. For this color triangle Maxwell determined that the fundamental sensation missing to the red blind must lie at point *D*. *Source*: Maxwell 1855, No. 2 (redrawn). Reproduced with permission of Dover Publications, Inc.

color blind. For dichromats the point *D* must be the point of intersection of many straight lines on the color plane, each one being the locus of color sensations of a constant hue that varies along the line in brightness and saturation. One of these, shown in Figure 6.4 as the line *DWa*, will pass through the white point. All points on the upper side of the line *DW* will appear to the dichromat as varieties of the blue fundamental sensation. Maxwell also insisted that those below it will appear as varieties of yellow, ignoring that the logic of his argument suggested that they should be seen as green (p. 141).

YOUNG'S THEORY AND THE *HANDBUCH* (1860)

Helmholtz must have read Maxwell's brilliant paper of 1855 with intense chagrin. Not only had Maxwell carried Helmholtz's own ideas further, but he had also created a theory of retinal action that sufficed, as Helmholtz must quickly have noted, to explain an even wider range of visual phenomena than Maxwell realized. By 1858 at the latest Helmholtz had adopted Young's theory in its Maxwellian form; he employed it in several preliminary papers on contrast, color blindness, and afterimages during 1858 and 1859; and he made Young's theory the leitmotif of the second volume of the *Handbuch*, which he published in 1860. So extensively and successfully did Helmholtz employ Young's theory to bring order to the chaotic field of color perception, that the theory was widely known thereafter as the "Young–Helmholtz" theory of color vision, despite Maxwell's undisputed priority.[4]

Richard Kremer noted that in the field of color theory (as in much of his other work) Helmholtz "acted as a creative borrower and synthesizer who clarified others' ideas, removed conceptual problems from others' experiments, collected scattered researches of others into unified programs of research, and sought to define orthodoxy by formulating an authoritative discourse for the field" (Kremer 1993a, 2). That genius for synthesis was nowhere more evident than in the second volume of the *Handbuch*, in which Helmholtz drew upon the work of Jan Purkinje, Johannes Müller, Thomas Young, Heinrich Dove, Ernst Brücke, Joseph Plateau, Heinrich Meyer, and especially that of Gustav Fechner and Clerk Maxwell to forge a new basis for the study of color perception. Two elements made possible the synthesis of these disparate bodies of works into a seamless theoretical whole. One was Young's theory, which emerged as an emphatic and protean leitmotif, woven through the disparate discussions of the *Handbuch*. The other was Helmholtz's ingenious and insistent bifurcation of visual phenomena into physiological and psychological realms.

Helmholtz opened the *Handbuch* with chapters that examined the kinds of stimuli that could evoke the sensation of light and the anatomical structures of the retina that could be most likely identified as light-sensitive. In 1860 he identified these as the cones alone, although by the 1867 reissue he was prepared to accept the rods as well. Helmholtz also considered the vexed and much-discussed question of whether the dimensions and density of these structures sufficed to explain the observed limits of visual acuity. In a chapter on "the simple colors" he analyzed the extent of the spectrum and its hues and discussed his previously used methods for obtaining pure spectra. In a chapter on compound colors Helmholtz set out again his distinction between additive and subtractive color mixtures, the results and methods of his previous experiments on color mixing, the determination of color sensations by the three variables of luminosity, hue, and saturation, Grassmann's laws, and the principles of the barycentric color plane. And—for the first time—he gave a short summary of Maxwell's experiments with color mixing and his derivation of color equations.

Helmholtz's low-key introduction of Young's theory directly followed the discussion of the experimental mixing and matching of primary colors and geometric constructions on the barycentric color plane (*POS* 2:141–46). This skillful juxtaposition tacitly conflated Young's fundamental sensations and their "mixing" in the sensorium with the operationally demonstrable mixing of other sets of primaries, and so rendered the concept less disconcerting. Helmholtz adopted Young's practice of speaking of the primary responses as associated with "three distinct sets of nervous fibers." He added that this assumption was wholly compatible with contemporary anatomical knowledge, but that Young's theory could equally well be understood as asserting the existence of three separate processes in each retinal fiber, provided that those processes remained wholly independent of each other before reaching the sensorium. Each version was compatible with Müller's law, and Helmholtz asserted his belief that "Young's hypothesis is only a more special application of the law of specific sense energies" (p. 145).

In that discussion, Helmholtz also introduced the much-reproduced, but entirely hypothetical spectral sensitivity curves shown in Figure 6.5. These heuristic curves show the separate response strengths of Young's three fundamental sensations (red, green, and violet as one, two, and three) for light of constant physical intensity but of all visible wavelengths (p. 143). The total color response at any wavelength will be the sum of the three fundamental responses. Because the three curves are represented as coterminous (in accordance with Maxwell's understanding of the theory), every wavelength must stimulate all three processes to some extent and so produce trace amounts of white sensation.

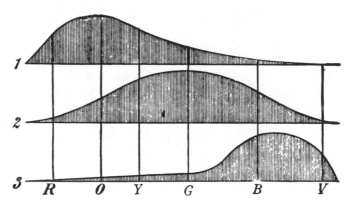

Fig. 6.5 Helmholtz's heuristic sketch of the spectral frequency response curves for Young's hypothetical red, green, and violet processes. *Source: POS* 2:143. Reproduced with permission of Dover Publications, Inc.

Helmholtz then applied Young's theory to color blindness (pp. 146–54). Like Maxwell, Helmholtz diagnosed color blindness as the absence of one of Young's fundamental sensations. Unlike Maxwell, Helmholtz was aware of the two classes of dichromats identified by Seebeck, and he unhesitatingly identified Seebeck's first and most common class as "red blind" (they lack the fundamental sensation of red) and Seebeck's other class as "green blind." Helmholtz reported experiments of his own, carried out on a local student diagnosed as red blind, using techniques very similar to those laid down by Maxwell. His results located the missing fundamental sensation on the barycentric plane as an extraspectral red very near the point experimentally determined by Maxwell.

Helmholtz enthusiastically reported that the interpretation of color blindness based upon Young's theory explained all the best-established facts about the disorder. It explains why the red blind see the red end of the spectrum dark and foreshortened; why the green blind see the spectrum the same length as normals; why the green blind (unlike the red blind) can readily distinguish between violets and reds; and why the red blind confuse white with the bluish-green of the spectrum.[5] As to what the color blind actually see, Helmholtz speculated that the red blind see all colors as violet, green, or mixtures of the two. They probably do not see white, he opined, although they use the term. He believed that dichromats reported reds, yellows, and greens all as yellow merely because of verbal confusion. Normals call the most luminous color of their spectrum "yellow," and the red blind learn to do the same, even though the most luminous hue in their spectrum would appear to normals as a brilliant and highly saturated green. By extension, they learn in the absence of other cues to call all colors that appear greenish to them "yellow." The green blind, Helmholtz speculated, probably see all colors as mixtures of violet and red. He called for further studies of the green blind, in order to locate the green fundamental sensation.

In Helmholtz's hands Young's theory proved no less successful in explaining the phenomena of afterimages (p. 228–63). They arise, Helmholtz speculated, as "variations of sensitivity" in the retina, induced by fatigue in Young's receptors. When we look at a bright object and suddenly turn our eyes away, the stimulated retinal receptors continue momentarily to respond, so that we see a bright outline of the object, which we call a "positive afterimage." When the positive afterimage fades and the retina is uniformly stimulated by a new illumination, then those retinal elements that were fatigued by the previous exposure will for a period no longer respond as vigorously as their neighbors. We then see a negative afterimage, that is, an outline of the bright object now substantially darker than the rest of the visual field. The occurrence of positive and negative afterimages depends upon the time and intensity of the original exposure, and especially upon the intensity of the new illumination that evokes the negative afterimages. The intrinsic light-chaos of the eye, which Helmholtz believed could be quite intense, suffices to evoke vivid negative afterimages in the absence of all external light. Similar reasoning based on Young's theory explains the well-known fact that negative after-images induced by staring at colored objects or fields appear in the complementary color.

Throughout this discussion Helmholtz drew extensively and explicitly on the work of Gustav Fechner, who had long championed a theory of afterimages based upon retinal fatigue (Turner 1987b). Indeed, Helmholtz's treatment of afterimages was little more than Fechner's explanations and experiments translated into the language of Young's theory. Accordingly, Helmholtz strongly opposed hypotheses like those of Belgian physicist Joseph Plateau, who held that any stimulation of the retina automatically triggers an antagonistic action, which commences immediately upon cessation of the initial stimulus (*PO5* 2:258–62).

Following up a pregnant suggestion by Maxwell, Helmholtz invoked afterimage phenomena as direct proof of Young's theory. Helmholtz stared at a small, monochromatic spectral field and then suddenly turned to look at a larger field illuminated with spectral light of the same intensity but of the complementary hue. The negative afterimage of the first field appeared in the complementary hue as expected, but in comparison to the surrounding field it appeared far more intensely saturated. The experiment showed, as Maxwell had predicted, that color sensations of extraspectral saturation can be experienced, when retinal fatigue allows one or two of the fundamental processes to work with reduced input from the third (p. 244).

Helmholtz also proposed that the response strength of the three separate processes might vary in distinct and nonlinear ways with the physical intensity of the illumination. That assumption allowed several puzzling visual phenomena to be modeled by Young's theory. One was the Purkinje effect, by which violets and blues on the one hand and reds and greens on the other seem to alter their relative levels of apparent brightness as the intensity of the total illumination changes. Another was the familiar observation that at increasingly high light levels, all colors become more whitish until finally hues cannot be distinguished at all. Finally, we can assume that the activity of each receptor type declines at a slightly different and nonlinear rate after an intense but brief stimulus. This offered explanatory purchase upon the recalcitrant phenomenon of chromatic fading, even though Helmholtz conceded that the model could not predict the actual sequence of colors (pp. 245–55).

SIMULTANEOUS CONTRAST

A second element, woven into the argument of the *Handbuch* alongside Young's theory, contributed to Helmholtz's formidable synthesis of color vision studies in 1860. This was his radical demarcation between sensory phenomena that allegedly arose from physiological causes and those from unconscious acts of judgment. That line sharply divided afterimages, which Helmholtz explained physiologically as results of retinal fatigue, from simultaneous contrast, which in his opinion resulted from erroneous judgments.

A typical situation of brightness contrast occurs when we juxtapose white and black fields and fixate a point on the boundary. The white then appears whiter, the black, blacker, than either would appear alone. Color contrast occurs when we fixate a light gray field against a colored ground. The gray field will then appear distinctly tinged with color, and specifically with a hue complementary to that of the ground. Most of the many theorists who had investigated these phenomena before Helmholtz had regarded afterimages and contrast as closely related effects; they frequently explained the latter by mechanisms of retinal induction. A stimulated retinal area was hypothesized to induce an opposite and opposing action in neighboring areas or somehow alter their sensitivity to light (*POS* 2:297). Joseph Plateau's was one theory of this sort; it treated both as the same phenomenon, the contrast expressing itself over time in afterimages, across space in simultaneous contrast (pp. 258–62).

Helmholtz rejected all such views and insisted that all true cases of simultaneous contrast, unlike successive contrast, arise from subjective, inferential judgments (pp. 264–99). They are like optical illusions, false conclusions that we draw in comparing the hue and brightness of juxtaposed fields. They illustrate our more general psychological disposition "to regard those differences which are distinctly and positively perceived . . . as being greater than those which either stand out indistinctly or must be estimated with the aid of the memory" (p. 270). If the role of this disposition had not been appreciated in earlier contrast experiments, Helmholtz suggested, it was because researchers had typically neglected to hold rigid fixation on the contrasting colored field being observed. This allowed afterimages to be engendered, and they confused physiological and psychological determinants (pp. 265–69).

That many color judgments are subjective and inferential was neither a new nor a controversial claim when Helmholtz made it. It appears, for example, in the writings of Michel Chevreul, Gustav Fechner, and Ernst Brücke, the two latter being individuals to whom Helmholtz owed heavy intellectual debts (Kremer 1993a, 51). But Helmholtz insisted on a sharper demarcation between physiological and inferential effects than had any writer before him. His motive for adopting this unusual and eventually controversial position seems to have lain less in philosophical assumptions about the eye's mind than in his early encounter with several phenomena that defied obvious physical or physiological explanations, yet seemed readily susceptible to "inferential" ones. These took on a formulaic role in Helmholtz's imagination, and he generalized them to many other cases and experimental situations. One of these, stereoscopic luster, was discussed in the previous chapter (*WAH* 3:4–5, no. 41; *PO5* 3:525–26). Another was the work of Gustav Theodor Fechner on the famous colored shadows experiment.

Before the 1850s simultaneous contrast was often discussed in terms of the two "colored shadows" cast by a stick or other small object onto a white wall when the stick is illuminated from two different sources with light of different colors, typically the yellowish light of a candle and white daylight. Under these circumstances, the shadow cast by daylight and illuminated by candlelight is seen yellow-tinged, just as expected from the nature of the illumination. But the shadow cast by the candle and illuminated by white daylight was seen as bluish, blue being the complementary color to the yellowish surround. Debate raged about why this contrast effect occurred, and many variations were done on the experiment. Gottfried Osann viewed the bluish shadow through a darkened tube that blocked all vision of the surrounding yellowish field. He observed to his surprise that the shadow persisted in its bluish hue even when the yellow surround could no longer be seen. Osann deduced from this that the blueness must somehow adhere in the objective light; it cannot be induced "subjectively" in the eye by the simultaneous presence of the yellow (Fechner 1838).

In a classic discussion of 1838, Fechner confirmed that the color complementary to the surround (blue in this case) does persist when viewed in isolation through a darkened tube, but he observed that it also persisted unchanged in hue when the color of the objective illumination was altered. If the first candle is blown out, or if a second candle is lit to illuminate the bluish shadow, the hue we see through the tube persists in its bluishness. Only when we remove the tube and view the shadow and its colored surround simultaneously does our perception of the color of the shadow alter significantly.

Fechner deduced from this experiment that contrast colors cannot originate "objectively" in the nature of the external stimulus as Osann had claimed. The experiment deeply impressed Helmholtz, who cited it frequently and drew a still stronger conclusion from it, namely, that neither physical nor physiological explanations sufficed to explain its outcome. On the contrary, he wrote, "no experiment shows more impressively or more clearly the influence of judgement on our determination of colour" (*PO5* 2:272).

Another crucial experiment done by Fechner reinforced this insight. Fechner showed that brightness contrast fades with time: juxtaposed black and white fields both fade toward a common gray as we stare fixedly at them for several minutes. The darkening of the white areas can readily be explained as due to a gradual fatiguing of the areas of the retina exposed to white (Fechner 1840). But since the retina cannot by definition be "fatigued for black," fatigue cannot explain why the black areas lighten to gray. To get around this difficulty, Fechner proposed that as the white field grows gradually darker due to retinal fatigue, we commit an unconscious "error of judgement" and falsely attribute the change in the relative brightness of the fields in part to a lightening of the black area. We commit this error, Fechner hypothesized, because the eye has no basis under these circumstances for an "objective" comparison of the black field to a true white (ibid.).

In the *Handbuch* Helmholtz generalized this suggestion far beyond anything Fechner imagined or approved. Drawing on similar conclusions reached by his friend Ernst Brücke in 1851, Helmholtz concluded that the assessment of true white is the most difficult and uncertain of all color judgments. In the absence of other whites for comparison, it involves being "able to recognize whether the relative intensities of the three fundamental colours of which it is composed have been altered or not" (*PO5* 2:274).

Helmholtz was sure that his earlier research on complementary spectral lights had illustrated the effects of our uncertainty in assessing objective white. He had found in 1855 that complementary pairs remained a steady and constant white, even as the overall physical intensity of the light entering the apparatus was increased over a wide range. This constancy struck Helmholtz as highly improbable on physiological grounds alone, since the Purkinje phenomenon showed that the subjective brightness of two different hues is very different at different levels of intensity. It suggested to Helmholtz that we have learned to sense, and unconsciously to compensate for, intensity changes in the components of white light that cause it to depart from objective whiteness. Specifically, we have learned to take sunlight as our standard of white and to psychologically correct for the daily variations in intensity that should make sunlight bluish at low intensities and yellowish at high ones (*WAH* 2:45–70, no. 35). Helmholtz pointed out that the most common (and important) manifestation of this inferential correction lies in our striking capacity instinctively to see objects we know to be white as white and not gray, regardless of the intensity of illumination that falls upon them (*PO5* 2:131, 287).

The last crucial experiment that shaped Helmholtz's thinking about contrast was that performed by Heinrich Meyer in 1855 and reported with many variants by Helmholtz (Meyer 1855). Take a piece of vivid green paper and lay upon it a small patch of gray paper of about the same brightness. A slight red tinge can sometimes be seen on the gray paper, but the contrast effect is relatively weak. Now overlay both with a piece of transparent white paper, which has the effect of desaturating the green ground. Now the red contrast color comes out very strongly on the gray patch seen through the transparent white. Meyer's experiment further proved to Helmholtz that contrast does not arise physiologically, from some retinal induction effect. If it arose physiologically, then vivid inducing colors ought to produce the strongest contrast effects, whereas Meyer's experiment shows that the strongest contrast colors are induced by whitish, desaturated colors (*POS* 2:276–78).

Brightness contrast can be plausibly attributed to our alleged tendency to exaggerate clearly seen differences, but that tendency scarcely explains color contrast, as it arises in experiments like Meyer's. Helmholtz's explanations of simultaneous color contrast were, in fact, rather involved. When we fixate a gray patch on a whitish green ground, our task is to assess the colors present. To do so we must take into account the level of brightness and the nature of the illumination. We do this by unconsciously comparing the colors present to white, but in this case that cannot accurately be done, because no pure white is present and the dominant color is a desaturated green. Under these circumstances the eye mistakenly adopts the green as its white standard (a mistake more readily made if the green is desaturated). In the language of Young's theory, the eye takes the ratio of the contributions of each primary process to the green sensation as the ratio that defines white. But by that standard of white, the process ratios characteristic of the gray field will contain an excess of red response over white. We correspondingly "see" the gray field as red, because this corresponds to our momentary and involuntarily adoption of the desaturated green as the white standard (pp. 270–78).

Helmholtz also offered a second, slightly different explanation of the contrast action in Meyer's experiment. He suggested that the overlay of transparent white paper creates the illusion that we are viewing the gray patch through a green veil, and that the gray patch lies behind the veil. In order to see objects in their true colors, we have learned to "correct" for the effects of intervening, transparent media, just as we have learned to "correct" for the prevailing illumination in assessing the intrinsic brightness of objects. In Meyer's experiment, we correct for the green veil by assuming that the gray patch must be redder than it appears, and we see it as such. If we draw dark borders around the outline of the gray patch, Helmholtz observed, then it appears to us as a distinct, separate object seen without obstruction; the contrast color immediately disappears, giving clear evidence of the "psychological" nature of the effect (pp. 282–87).

Other writers did not agree with Helmholtz that phenomena like this demanded an exclusively psychological theory of simultaneous contrast. Fechner, for example, continued to insist that contrast involves both physiological and psychological moments, and in 1861 he published a respectful but pointed critique of what he saw as Helmholtz's exaggerated psychological interpretation (Fechner 1860a, 1861; Turner 1987b). Fechner's dissent suggests that some additional factor motivated Helmholtz's strong attachment to that interpretation. That factor may well have been Helmholtz's strong commitment to Young's theory. To Helmholtz, Young's theory required that every retinal receptor be isolated from all others and be linked to the sensorium by an individual nerve fiber. But if simultaneous contrast were to be explained as other than a central effect, or if retinal induction were to be invoked, then the retinal receptors would have to possess complex networks of lateral neural connections. This anatomical image was exactly opposite to that required by Young's theory, with its insistence on discrete receptors and private lines to the brain. For Helmholtz, interpreting contrast as a central, psychical process removed the anatomical challenge it offered to Young's theory.

CONCLUSION

In 1850 the research field of color and color sensations was scarcely a "field" at all. Knowledge of color phenomena derived from separate and isolated traditions, and there was a lack of common methods of investigation, strong integrating theories, or an agreed-upon research front. In 1860 Helmholtz provided the basis for all these things, primarily through his creative and highly selective synthesis of the work of others. The center point of this synthesis was the theoretical integration offered by Young's theory in its Maxwellian guise, but the *Handbuch* created a unified basis for future research practice in other ways as well.

Out of theoretical integration came a new set of problems now nested at the heart of physiological optics. To consolidate the achievements of the *Handbuch* the field needed to determine the spectral locus through precise colorimetric measurements, to identify the fundamental sensations and calculate their frequency response curves, and to extend the interpretation of color blindness to the green and blue blind as had already been done for the red blind. Precise colorimetric photometry would make it possible to determine the intensity response curves of the three fundamental processes on which so many visual phenomena depended, and so show precisely how these relationships differed from Fechner's logarithmic psychophysical law. This set of problems, all laid out explicitly in the *Handbuch*, was now established as the core program of the Helmholtzian synthesis.

The *Handbuch* also laid down a basis for future practice through its long excursions into instrumentation and research methods. Helmholtz sketched in much detail techniques for obtaining pure spectra, investigating the ultraviolet regions, observing florescence, and mixing spectral colors. Especially noteworthy were his well-illustrated designs for adjustable slits, fashioned in brass, for collimating light beams, isolating homogeneous colors, and producing overlapping spectra (*PO5* 2:108–13, 157–61). Also important were his methods for eliminating diffusion and internal reflection in prisms, and his discussions of the theory, construction, and use of simpler experimental devices like the color tops and stroboscopic disks (pp. 215–24). Although Helmholtz usually developed the mathematical theory of his instruments at length, the focus of his methodological discussions was on practical manipulation. Few of the problems, instruments, or methods he discussed were entirely original, but the *Handbuch* offered for the first time a one-volume, practical manual on most of the experimental techniques used in color vision studies until well into the twentieth century.

The *Handbuch* also imposed terminological standardization on discussions of color vision. After 1860 German writers seem to have unanimously followed Helmholtz in describing the extreme ends of the visible spectrum as red and violet and reserving "purple" to denote nonspectral mixes of these. It became standard to describe a color sensation in terms of *Helligkeit*, *Farbenton*, and *Sättigungsgrad*. More slowly, *Nachbilder* and *Kontrast* replaced older terms like *Ergänzungsfarben* and *subjektive Farben*, and later threatened the newer terms *successiver* and *simultaner Kontrast*.

The *Handbuch* set the future practice of color research in one further way. The researchers upon whom Helmholtz drew predominantly in his great synthesis—Young, Maxwell, Fechner, Grassmann—were physicists. The methods Helmholtz borrowed from these men and made de rigueur for color vision studies henceforth were physical methods. They included precise colorimetry, psychophysical measurement, photometry, mathematical formulas, and a knowledge of physical optics at least sufficient to manipulate instruments for obtaining and mixing pure spectral lights. What Helmholtz brought to his own synthesis was a physiologist's knowledge of the structure and function of the eye and of the large literature on subjective visual effects and pathologies. He was ideally suited to create a tradition of color vision research that would integrate the methodological approaches of the physicist and the physiologist, or—as Ewald Hering and his followers were soon to claim—to subordinate physiological to physical understanding altogether.

CHAPTER SEVEN

Hering on Light and Color

THE RECEPTION OF YOUNG'S THEORY
IN GERMANY, 1860–75

Within a few years Young's theory had been enshrined in a series of important elementary texts on physiology. Helmholtz's assistant Wilhelm Wundt incorporated it unhesitatingly into his semipopular survey, *Vorlesungen über die Menschen- und Thierseele* (1863), and physiologist Adolf Fick, who had been a fellow student with Helmholtz at Berlin, adopted it without reservation in his brisk and business-like *Lehrbuch der Anatomie und Physiologie der Sinnesorgane* (1864) (Wundt 1863b, 138–201; Fick 1864, esp. 291). A decade later Helmholtz's friend Ernst Brücke placed his imprimatur upon the theory in his *Vorlesungen über Physiologie* (1873), abandoning his former advocacy of retinal induction to explain simultaneous contrast in doing so. Ludimar Hermann, the former student of du Bois-Reymond, presented Young's hypothesis as a theory confirmed beyond reasonable doubt in his *Grundriß der Physiologie des Menschen*, a work that went through twelve editions between 1863 and 1899 and was one of the most successful elementary texts of the era.

In the more specialized literature, however, Young's theory met a cooler reception. Hermann Aubert showed deep ambivalence about the theory in his influential *Physiologie der Netzhaut* (1865). He accepted the theory on pragmatic grounds as a working hypothesis for physiological optics, but he criticized it as indifferent to or even inconsistent with Müller's law of specific nerve energies. Maxwell and Helmholtz had both failed, he wrote, to clarify how three distinct sensation energies get somehow "psychologically mixed" in the sensorium (p. 179). Indeed, we have no basis for assessing the exact number or the nature of the fundamental sensations, and there may well be four rather than three, since red, green, blue, and yellow appear to most observers as intuitively simple and primitive. Aubert also felt that physiological and psychological factors were more closely interwoven in contrast effects than Helmholtz had admitted, although he accepted most of Helmholtz's specific accounts of these phenomena (p. 184).

In 1866 Bonn anatomist Max Schultze published a major study of the microanatomy of the rods and cones that owed much to Aubert.

Schultze's work powerfully shaped the reception of Young's theory among physiologists, for it presented the first alleged anatomical evidence for the theory (Schultze 1866). Schultze claimed to have established the "nervous nature" of the "radial fibres" that intervene in the retina between the rod-cone and ganglion cell layers (p. 5). Because the radial fibers originate from rods as well as cones, Schultze argued that both must be light-sensitive elements, although only the cones are capable of mediating the color sense. As evidence for this restriction of color vision to the cones, Schultze noted that animals that live and forage primarily in the dark normally have rods but few or no cones. Humans retinas possess exclusively cones in the foveal region, where color vision is most acute, but a low cone-to-rod density on the retinal periphery, where (as Aubert had shown) color perception is greatly reduced or altered (pp. 73–87).

Schultze's anatomical evidence in support of Young's theory came from the cone-rich retinas of birds. In these retinas he was able to distinguish three types of cones, two of which possessed small yellow or red spheres in the cone tip. Schultze interpreted this as the threefold differentiation of cones for color sensitivity required by the Young–Helmholtz hypothesis. Unfortunately for that hypothesis, Schultze found no similar differentiation among human cones. He did, however, detect internal structures, which he believed endowed human cones with the capability of coding for at least three colors (pp. 81–82).

These structures consisted, according to Schultze, in the differentiation of human cones along their midsection into an "outer member" and an "inner member." While the outer member is entirely transparent, the inner member shows internal striations along its length and seems to consist of parallel laminae, each of which appeared to be associated with the termination of one striation. Noting that the radial fiber extending from the inner member of a typical cone is thick and apparently "composed of fibrils," Schultze speculated that the internal striations are extensions of the nervous fibrils and so constitute a series of distinct, light-sensitive elements within the cone body (pp. 73–75). He hypothesized that the inner member of a cone functions only as a "purely reflective optical apparatus." The series of laminae within the inner member somehow function as tuned resonators, which physically sort light of different wavelengths and allow it to activate the nervous receptor associated with each lamina (pp. 83–87). If rods, unlike cones, respond to the physical intensity of light but not to wavelength, then they should lack this internal structure. Sure enough, Schultze reported that the inner members of rods are unstriated and that the radial fibers emanating from them are thinner and do not seem to be composed of separate fibrils (p. 83).

Schultze's work created a mild sensation among German physiologists, and by the end of the 1860s, some had come to see Young's theory largely through the eyes of Schultze's findings. In 1869 Helmholtz's student Albrecht Nagel gave Schultze almost equal time with Helmholtz and Young in a discussion of contemporary color theory (Nagel 1869). Ludimar Hermann discussed Schultze extensively in his 1872 text edition, and went so far as to speak of the *Young-Helmholtz-Schultze'sche Theorie*. The problem with Schultze's observations, however, was that the inner members of cones show substantially more than three striations each, even though each separate fibril and striation was supposedly associated with a fundamental sensation. Accepting this result, Hermann informed students that Young's theory actually postulated a "multiplum" of tuned color receptors, and that while three was traditionally assumed for simplicity, "in truth the number is perhaps much greater" (Hermann 1872, 364).

If the theory's supporters disagreed about the number of receptor processes, they also disagreed about their sensory correlates. Helmholtz in 1860 and Maxwell in 1855 had considered Young's physiological primaries to be most likely highly saturated, extraspectral hues of green, violet, and extreme spectral red. In 1860 Maxwell changed his opinion and suggested that the third physiological primary is more probably blue than violet. Helmholtz, supported by investigations of his student J. J. Müller, adhered to violet.[1] In 1868 Sigmund Exner pointed out that the Fechner–Helmholtz theory of afterimages offered a way to determine the fundamentals approximately. If the retina is exhausted by a homogeneous light of some hue, the exhaustion effects (observable in afterimage experiments) will be less pronounced if the hue closely matches that of a primary sensation. Exner's experiments, done in Helmholtz's Heidelberg laboratory, showed that violet exhaustion produced the strongest afterimage effects, indigo blue the least (Exner 1868). On this and other evidence, Exner, Fick, Brücke, and William Preyer at Jena all adopted blue as the hue of the third fundamental sensation (Fick 1864; Brücke 1873; Preyer 1868; Preyer 1870, 67–68; Preyer 1870–88, no. 2 [05.01. 1871]).

A few contemporaries flatly rejected the Young–Helmholtz theory or at least opposed central elements of it. Fechner, as already noted, immediately challenged Helmholtz's exclusively psychological interpretation of simultaneous contrast (Fechner 1860a). Physicist Conrad Bohn at Giessen called the theory suggestive, but at the same time unproven and inconsistent with observations on visual acuity in cone-rich retinal regions (Bohn 1865). Most important, the young Ernst Mach, newly named professor of physics at the University of Graz, recanted his earlier acceptance of Young's theory and in 1865 denounced it as incompatible with the phenomenological fact that we perceive at least six fundamental or unmixed colors: red, green, blue, yellow, black, and white. To do justice to this fact, Mach claimed, a color theory must postulate at least six independent retinal processes. Mach had already concluded from experiments on rotating disks that lateral interaction among retinal receptors is necessary to explain contrast and the phenomena now known as Mach bands. These positions may have significantly influenced his colleague Ewald Hering at Prague (Mach 1866; Kremer 1993b).

The reception of Young's theory turned primarily on the theory's adequacy to explain color blindness. Helmholtz and Maxwell both considered that the theory's great triumph, and in the early 1870s Preyer, Brücke, and the young Eduard Raehlmann still took the theory as the indispensable starting point for any understanding of that affliction (Preyer 1868; Brücke 1873; Raehlmann, 1873). Preyer used data from dichromats to locate the respective peaks and intersections of the spectral-response curves of Young's fundamentals, and found that his results agreed closely with those J. J. Müller and Exner had obtained by different methods (Preyer 1868, 324–29). For him, that kind of reciprocal elucidation showed that Young's theory alone made possible a "scientific theory of color" (Preyer 1870, 37).

Others had doubts. In 1865 Berlin surgeon Edmund Rose published a major clinical study of thirty-five cases of color blindness. Rose's study was thorough and instrumentally sophisticated, but its conflation of congenital, pathological, and drug-induced cases practically guaranteed his main conclusion: that color deficiencies were too diverse in kind and too individually variable to be reduced to three categories corresponding to the loss of red, green, or violet processes (Rose 1865, 86–87). Rose's study triggered a wave of intense European interest in pathologically induced color blindness. Henri Dor, assessing the results in 1872, concluded that the condition was nearly always associated with cerebral or spinal disorders or with atrophy of the optic nerve; it was rarely or never associated with peripheral afflictions like retinitis or retinal degeneration, as would be expected from the Young–Helmholtz theory.

Interest also attached to the temporary abnormalities in color vision induced by the drug santonin, commonly used against intestinal worms. This drug was known to make bright objects temporarily appear greenish-yellow and the violet end of the spectrum to disappear. That effect, Helmholtz suggested in 1867, was readily explicable as a temporary loss of sensitivity in Young's violet receptors (*PO5* 2:170–71). On the other hand, dark objects appear violet under the effect of santonin, necessitating the additional assumption that the drug paralyzes the violet receptors but still somehow stimulates the violet response at a higher neural level. Making a virtue of necessity, J. J. Müller argued that this effect at least proved that the third physiological primary is violet rather than blue (Müller 1870, 610–11; Raehlmann 1873, 97–106).

Peripheral color blindness proved still more troublesome to the Young–Helmholtz theory. Despite confusion surrounding the issue, it was generally agreed that reds and greens pass into yellow, purples pass into blues, and finally all colors fade to white or gray as they are viewed increasingly far out upon the retinal periphery. Helmholtz suggested in 1867 that the phenomenon is easily explained by assuming the density of red receptors to decrease toward the periphery, and that finally all the color receptors gradually vanish (*POS* 2:154–55). But that suggestion was hard to reconcile with Max Schultze's anatomical evidence that a single human cone contains all three receptors. More troublesome, it could not explain how yellow sensations can be produced on the retinal periphery in the absence of the red process. The congenitally color blind might incorrectly describe their green color sensations as yellow, but normals could hardly be expected to make such an error about their peripheral color vision. And, as a last minor embarrassment, peripheral color blindness pointed to a blue fundamental while the santonin effect pointed to a violet one.

William Preyer had these and other phenomena in mind in 1868 when he called color blindness a "labyrinth" (Preyer 1868, 311). Both Preyer and Raehlmann, though supporters of the Young–Helmholtz theory, agreed that color blindness effects could not be adequately explained as the simple absence of one, two, or three receptors (Preyer 1868, 310–11; Raehlmann 1873, 103–6; Aubert 1865, 184). Other critics found the new color blindness phenomena grounds on which to reject the Young–Helmholtz theory altogether. The University of Greifswald emerged as the center of opposition. The physiologist there was Julius Budge, who had left his *Ordinariat*-position in Bonn in 1856 partly because of the opposition, and the competition, offered by the newly arrived Helmholtz. Open criticism of the theory, however, came not from Budge but from Rudolf Schirmer in the medical faculty, one of Prussia's pioneer ophthalmologists. Having already set his students upon the theory, Schirmer himself weighed in with an influential article in Graefe's prestigious *Archiv für Ophthalmologie* (Schirmer 1873).

Like many other ophthalmologists, Schirmer based his critique mostly on the evidence of pathological color blindness. In his view that evidence, plus the sheer diversity of visual color deficiencies, proved conclusively that there are no discrete categories of color blindness, only stages in a fixed sequence of color loss that may become hereditarily fixed at some stage in some individuals. Above all, Schirmer zeroed in on the central weakness of the Young–Helmholtz theory. All classes of the color blind, both hereditary and pathological, commonly report yellow and blue sensations. There are, Schirmer insisted, no adequate grounds on which to doubt these color reports, yet the perception of any yellow by those identified as red or green blind is fatal to the Young–Helmholtz theory. Schirmer gave the names of four prominent ophthalmologists, who, he claimed, had publicly attacked the theory or had recanted their former acceptance of it (p. 235).

HERING ON THE ORGANISM

These early debates over Young's theory had gone on without Ewald Hering. During the 1860s his research and his polemical exchanges with Helmholtz dealt exclusively with binocularity, eye movements, and the visual perception of space. But Hering was still a young man at the end of the 1860s, and his scientific style and his own understanding of his differences with Helmholtz were evolving rapidly. Hering was also thinking deeply about the nature of the organism and of sensory perception. His popular lecture of 1870, "On Memory as a General Function of Organized Matter," reaffirmed Fechner's psychophysical parallelism, applied it to the realm of organic evolution, and without mentioning Helmholtz explicitly, merged Helmholtz's associative processes and unconscious inferences into Hering's own more evolutionary and organismic conception of perceptual events (Hering 1870, 1902/1870, 1921).

In that lecture Hering further took upon himself the mantle of true successor to Johannes Müller. Hering charged that Müller himself had seen his "specific nerve energies" as sensory energies, modes of sensation in the nerves, and so specific to the type of nerve considered. But Müller's own disciples had corrupted or suppressed this idea in their claim that all nerves passively transmit identical kinds of impulses to the brain and that only in the brain do these impulses evoke particular types of sensations. To Hering, this led only to useless, infinite regress. He speculated that the chemicophysical action in the nerves differs according to the type of sensation that the nerve produces, even though physiology is not at present able to detect those differences.

The philosophical views expressed by Hering in 1870 reflected both old intellectual debts and the fruits of new research interests. The position at the Josephinum in Vienna that Hering assumed in 1865 offered him facilities, poor though they were, for physiological research that he had never enjoyed before (Ullmann 1970, 4–5). Between 1866 and 1872 the main focus of his research shifted to pure physiology. In 1866 he published on the structure of the mammalian liver and in 1867 and 1868 on the physiology of the blood cells. Sometime in 1867 Hering made the acquaintance of Josef Breuer, later Freud's collaborator and one of the pioneers of psychotherapy, then an assistant in one of the university medical clinics. They collaborated on a series of vivisectional experiments in which Breuer demonstrated the "self-regulation" (*Selbststeurung*) of the respiratory function, later called the Hering–Breuer reflex. Working on his own, Hering showed in 1870 that inflation of the lungs accelerated the activity of the heart and also stimulated the vasoconstriction centers of the brain, giving rise to the so-called Traube–Hering pressure waves in the blood and explaining their correlation with respiration. Study of the "self-regulation" of the organism later rivaled the study of vision as the main research focus of Hering's school (Ullmann 1970).

This research, especially that done with Breuer, strongly influenced Hering's biological views (Ullmann 1970, 12–13; Hurvich 1969). The two men had speculated (on analogy with the sensation of temperature) that the same fibers of the vagus nerve carry both inspiratory and expiratory impulses. Hering drew upon this finding in his suggestion of 1870 that the response of sensory nerve fibers (their specific energy) might also be a "multi-form potency," which could be innervated in different ways and so produce its characteristic sensation *or* its opposite (Hering 1902/1870, 40; Breuer 1970/1868, 384–85). They had also discovered that electrical stimulation of the sectioned vagus nerve stump failed to elicit the same pattern of response as the "natural innervation" produced by the inflation of the lungs. Hering concluded that within the body nerves do not respond like passive telegraph wires, independent of the nature of the stimulus or the organic context of their action.

The research on self-regulation cemented Hering's lifelong opposition to any conception of the living organism as a machine waiting passively for an external stimulus to elicit organic response. He held on the contrary that life is a dynamic equilibrium of antagonistic processes. External stimuli can disturb this equilibrium, but the processes themselves contain self-regulating mechanisms that act to restore it (Hering 1888a). Organic response to a stimulus therefore depends as much upon the state of the organism itself as upon the nature and intensity of the stimulus. Hering only formalized these views later, but they led him immediately to a new assessment of his differences with Helmholtz over sensory perception and a new basis for attacking the Helmholtzian view. That attack came in the first installment of his *On the Theory of the Light Sense* (1872).

THE "SPIRITUALISTIC" DIRECTION IN PHYSIOLOGY

The foreword to Hering's 1872 treatise set out his first and polemically most effective reply to Helmholtz's criticism of the nativist position. It occupied only five pages, yet it was calculated for maximum polemical effect and—always important to Hering—maximum provocation of his opponents. Hering adroitly employed the rhetorical strategy of inversion, turning Helmholtz's arguments back upon him. Where Helmholtz had tried to link Hering and nativism to idealism and speculative philosophy, Hering hammered home an alleged similarity between Helmholtz's approach and the very vitalism Helmholtz and his reductionist allies had anathematized. Whereas Helmholtz had defended empiricism for the scope it granted to learning, intellect, and self-mastery, Hering rejected the approach as abandoning the search for naturalistic understanding. Whereas Helmholtz had sought to occupy the methodological high ground by stressing the powerful topoi of simplicity and conceptual parsimony, Hering countered with the equally potent topoi of explanatory power and consistency with the commitment to naturalistic explanation that prevailed elsewhere in physiology.

Hering opened with a direct challenge. Since his earlier work on spatial perception, he wrote, he had become increasingly convinced "that that modern tendency in sensory physiology, which has found its most acute expression in the *Physiological Optics* of Helmholtz, is not leading us to the truth, and whoever wishes to open up new avenues of research in this area, must first free himself from the theories which now prevail" (Hering 1878/1874, 1). Hering branded that "modern tendency" the "spiritualistic" direction in sensory physiology, or "as it is euphemistically designated, the 'psychological' [one]" (p. 2). Just as earlier physiologists explained away troublesome phenomena by appeals to "vital forces" (*Lebenskraft*), so today one meets everywhere in treatises on physiological optics invocations of "the soul" (*Seele*), the spirit (*Geist*), the judgment (*Urteil*), or "inference" (*Schluß*) as deux ex machina to eliminate all difficulties. The many sensory phenomena that at present cannot be explained through physics and chemistry give this "spiritualistic physiology" a wide range for potentially legitimate application. Unfortunately, wrote Hering, psychological platitudes are also invoked today to dispose of many phenomena that are susceptible to physiological investigation and explanation.

Against this "spiritualistic" tendency in sensory physiology Hering opposed the direction that he claimed always to have espoused himself, the "physiological" direction. From this perspective, "the phenomena of consciousness are seen as conditioned and sustained by organic processes, and the sequence and interrelationships of the former are to be interpreted in terms of the unfolding of the latter, insofar as this is generally possible at the present" (p. 4). This "physiological direction," Hering claimed, benefited both physiology and psychology. It promoted intense, reciprocal study of consciousness and its organic substrate, and so made possible a "physiological psychology" (or, as Hering preferred, a "physiology of consciousness"). Physiological psychology would replace the older, descriptive tradition of "philosophical psychology," which had investigated the phenomena of consciousness without regard for its organic basis (pp. 4–5).

Hering insisted that the importance of these two tendencies in contemporary physiology made the distinction Helmholtz had drawn between "nativistic" and "empiricist" directions basically irrelevant: Helmholtz simply tried to make a subordinate issue into the main one. The distinction between "nativism" and "empiricism" is purely one of degree. No empiricist denies that some sensory functions are innate and inborn. No nativist denies the powerful influence of custom and exercise on the functions of our sense organs. Hence, "insofar as they are real physiologists," the only possible debate between nativists and empiricists can be over where the line between inborn and acquired capacities is to be drawn (p. 3).

Hering held the differences between nativists and empiricists to be merely ones of emphasis and degree, but he insisted that the gap between "spiritualist" and "physiological" directions is fundamental. One direction painstakingly deduces the laws of consciousness out of organic and material processes, the other takes the easy way and explains them from the hypothetical particularities of the spirit or the soul (ibid.). But the two divisions are not entirely unrelated. "The spiritualist," wrote Hering, "will always be inclined to restrict the realm of the innate, in order to win a fuller and freer scope for the human spirit, and to be able to portray the spirit as being as independent as possible from its organic basis." Therefore, Hering concluded, "spiritualists are empiricist by preference" (ibid.).

SIMULTANEOUS AND SUCCESSIVE LIGHT INDUCTION

The special target of Hering's attack was Helmholtz's radical and "spiritualistic" demarcation of simultaneous from successive contrast. On the contrary, Hering insisted, the two are closely linked, as can be seen in the so-called *Lichthof* or light border that surrounds dark negative afterimages. If we fixate a small, moderately bright disk on a black background for fifteen to sixty seconds and obtain the afterimage against a dark field, for example, by shutting the eyes, then the dark afterimage of the bright disk will be surrounded by a border (the *Lichthof*) that is brighter than the afterimage or the rest of the field. Helmholtz, of course, had explained the afterimage as a result of retinal fatigue, the light border as a psychological effect arising from our tendency to exaggerate clearly perceived differences of brightness (Hering 1878/1874, 6–8).

Hering attacked this explanation. If the effect is really an "error of judgement," then we should see the whole background as lighter than the afterimage, not just the border. Also, when we fixate a field like that shown in Figure 7.1 and obtain the negative afterimage, so that the two light borders along the sides overlap, then they reinforce each other and the area *AA′* is seen brighter than other segments of the light border and brighter than anything else in the field. The reinforcement suggests a physiological rather than psychological effect (pp. 8–10). Finally, Hering noted, when we obtain the negative afterimage of a black disk on a white field, the dark border we might expect does not appear. Yet the juxtaposition of opposites, and so all the conditions Helmholtz required for a psychological contrast effect, are fully met.

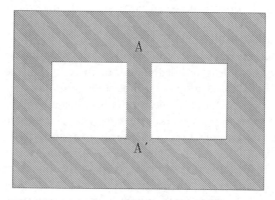

Fig. 7.1 Afterimage experiment by Hering, to demonstrate that the two "light border" segments *AA′* reinforce one another, contrary to what is expected from inferential accounts of contrast like that of Helmholtz. *Source*: Hering 1878/1874, 9 (from the description).

Hering also denied that afterimage phenomena, and especially the patterns of brightness they display, can be explained by retinal fatigue alone. Suppose we fixate a black disk on a white field for several seconds and then shut our eyes. We are then looking at the intrinsic retinal light. Because the original white field has fatigued most of the retina for white, the intrinsic retinal light will be reduced on those areas and they will seem dark. The original black disk, however, does not fatigue the retina at all, and so in the afterimage we see intrinsic light in the region of the disk undiminished and hence brighter than the rest of the field. But, Hering noted, this appeal to retinal fatigue fails to predict the relative intensities correctly: the bright afterimage always appears much brighter than the intrinsic retinal light ever appears under any circumstances (p. 14).

Helmholtz, also, had recognized the anomalous brightness of this afterimage and had explained it as an illusion of comparison. Because we cannot remember how bright the intrinsic light usually is, we take the brightness of the afterimage background to be its usual value, and so are compelled by comparison to "see" the brightness of the afterimage disk as comparatively much greater. Hering reviewed this account with considerable sarcasm, and offered a whole series of experiments in refutation of it. Some of these involved contrast effects observed in patterned negative afterimages that contained some very bright portions of "objective white." Contrast still occurred, even though these true white sections presumably eliminated the possibility of illusion due to a false white standard (pp. 15–17). In other experiments Hering allowed the negative afterimage to fade, yet he observed the contrast effect to persist in parts of the image, even after the inducing field supposedly responsible for it had vanished. Like Fechner and others before him, Hering noted that on long and continual fixation contrast effects weaken, with both dark and light fields changing to a neutral gray (an effect Hering called *simultane Lichtinduktion*). If we fixate a black patch on a white field so long and so intensely that it brightens to a gray, and then suddenly dim the objective light in the room, then the patch can actually appear lighter than the ground (*successive Lichtinduktion*) (pp. 21–30).

Taken together, Hering concluded, these experiments proved that every "subjective" light sensation has a "physiological basis in the organ of vision, and cannot arise merely out of false judgements" (p. 18). Not only is Helmholtz's psychological theory of simultaneous contrast incorrect, but his theory of afterimages is incomplete. While many afterimage phenomena do arise from retinal fatigue, Hering conceded, that theory cannot explain afterimage phenomena such as the light border effect or the anomalous brightness of the negative afterimage of a dark field. These phenomena prove that "any part of the retina determines the activity of the others, and [that] not every retinal element represents an individual independent of its neighbors, a claim which has been repeatedly put forward but never generally acknowledged" (p. 19). But Hering cautioned explicitly that by "retina" he meant not just the parts of the visual nervous apparatus in the eyeball, but also the fibers and areas of the brain in nervous contact with them. Thus he left open the question of whether contrast and other effects arise peripherally or in the central nervous system (pp. 8–9).

Hering also made several strategic terminological choices. What Helmholtz had called afterimages and contrast, Hering called successive and simultaneous contrast, terms that suggested the underlying similarity of the two phenomena. Hering coined two new usages, "simultaneous light induction" (*simultane Lichtinduction*), and "successive light induction" (*successive Lichtinduction*), to denote these effects. The terms reflect Hering's unhesitating readiness to use the term "light" to describe what Helmholtz in most cases would have called "the sensation of light." "Light," for Hering, was a sensation by definition, and it was not to be confused with the "light" of the physicist.

HERING ON BLACK

The 1874 installment of *On the Theory of the Light Sense* opened with a phenomenological manifesto:

> When it comes to deriving suitable and rigorous concepts and designations for the various characteristics of our sensations, the first requirement is that these concepts should be derived entirely out of the sensations themselves. We must rigorously avoid confusing sensations with their physical or physiological causes, or deducing from the latter any principle of classification. (Hering 1878/1874, 51)

To illustrate how physiologists ignore this principle, Hering offered the example of black. Physiologists almost universally treat black as different from other color sensations, Hering complained, and describe it as a "resting condition" of the eye, or as a sensation corresponding to no stimulus. In fact, Hering insisted, black is a distinct sensation that differs little from white or red or green. The series of grays leading from the blackest black to the whitest white is not an "intensity series" in which a single sensation we call brightness changes in a quantitative sense, but a "qualitative series" of distinctly different gray sensations, each a different mixture of black and white (pp. 55–56). True black, as Aubert had already insisted, must not be confused with the neutral gray of the intrinsic retinal light or with the sensation we have with rested eyes in a totally dark room. True black is as much induced by an external light stimulus as is white, only light evokes the black sensation indirectly, through simultaneous or successive contrast effects (p. 64).

Hering blamed the theory of retinal exhaustion partly for physiologists' failure to recognize black as a legitimate color sensation. This theory has confused the relationship of the external stimulus to the deep-black sensations obtainable in afterimages. He blamed the failure partly on the "spiritualistic theory" that dismissed the true-black sensations available through simultaneous contrast as "illusions of judgement" (pp. 65–66). But he attributed the mistake primarily to the predominant concern of researchers with the physical stimulus of external light itself rather than with the sensations to which it gives rise. Hering wrote that we have always falsely thought of the visual field as a "blackboard" on which physical light writes in white and in colors; we have studied the physical light and neglected the board itself (p. 66).

Of course, Hering found this error most flagrant in the writings of Helmholtz. In Helmholtz's *Handbuch*, Hering mocked, we find chapter titles like the "homogeneous colors" the "compound colors," and the "three primary colors"—all under the general heading of "the theory of visual sensations"! But color sensations in themselves are neither homogeneous, nor compound, nor primary; to impose that terminology upon them is to confuse aspects of the physical stimulus with sensations themselves. It is absurd, Hering objected, to regard spectral violet as a "primary" color, as Helmholtz asks us to do, when it clearly contains red and blue; or to think of white as compounded from red, green, and violet sensations; or to think of black as somehow resulting from a state of zero intensity of these sensory elements. That presentation suffices for physicists, who are primarily interested in the physical stimuli, "but for physiologists to accept that classification also would be a great mistake" (p. 57).

At the heart of the "spiritualistic" view, Hering went on, is the distinction it draws between "sensation" on the one hand, and "perception" or "representation" on the other. The former it regards as direct and organic, the latter as an "intellectual" product because it supposedly results from an "interpretation" or "unconscious inference" carried out on the sensation. In reality, Hering wrote, whenever similar stimuli lead to different perceptions, then the intervening sensations must have been different. That result will seem paradoxical only to those who forget that the effect of a stimulus depends not only on the stimulus itself, but on the momentary state of the organism on which it acts. That state will be a result, in part, of the organism's entire optical experience throughout its life. The sensation excited by any single stimulus must be regarded as "a resonance of our whole sensorium" (p. 67–68).

Hering admitted that some phenomena, like our ability to perceive objects in a constant color or constant intrinsic brightness over broad ranges of illumination, *seem* to manifest unconscious inference. Nevertheless, the task of sensory physiology is to provide, insofar as possible, purely biological accounts of these phenomena while adhering to the phenomenological manifesto laid out earlier (p. 69). In one of his striking similes, Hering compared the task of sensory physiology to the construction of a tunnel, simultaneously bored from both ends. One approach begins on the chemicophysical side with the external stimulus or with externally accessible neural processes; the other approach begins with our own, introspective awareness. The point at which the two tunnels must meet is the neural event or structure corresponding to the psychophysical interface. That interface is inaccessible to direct investigation. Nevertheless, by assuming the lawfulness of both realms surrounding it, and by a joint approach from both realms, we can draw valid if indirect conclusions about the nature of that event and the structures that mediate it (p. 106).

A THEORY OF THE VISUAL SUBSTANCE

In the fifth installment Hering rose to the challenge he had set for sensory physiology as a whole (Hering 1878/1874, 70–106). Hering returned to the foundation of his psychophysical worldview. We must regard black and white as separate, elemental sensations; the fact that one must mix lights of different wavelengths to stimulate the sensation of white is compatible with many different physiological hypotheses and in no way contradicts the phenomenological claim for the elemental nature of white and black (p. 71). As distinct and elemental sensations black and white or darkness and brightness must be associated with two different psychophysical processes going on in the visual substance. From our introspective knowledge of the relationships of black and white, we can directly and reliably infer the nature of the material processes to which the psychophysical event is coupled.

Hering drew on contemporary analogies from metabolic chemistry for a model of the visual substance. The observed facts of the black-white series compel us to assume that the sensation of whiteness is associated with a dissimilation (*Dissimilierung*) of the visual substance (or a specific part of it) under the action, direct or indirect, of a light stimulus. The sensation of blackness is associated with a spontaneous assimilation (*Assimilierung*) of the visual substance out of materials supplied by the blood. These complementary and antagonistic processes differ only in that light stimuli do not accelerate the assimilation process directly, as they do the dissimilation process. When the rate of dissimilation exceeds that of assimilation, the net psychophysical effect is the sensation of brightness, and the converse (pp. 74–80).[2]

Hering reasoned that the rate of dissimilation induced by a light stimulus will depend upon two things: the strength of the stimulus itself, and the momentary "susceptibility" (*Erregbarkeit*) of the visual substance to the stimulus. A stimulus evoking the dissimilation effect (a "*D*-stimulus") will reduce the quantity of the visual substance available for further dissimilation, gradually slow down the *D*-effect, and lower the "*D*-susceptibility" (*dissimilierungs-Erregbarkeit*) of the affected retinal area. Exactly the same is true of the assimilation process, except that light does not act as a direct stimulus to cause it. Hering also assumed a constant "internal stimulus" at work in the visual substance, sustaining base levels of both assimilative and dissimilative activity.

These assumptions, Hering noted, led to interesting and elegant explanations of several visual effects. When the rested eye is exposed to a strong light, the light at first seems intensely bright; but, as adaptation ensues, the brightness effect grows weaker. In terms of Hering's mechanism, the light at first induces a strong D-action, but as the D-susceptibility of the retina is reduced, the D-action itself falls and with it the ratio of D to the basal A-activity. Similarly, in the continued absence of any light stimulus, the basal levels of A- and D-action will come to an equilibrium with one another and produce the "midgray" we see after being in total darkness for several hours (p. 89).[3] The same processes explain the phenomenon Hering had called "simultaneous light induction": when we stare fixedly at an image for a long period, the bright and dark regions fade toward a common neutral gray (pp. 95–96).

Hering's mechanism yields the result that the net sensation of brightness evoked by a light will not depend upon the absolute level of D it causes, but upon the ratio of D to A. We are to measure the "brightness" of a sensation as the ratio $D/(A + D)$, where $A + D$ is the absolute magnitude or "weight" of psychophysical process occurring. The increase in brightness that follows from a unit increase in the strength of the stimulus will depend upon the total psychophysical activity (pp. 83–85). This allows the mathematical derivation of a psychophysical law, though one different from the Weber–Fechner formula.

To explain simultaneous contrast, Hering assumed that D-activity in one area of the retina will enhance the A-susceptibility of surrounding areas, the effect decreasing with distance from the region of the D-stimulus. Enhanced A-susceptibility (and with it reduced D-susceptibility) will raise the basal level of the intrinsic A-activity, and so cause the parts of the visual field contiguous to a light area to appear darker (pp. 89–95). Sounding a theme that he would later emphasize much more strongly, Hering claimed that simultaneous contrast plays a crucial and hitherto unrecognized role in counteracting the effect of irradiation. Irradiation is the tendency of light in the eye to spread from illuminated retinal areas onto contiguous dark areas; Hering agreed with Helmholtz that this is a dioptric effect arising from strictly physical causes. If uncompensated, however, irradiation would blur all contours and sharply reduce visual acuity. Simultaneous contrast corrects for irradiation by reducing the susceptibility to light of dark areas contiguous to light ones, and so restoring the sharpness of visual contours (p. 91).[4]

Successive contrast effects required a slightly different explanation and an additional assumption. The action of a D-stimulus will gradually lower the D-susceptibility of the region on which it acts; Hering called this effect "D-exhaustion" (D-*Ermüdung*). If the light stimulus ceases, the D-activity will stop altogether, and, given the reduced D-susceptibility, the basal level of the intrinsic A-activity will yield a very high D/A ratio. The previously bright region will appear excessively dark after the end of the external stimulus, thus producing a negative afterimage. Hering explained positive afterimages (rather weakly) as the result of a D-

stimulus so intense and so destructive of the visual substance that the blood circulation can momentarily no longer supply enough substance for *A*-activity even at the basal level (pp. 99–103).

Having postulated these basic mechanisms in the visual substance, Hering retraced his steps through the various afterimage and contrast experiments he had discussed in earlier sections, showing how their outcomes were to be interpreted in terms of the opponent process theory of assimilation and dissimilation. While Helmholtz's theory could often explain the pattern of relative brightness in various afterimages, his own alone, Hering claimed, could explain the absolute levels of brightness we observe.

THE OPPONENT PROCESS THEORY OF COLOR VISION

Having laid the foundations, Hering presented to the Vienna Academy in May 1874 the theory of color vision that he and his school would develop and defend for the next half-century. He began with consideration of what he called the "natural" system of color sensations—the impressions of color and color relations that allegedly present themselves to the eye prior to all analysis of color theory or physical stimulus. The first consideration, according to Hering, is that just as all grays constitute a "nuanced series" (*Nuancenreihe*) running from deepest black to purest white, so do all possible colors arrange themselves in four other nuanced series: red-blue, blue-green, green-yellow, yellow-red. Every color sensation lying in one of these series will appear to be a mixture of the purer colors defining its extreme points. The four sensations constituting the end points of these series, however, have a special status. It is possible for these "simple" or "primary colors" (*einfache* or *Grundfarben*) alone to appear as absolutely pure colors, unmixed with any other color, or if they do appear as a mixture, only of themselves and one other primary color, never of two (Hering 1875[42], 169–73).

These four simple or primary colors, Hering went on, have the additional property of being organized as "opponent" or "antagonistic" colors (*Gegenfarben*). Thus green can appear mixed with blue or yellow, but never with its opponent color red; reddish-greens are phenomenologically unknown and unthinkable. Blue and yellow are opponent colors likewise. This relationship is captured schematically in Newton's color circle, if the four primary colors are located on perpendicular diameters. But the relationships have nothing to do with light or the spectrum; the red which (according to Hering) appears unmixed with blue or yellow does not appear in the spectrum at all, and the most extreme spectral red still appears yellowish. In fact, Hering concluded, we do not know why these color relationships are true, but we know from experience that they are (p. 171).

Hering recognized, of course, that more than hue contributes to color sensation. He wrote that any hue, whether simple or mixed, can be further "nuanced" by the admixture of black, white, or any intermediate gray of the black-white series. To illustrate this notion, Hering proposed a color triangle of his own very different in concept and representation from those of Helmholtz and Maxwell. He offered the triangle *CWB* (see Figure 7.2), where *C* represents any color, *W* extreme white, and *B* extreme black. Each point of the triangle, Hering explained, will represent a possible "nuance" of the color C. Every point/color of the triangle will display the same hue or color tone (*Farbenton*), but its purity (*Reinheit*)—defined as the proportion of gray admixture—will, in general, vary from point to point. The line *CM* represents the color of tone *C* mixed with varying proportions of the neutral or midgray *M* of the dark-adapted eye. All lines parallel to *CM* display nuanced series of the color *C* of the same "whiteness" or "brightness" but of varying purity. As for the color sensation represented by the point *C*, Hering noted that it does not actually occur. But if it could, it would have the degree of brightness of *M* (because it lies on the line *CM*), and thus all such pure color sensations would have identical degrees of brightness (pp. 173–78).

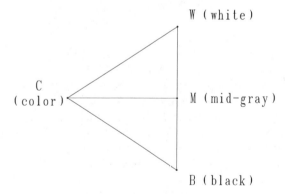

Fig. 7.2 Hering's equilateral color triangle, a vertical cross-section of the color solid. *Source*: Hering 1875(42), 173–75 (from the description).

This simple geometrical representation vividly expressed the difference between Hering's program and the Young–Helmholtz tradition. Hering's color triangle represented a vertical section through a color space bounded not only by convergence to absolute blackness below, but also by convergence to absolute brightness above. Helmholtz–Maxwell color triangles more nearly represented horizontal sections through a color space that converged to blackness below but was unbounded above (because, as Hering put it, they confused brightness with the [potentially unlimited] physical intensity of the stimulus). Horizontal sections ideally represent mix relationships among hues and so express the colorimetric commitments (obsession, Hering would have said) of the Young–Helmholtz tradition. Vertical sections as Hering drew them more nearly express subjective brightness relationships, the equivalence of brightness and darkness as true sensations, and the reality of an achromatic sensory response wholly separate from any chromatic ones. The struggle between programs was also to be a struggle over the representation of color space itself.

Geometry led Hering to arithmetic. Imagine a sensation composed of two primary colors plus white and black, in relative proportions given by the variables C, W, and B. The purity (*Reinheit*) of the chromatic part of the sensation, then, is given by $C/(B + W + C)$. The brightness of the chromatic part is given by $(W + (C/2))/((W + (C/2)) + (B + (C/2)))$. The chromatic part contributes to the "brightness" and the "darkness" of the sensation in equal amounts, since its intrinsic brightness is that of midgray. These numerical relationships can also be derived from center-of-gravity constructions carried out on the triangle CWB, Hering noted, though he warned his readers sourly that center-of-gravity constructions in general "were responsible for much confusion in the theory of colors" (pp. 178–80, on 180).

Arithmetic led Hering back to physiology and to psychophysics. Like white and black, red and green and blue and yellow are all primary sensations; in accord with the principles of psychophysics each pair of opponent colors may be associated with a specific dissimilation-assimilation process occurring in the visual substance (pp. 180–84). Just as there is a black-white sensitive substance, so we can infer the existence of a blue-yellow sensitive substance and a red-green sensitive substance, each undergoing dissimilation and assimilation under the stimulus of light. We cannot be sure, however, whether there exist three kinds of visual substance, or a single visual substance capable of sustaining three distinct kinds of metabolic process. While we can associate white with dissimilation, we cannot know whether blue or yellow, red or green, play that role in the chromatic processes. Finally, we cannot be sure whether these visual substances are located on the periphery in the eye, or in the brain. Observation, however, proves that the three assimilation-dissimilation processes and the associated psychophysical events operate wholly independently of each other.

Hering emphasized the differences between the black-white and the chromatic processes. The most important one is that all light must stimulate dissimilation in the black-white substance, but in the two chromatic processes some wavelengths must stimulate dissimilation and others assimilation. Thus half the solar spectrum stimulates the yellow-blue process to the sensation of yellow, the other half to the sensation of blue. Wavelengths around the middle of the spectrum must stimulate the red-green process to green, those on either extremity must stimulate red. All wavelengths stimulate the black-white process to white, but the intensity of the resulting white and so the brightness of the sensation will vary across the spectrum and have a maximum in the "yellow" wavelengths. The sensation that comes to consciousness will be the sum of the inputs from all three processes (pp. 182–83). Since any light that stimulates a chromatic response will also stimulate the black-white process, all colors (including those stimulated by homogeneous lights) come to consciousness mixed with white and hence are not seen in their full purity.

The chromatic processes show other importance differences from the black-white process. A properly chosen mixture of physical wavelengths can stimulate equal measures of both assimilation and dissimilation in one of the chromatic processes, thus leaving the ratio of A- and D-action equal to one and producing no chromatic response at all (pp. 181–83). When light of such "complementary" wavelengths acts on the chromatic processes, Hering insisted, the effect of the resulting cancellation is not to produce white, but no sensation at all (p. 183). In the dark-adapted eye, where the ratio of A- and D-activity has approached unity in all three processes, the resulting sensation is a midgray emanating from the black-white process. Under this circumstance, the chromatic processes make no contribution to sensation, for the level of activity in them has dropped below the threshold of sensory awareness (pp. 181–82). Since physical light too weak to excite color perception still can be readily seen, the chromatic threshold must be substantially higher than the black-white threshold.

These differences aside, Hering insisted, the similarities between the black-white and the chromatic processes explain many phenomena of color vision. If one postulates the same properties in all three processes regarding induction and exhaustion, then the mechanism accounts for color effects in successive and simultaneous contrast in ways analogous to those for brightness effects (p. 192). Above all, the theory accounts elegantly for what Hering called *Umstimmung*, or adaptation (pp. 188–94). Any A- or D-action in either opponent process reduces the A- and D-susceptibility for that action, and so, if the stimulus remains constant, reduces the eye's ability to respond to it. When brought out of equilibrium by the action of light, the metabolic mechanisms constantly move back toward equilibrium, equilibrium in the chromatic receptors yielding no sensation at all. Thus, the eye constantly and quickly adapts to the bluishness of light from the sky, or the yellow-tinge of artificial illuminants, so that both appear white (p. 196). No psychological illusion produces this adaptation, Hering insisted, but rather the equilibrium-seeking, self-directing action of the opponent process mechanisms of the retina.

Physiology and psychology were to debate long and furiously the relative merits of the opponent process and Young–Helmholtz theories. Hering in 1875 also assessed the strengths and weaknesses of the two; predictably, he found few weaknesses in his own theory and many in Young's. Young's theory, he admitted, represented a major step forward in its attempt to "reduce the great multiplicity of light and color sensations to a few physiological variables" (p. 198). It had stumbled, however, in failing to recognize the existence of four phenomenologically simple colors and the independent existence of black and white, as Ernst Mach had pointed out in 1865. Yellow, as a simple sensation, can never be mixed from simple red and simple green. Young's followers delude themselves that they have done so, when in fact they use spectral reds that already contain trace amounts of yellow.[5]

Beyond its sound fundamental premise, judged Hering, there "remains not much more good in [Young's theory] to report" (p. 199). As a theory of retinal exhaustion it provides gross explanations of afterimages, but it cannot explain their precise hues or levels of relative brightness without unacceptable appeals to illusions of judgment. Because Young's theory recognizes only the kind of psychophysical action corresponding to dissimilation, it could form no conception of the antagonistic physiological processes fundamental to vision. Hering criticized Young's theory for failing to recognize that "complementary" light rays cancel or neutralize one another, and for erroneously holding instead that they "complement" or "complete" one another to make white. Thus, for Young the white process arises from and is dependent on the chromatic ones, while Hering insisted that it is clearly separate and more fundamental (p. 198). Most serious, the new literature on color blindness proves that there are no "red blind" or "green blind" individuals, but only subjects who are simultaneously "red and green blind." These must lack the red-green opponent process, not the hypothetical red or green receptors of Young's theory. Hering did not elaborate his discussion of color blindness, but promised to return to it (p. 201).

REPRISE: THE UNIFICATION OF PHYSIOLOGICAL OPTICS

Hering's insistence on all that separated his theory of color vision from that of Helmholtz and Maxwell ought not to obscure their extensive common ground. Both were theories that sought theoretical economy by postulating a limited number of fundamental sensations and distinct physiological processes. Both explained color blindness in the first instance by the loss of one or more components, and both accepted the notion of psychological mixing. Each described color sensations in terms of precisely three variables, and each accepted and built upon the operational trichromacy of the eye, the techniques of colorimetry as developed by Maxwell, and the barycentric properties of the color plane. That broad agreement about the theoretical foundations of color vision, like the broad agreement between Helmholtz and Hering on spatial perception that the nativist-empiricist controversy so obscured, was fundamental to the integration of physiological optics that occurred at the middle of the nineteenth century.

It is sometimes possible to agree about everything except the fundamentals. By the conclusion of *On the Theory of the Light Sense*, Hering had largely abandoned the polemical rhetoric with which the tract had begun, and had turned to higher programmatic objectives. The opponent process theory of vision, he insisted, expressed overarching psychophysical principles as well as the kinds of self-regulating, equilibrium-seeking physiological principles that permeate all organic life:

> The theory presented here, although grounded in the first instance on the most unprejudiced analysis of visual sensations possible, is nevertheless most essentially rooted in certain fundamental laws which I have abstracted from the manifestations of organic and psychical life. [These include] on the one hand . . . the fundamental psychological laws which yielded the important concepts of the quality and weight of sensations. On the other hand . . . [they include] the proposition that every living and irritable substance possesses one or more specific D-susceptibilities and also various A-susceptibilities according to the dissimilation and assimilation processes occurring simultaneously within it. . . . My view as to the integration (*Zusammenhang*) of numerous physiological themes, and especially those of nerve and muscle physiology, came out of this conception—just as in some respects light [emerges from] the manifestations of mental life. (Hering 1875[42], 201–2)

For Hering and for his school, the subsequent controversies with Helmholtz and his followers were not merely to be about a theory of color perception or about the genesis of spatial awareness. They were to be about a particular conception of organic life and of mind, and about the disciplinary commitments prerequisite to understanding them.

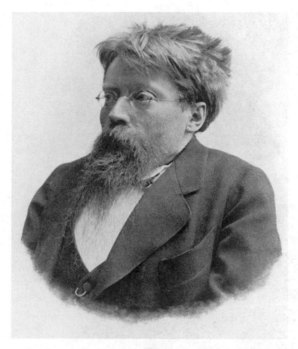

1. Arthur König (1856–1901).

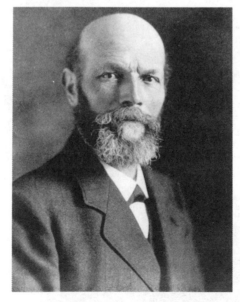

2. Johannes von Kries (1853–1928).

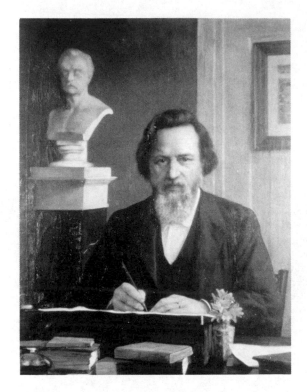

3. Franciscus Cornelis
Donders (1818–1889).

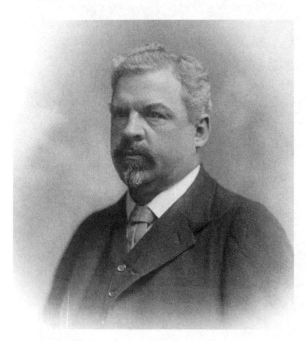

4. Franz Hillebrand
(1863–1926).

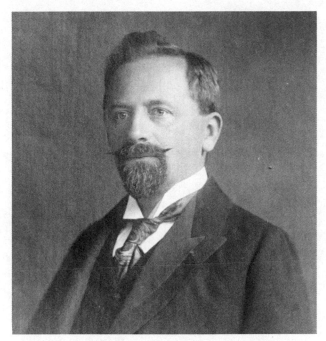

5. Armin von Tschermak-Seysenegg (1870–1952).

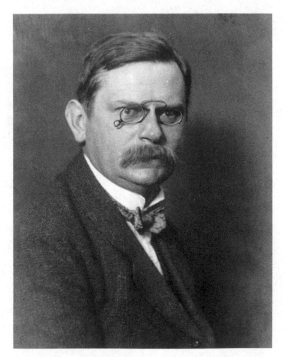

6. Ernst Heinrich Siegfried Garten (1871–1923).

Part Three

THE WIDER CONTROVERSY

CHAPTER EIGHT

Core Sets and Partisans

By 1875 THE direct exchanges between Helmholtz and Hering were over. Helmholtz had abandoned sensory physiology for physics, and his position in the subsequent controversy was publicly defended mainly by others. Hering, in contrast, continued to play the leading role in the controversy well into the twentieth century, even though most of his original research contributions had been made by 1875. Increasingly he was assisted by a small but formidable circle of students and scientific allies, who by 1900 had taken the controversy largely onto their shoulders. Who were the men and women who rallied to these scientific causes, and what factors shaped their commitment?

THE CORE SET

The recent literature of science studies has typically analyzed controversies in terms of the social units Harry Collins called "core sets" (Collins 1979; 1981; 1985, 142–47). Martin Rudwick subsequently identified the core set as "the social correlate of the cognitive category 'focal problem,'" and defined it as

> the small set of individuals through whose changing opinions a focal problem is ultimately treated by the rest of the "scientific community" as having been settled. Once those few individuals have concluded that the problem has been solved satisfactorily, then it *has* been solved: not in any prescriptive sense, but in the sense that it is treated de facto as solved. Thus as soon as conflict and controversy within the core set for any focal problem are replaced by virtual consensus, the focal problem is at an end and the core set dissolves. Like the zones of competence and involvement, a core set is a weak-boundaried grouping. (Rudwick 1985, 427)

Rudwick and Collins both emphasized the typically complex and fluid nature of the alignments within a core set. Rudwick, especially, insisted that identifying a core set involves tracing diachronic and synchronic lines of development and pressure within that set. He stressed that the polemical exchanges conducted among the members of a core set normally constitute a tacit negotiation, which usually (although not invariably) results eventually in closure.

The Helmholtz–Hering controversy poses several obstacles to core set analysis of this kind. First, it was not actually a single controversy, but a complex, sprawling array of separate focal problems, for each of which a distinct core set might legitimately be identified. Many participants weighed into the dispute over spatial perception who did not do so for the color theory debates, and vice versa. Second, and more important, this dispute was not only a scientific controversy but also a confrontation of scientific schools. The core set consisted on the one hand of "partisans" associated with one school or its rival, and on the other of a relatively small group of "nonaligned" who tried to moderate between the two positions or to define alternate approaches, and who were in turn intensely courted by the partisan groups. Core set analysis must take that tripartite division into account, even though the boundary between partisans and nonaligned was fluid and indistinct.

Table 8.1 presents one possible core set reconstruction of the Helmholtz–Hering controversy. It shows that set partitioned into three distinct groups: the partisans of Helmholtz, the partisans of Hering, and nonaligned participants. Peer acknowledgment constitutes the chief criterion for inclusion on that list. While the forty-two individuals shown represent only a fraction of those who wrote on the issues of the dispute, all those individuals, or their research results, were cited by other participants as particularly significant to the controversy. The large subset of participants who are listed as partisans met several additional criteria. They either publicly espoused one side of the dispute or wrote in such a way that no informed contemporary could doubt their alignment or purpose. They carried on their advocacy in the research literature of the day or in advanced discussions of that literature, and not merely in elementary textbooks, reviews, or lecture halls. On the other hand, individuals did not have to agree slavishly with Helmholtz or Hering in order to be considered partisans for the purposes of Table 8.1. Both Ernst Mach and G. E. Müller, for example, proposed theories of color vision rather different from Hering's own, yet both were clearly aligned with Hering and his students in the larger controversy. Similarly, Johannes von Kries modified Helmholtz's original position on many points, without ceasing to be his staunchest defender.

The selection and categorization of the nonaligned participants shown in Table 8.1 are inevitably more tentative and arbitrary than that of partisans. The list of nonaligned includes participants who in the public judgment of their peers took a significant part in the controversy, but who refused to identify exclusively with one side or the other, who espoused definite intermediate positions, or who defended distinct programs of their own. That criterion leaves the boundary between partisans and the nonaligned subjective and indistinct in many cases, particularly when

TABLE 8.1
The Core Set of the Helmholtz–Hering Controversy

Helmholtz Partisans	*Hering Partisans*
Bezold, Wilhelm von (1837–1907) Physics	Bielschowsky, Alfred* (1871–1940) Ophth.
Brodhun, Eugen* (1860–1938) Physics	Brücke, Ernst T.* (1880–1941) Physl.
Brücke, Ernst (1819–92) Physl.	Garten, Siegfried* (1871–1923) Physl.
Dieterici, Conrad* (1859–1929) Physics	Hess, Carl von* (1863–1923) Ophth.
Exner, Franz (1849–1926) Physics	Hillebrand, Franz* (1863–1926) Psych.
Exner, Sigmund* (1846–1926) Physl.	Hofmann, Franz* (1869–1926) Physl.
Fick, Adolf (1829–1901) Physl.	Mach, Ernst (1838–1916) Physics/Physl.
Fleischl von Marxow, Ernst (1846–91) Physl.	Müller, Georg E. (1850–1934) Psych.
Graefe, Alfred von (1830–99) Ophth.	Sachs, Moriz* (1865–1930) Ophth.
Holmgren, Frithiof (1831–97) Physl.	Stilling, Jakob (1842–1915) Ophth.
König, Arthur* (1856–1901) Physics	Tschermak-Seysenegg, Armin* (1870–1952) Physl.
Kries, Johannes von* (1853–1928) Physl.	Zoth, Oskar (1864–1903) Physl.
Leber, Theodor* (1840–1917) Ophth.	
Lummer, Otto* (1860–1925) Physics	
Müller, J. J.* (1846–75) Physics/Physl.	
Nagel, Willibald (1870–1911) Physl.	
Raehlmann, Edward (1848–1917) Ophth.	

Nonaligned Participants

Aubert, Hermann (1826–92) Physl.	Katz, David (1884–1953) Psych.
Du Bois-Reymond, Emil (1818–96) Physl.	Ladd-Franklin, Christine (1847–1930) Psych.
Donders, Franciscus (1818–89) Ophth., Physl.	Lipps, Theodor (1851–1914) Psych.
Ebbinghaus, Hermann (1850–1909) Psych.	Preyer, Thierry William (1841–97) Physl.
Hippel, Arthur von (1841–1916) Ophth.	Stumpf, Carl (1848–1936) Psych.
Jaensch, Erich (1883–1940) Psych.	Wundt, Wilhelm (1832–1920) Psych.
Javal, Louis-Emile (1839–1907) Ophth.	

* = student or laboratory assistant

participants changed their opinions and alignments. Contemporaries, for example, probably thought of Hermann Aubert as drifting away from a neutral or slightly pro-Helmholtz position at the beginning of his career, to become a Hering supporter later. Arthur Hippel produced key evidence on behalf of Hering's theory of color vision, but seems never to have been treated by Hering or his students as an open ally.

The major criterion for inclusion among the significant nonaligned was that partisans themselves must have invoked these individuals as allies, enemies, or alleged spokespersons of some scientific consensus. One indirect consequence of that criterion is that prominent non-German scientists writing on the issues of human vision fail to appear on the list if their positions were not cited by German partisans. And in fact, only four non-Germans appear at all in Table 8.1: French ophthalmologist Louis-Emile Javal, American psychologist Christine Ladd-Franklin, Dutch ophthalmologist Franciscus Donders, and Swedish physiologist Frithiof Holmgren. In 1880, when German research dominated physiological optics, the absence of significant non-German voices legitimately reflected the comparative state of the field. By the early twentieth century, when vision studies had become a more nearly international endeavor, that absence had become a sign of parochialism.

SIGNIFICANT PARTISANS: HERING

Among the significant partisans on behalf of Ewald Hering, one factor especially stands out as significant in shaping the common theoretical commitment: personal connection with Hering himself. At least eight of the twelve individuals listed had been students of Hering and in most cases his institute assistants. Carl von Hess and Franz Hofmann, both ophthalmologists, served as assistants to Hering and his colleague Hubert Sattler at the University of Prague and both followed Hering to Leipzig in 1895. They were joined there by Alfred Bielschowsky, student of Hering and assistant to Sattler. Siegfried Garten studied at Leipzig, where Ludwig introduced him to physiology. When Hering succeeded Ludwig in 1895, he turned Garten's interest to sensory problems. Garten spent his career at Leipzig and followed Hering in the chair for physiology there. Psychologist Franz Hillebrand and ophthalmologist Moriz Sachs studied with Hering at Prague, and physiologist Ernst Theodor von Brücke served as assistant to Hering at Leipzig and habilitated there in 1907.

Not all Hering's defenders were his students and assistants. At least one of the others had a personal affiliation with him. Ernst Mach was a colleague of Hering's at the German university in Prague for twenty-five years, and the two men remained warm scientific allies. Ophthalmologist Jakob Stilling apparently never studied with Hering, but may have had contact with him in Vienna. Göttingen psychologist G. E. Müller and physiologist Oskar Zoth also had no institutional connection with Hering during their careers. Both, however, had strong Austro-Hungarian connections like many of Hering's defenders. Müller was briefly professor at Czernowitz, and Zoth was student of and successor to Alexander Rollet at Graz.

The lists of significant partisans contain the names of a few individuals whose careers and reputations revolved about the Helmholtz–Hering controversy. Among Hering's defenders, one such individual was Franz Hillebrand. In the late 1880s he became a student in Hering's institute at the University of Prague; in 1893, privatdozent at the University of Vienna; and in 1896, professor of philosophy at the University of Innsbruck. As an experimental psychologist, Hillebrand held academic posts in philosophy as was then customary, and he was important for developing the psychological dimensions of Hering's physiological program. Hillebrand published only eleven papers on sensory psychology and vision, most in the *Zeitschrift für Psychologie*, but all were formidable experimental elaborations and defenses of Hering's basic doctrines.

Armin von Tschermak-Seysenegg (1870–1952) was also Austro-Hungarian by extraction and came from a prominent Viennese academic family. He studied with Hering at Leipzig between 1896 and 1899, and then with Helmholtz's former assistant Julius Bernstein at Halle in 1900. In 1906 Tschermak became professor of physiology at the Vienna Tierärztliche Hochschule, and in 1913 took Hering's former post at the German university in Prague. When the German university vanished at the end of World War II, Tschermak moved to the University of Ravensberg. He published in many areas of physiology, and after the deaths of Hillebrand, Carl Hess, and Franz Hofmann during the 1920s, was left as Hering's last major disciple.

From the mid-1880s Hering's partisans clearly constituted a "research school." Contemporary science studies uses that term to denote a (usually) local group of researchers under direction of a leader who systematically develop a particular research program or theoretical line, exploit a newly invented research method, or investigate a new problem or subfield (Servos 1993). Members of the research school may come and go (always the case in a graduate school or university setting), but the leader provides the focus and continuity necessary to give the group and its program a distinct character. In a well-known discussion of 1981, historian Gerald Geison stressed the role of research schools as the loci of conceptual innovation in modern science (Geison 1981). He also noted that the existence of research schools depends upon conditions of institutionalization that allow systematic recruitment, continuity of program, an integrated and hierarchical ordering of research, and a relatively generous and constant allocation of resources. These conditions were rarely satisfied in European science before the nineteenth century, making research schools an organizational form of recent historical vintage.

In that discussion Geison also offered fourteen empirically derived criteria (borrowed from J. B. Morell [1972]) for the success or failure of research schools. These criteria are listed in Table 8.2. An evaluation of Hering's group in terms of these criteria suggests that it was a highly successful one, satisfying as many as twelve of the fourteen requirements.

TABLE 8.2
Factors in the Success or Failure of Research Schools

1. Charismatic leader(s)
2. Leader with research reputation
3. "Informal" setting and leadership style
4. Leader with institutional power
5. Social cohesion, loyalty, esprit de corps, "discipleship"
6. Focused research program
7. Simple and rapidly exploitable experimental techniques
8. Invasion of new field of research
9. Pool of potential recruits
10. Access to or control of publication outlets
11. Students publish early under own names
12. Produced and "placed" significant numbers of students
13. Institutionalization in university setting
14. Adequate financial support

Source: Gerald L. Geison, "Scientific Change, Emerging Specialties, and Research Schools," History of Science 19 (1981):20–40, on 24.

Especially important to the school's success was Hering's charismatic leadership, the sense of 'discipleship' he inspired, and the highly focused research program he superintended. If Hering founded no journal of his own, he and his students had ready access to E. F. W. Pflüger's Archiv für die gesammte Physiologie and to the important Zeitschrift für Psychologie und Physiologie der Sinnesorgane. Pflüger's physiological views coincided closely with Hering's, and Hering and his students were well represented on the editorial board of the Zeitschrift, even though editorial control was nominally in unfriendly hands.

The fate of the Hering school hinged upon the two Geison–Morell criteria that the group did not satisfy. First, the work of the school was not based upon "simple and rapidly exploitable experimental techniques." On the contrary, Hering's preferred techniques were often ingenious adaptations of traditional methods, most of which required such considerable observational skills that only a few specialized students could master them. Second, Hering's group invaded no new field of research; rather they focused their investigations upon some of the most intensely studied and fiercely disputed territory of nineteenth-century science.

Not all scientific "schools" need be "research schools" in the sense of modern "research groups." Nineteenth-century contemporaries used the term "school" in its looser and more general sense, to denote a particular intellectual alignment distinguished from other competing alignments. The list of Hering's significant partisans shows that his followers also constituted a "school" in this more inclusive sense. A few individuals lacked all institutional affiliation with Hering and were never formally his students. The others did not merely develop and defend Hering's views while working under his direction; in most cases they continued to do so long after they had left his institute and his intellectual circle. The appeal of Hering's program flowed from the theoretical and philosophical stances he adopted, rather than from particular research methods or new fields of research he exploited. Partly for this reason, those who had never experienced his charismatic leadership could nevertheless feel that appeal, and so participate in a school alignment that extended beyond the institutes at Prague and Leipzig.

SIGNIFICANT PARTISANS: HELMHOLTZ

Helmholtz's partisans differ considerably from Hering's. The proportion of those who had actually been Helmholtz's students or assistants is much lower than for Hering's supporters. His direct students included Theodor Leber and J. J. Müller, who took Ph.D.s with Helmholtz at Heidelberg. Leber went on to become professor of ophthalmology at Göttingen and Heidelberg and master of a large and influential school; Müller died at thirty-one on the threshold of a promising career in what he called "physiological physics." Better-known students of Helmholtz included the famous Johannes von Kries, who worked with Helmholtz in Berlin in 1877; and Helmholtz's protégé, physicist Arthur König, who conducted color vision experiments in loose affiliation with Helmholtz during the decade before his death. Eugen Brodhun, Conrad Dieterici, and Otto Lummer were young physicists who collaborated with Helmholtz and König on that same experimental program. A few other partisans had personal contact with Helmholtz, although not as his students. Ernst Brücke and Adolf Fick had been his fellow students, and J. F. W. von Bezold a colleague at Berlin from 1885 to 1894.

More markedly than the list of Hering's supporters, the significant partisans of Helmholtz range from individuals only marginally associated with the controversy to those who built careers upon it. Foremost among the latter is the unusual and oddly tragic figure of Arthur König (Engelmann 1903). König suffered throughout his life from a progressive and painful spinal deformity that led to his death at age forty-five. Scarcely less debilitating were his social and educational liabilities: König's father was a primary school teacher, his secondary education from a *Realschule* rather than a gymnasium, and he passed several years early in life as a merchant's apprentice. Despite these liabilities, König entered the University of Berlin in 1879 and, in what was certainly the turning point of his career, attracted the attention and patronage of Helmholtz. He became

Helmholtz's assistant in the physics institute, editor of his collected papers and lectures, and with Helmholtz's support, associate professor in the philosophical faculty. In 1889, following the death of the incumbent Arthur Christiani, Helmholtz's friend du Bois-Reymond appointed König director of the "physical" division of the university physiological institute in the medical faculty, with special teaching responsibilities in physiological optics. König clearly owed this appointment to Helmholtz's patronage, as he had neither physiological training nor a medical degree. He held this post until his death in 1901.

Above all König was a measurer. From the mid-1880s on he conducted precision colorimetric determinations of optical response to complex variations of physical stimuli in normal and color blind eyes. Helmholtz drew on these results in his mathematical studies of color vision in the 1890s and incorporated many of them into the second edition of the *Physiological Optics*, in the preparation of which he was assisted by König. In 1886 König and Conrad Dieterici published the first systematic determinations of spectral response curves for experimental primaries that had been made since Maxwell's (König and Dieterici 1886[14]). This work led König into direct conflict with Hering; König's publications between 1884 and 1897 constituted a running series of exchanges with Hering.

How actively Helmholtz himself controlled or influenced König's research at Berlin is impossible to know, but Hering's school regarded König as little more than a surrogate. The young men who collaborated with him were often physics students from Helmholtz's institute, and they usually drifted back into Helmholtz's orbit, sometimes to take positions in the *Physikalisch-technische Reichsanstalt* of which Helmholtz was president. When the *Zeitschrift für Psychologie und Physiologie der Sinnesorgane* was founded in 1890 (to compete with Wilhelm Wundt, it was rumored), König was made editor alongside Hermann Ebbinghaus, the Berlin *Ordinarius* for psychology. That such a sensitive position should have gone to an individual with relatively little personal standing and limited credentials suggests again the influence of Helmholtz. Whether König himself felt stifled by Helmholtz's paternalistic hand is also impossible to know. Almost immediately following Helmholtz's death, however, König's theorizing began to move along radically new lines, which drew the ridicule of Hering and disconcerted Helmholtz's other supporters.

By far the most influential of Helmholtz's defenders was Johannes von Kries (1853–1928). A Prussian noble by birth, Kries studied medicine at Halle with the venerable A. W. Volkmann and then physiology at Leipzig with Carl Ludwig. Kries worked briefly with Helmholtz in the physics institute at Berlin in 1876–77, and then returned to Ludwig at Leipzig to habilitate in physiology (Kries 1925; Rothschuh 1973, 217–19). In 1880 he moved to the University of Freiburg and made his career there. Kries specialized in sensory physiology and trained some important students, including his collaborator Willibald A. Nagel (who succeeded König at Berlin), Wilhelm Trendelenburg, and Rudolf Metzner. Kries had deep philosophical interests and later in his career became an exponent of Neo-Kantianism and interpreter of its significance for natural science. Scientifically, Kries is best known for his 1894 formulation of the duplicity theory of vision, a theory that grew directly out of the Helmholtz–Hering controversy.

Kries' first polemical exchanges with Hering occurred as early as 1879, and they increased in frequency and ferocity until the turn of the century, when age and infirmity forced Hering to curtail his polemical writing. Kries and Nagel were then forced into exchanges with Hess, Hillebrand, and Tschermak, to defend Helmholtz's views as well the duplicity theory. In all his writings Kries presented himself, not insincerely, as a mediator between the schools of Helmholtz and Hering, and as an impartial judge weighing the merits of both positions. With Frans Donders he was Europe's first and foremost advocate of a "zone theory" compromise, which would see the Young–Helmholtz trichromatic mechanism active in the retinal receptors and a four-color, opponent process mechanism active at some higher neural level.

The third partisan who requires special notice is Adolf Eugen Fick (1829–1901). Fick was a near-contemporary of Helmholtz. The two men studied medicine together at Berlin, and Fick went on to a successful career in physiology spent largely at the University of Würzburg. His scientific interests also paralleled Helmholtz's closely: muscle energetics, metabolic exchanges, the nerve stimulus, the eye muscles, and sensory physiology in general (Schenck 1903; Rothschuh 1973, 248–50). In 1873 Fick proposed a major revision of the Young–Helmholtz theory to allow it to cope with the puzzling phenomenon of color blindness, and he became the foremost critic of Hering's concept of brightness (Fick 1873, 1900). These initiatives led to confrontations with Hering that continued until Fick's death in 1901.

Ernst Brücke, a close and lifelong friend of Helmholtz, played an unusual role among the partisans. His early research on vision, and his terminological innovations, strongly influenced the young Helmholtz. Later Brücke's research began to move in different directions and it had little direct influence on the controversy. But Brücke preserved the physiology institute in Vienna as an important Helmholtzian outpost in the Hapsburg territories, where Hering's views elsewhere enjoyed considerable influence. Brücke introduced Sigmund Exner and Fleischl von Marxow to Helmholtz and his ideas, and he is said on two occasions to have assisted in blocking Hering's appointment to the University of Vienna. The first occasion arose in 1872, when the creation of a second chair for physiology was proposed; the second in 1890, when Hering was nominated to succeed Brücke himself. On both occasions Hering's nomination enjoyed majority support in the medical faculty (Lesky 1976, 481–98).

The careers of Helmholtz's supporters show that the master-student relationship was less important in determining partisanship for Helmholtz than for Hering. The eight partisans who had nominally studied with Helmholtz did so in most cases very briefly, and he was not always the primary influence upon them. Johannes von Kries, for example, came to Berlin to work in Helmholtz's institute in 1876–77 and praised the "sureness and clarity" of Helmholtz's thought, his experimental skill, and the "deep and imposing impression" Helmholtz made upon him. But he added that "the nature of my activity in the institute afforded little opportunity for the deeper discussion of scientific questions," and he quickly decamped back to Leipzig to resume work with Carl Ludwig, who had been the main personal influence upon his scientific career (Kries 1925, 129–30).

Similarly, Albrecht von Graefe and not Helmholtz was the main scientific influence on Theodor Leber, even though Leber had been briefly Helmholtz's student. Brodhun, Dieterici, and Lummer took their Ph.D.s with Helmholtz and acknowledged him as their master, but their actual research seems to have been directed by König, to whom they were seconded. Sigmund Exner and Fleischl von Marxow were as much the students of Ernst Brücke as of Helmholtz; Edward Raehlmann studied primarily with Adolf Fick and Helmholtz's former assistant Edward Bernstein. In comparison to Hering's supporters, Helmholtz's partisans constituted a looser, more diverse group whose personal ties to the master were more indirect.

All this suggests that Helmholtz's supporters did not constitute a research school in the strong sense of the term used by Geison and Morrell (cf. Cranefield 1966). Indeed, their criteria for a successful research school (Table 8.2) cannot unambiguously be applied to the partisans listed in Table 8.1. Those criteria can, however, be applied to the group that worked under König's direction at Berlin between 1884 and 1898, first in Helmholtz's laboratory and then in König's own laboratory in the physiology institute. This research group numbered about fifteen individuals over the period studied; four (Brodhun, Dieterici, König, Lummer) are counted as significant partisans. Wilhelm Bezold also collaborated with the group during this period, as did the nonaligned participants Hermann Ebbinghaus and Christine Ladd-Franklin.

König's small and diverse circle satisfied approximately eight of the fourteen Geison–Morrell criteria. König freely opened his laboratory to women (Else Köttgen, Christine Ladd-Franklin), tolerated considerable disagreement among his co-workers, and regularly published joint papers with them. The laboratory activity revolved about a focused research program based upon Helmholtz's ideas and upon exploitable experimental techniques and sophisticated instrumentation drawn mostly from physical optics. Helmholtz and König enjoyed an adequate pool of recruits (many of them physics students) and encouraged them to publish early and in their own name. The research done at Berlin, however, attracted only occasional students of physiology, ophthalmology, or psychology, and it seems unlikely that König or even Helmholtz could have exercised the patronage necessary to have successfully "placed" students in those disciplines. There is little evidence that either leader was especially charismatic or that the group cultivated much esprit de corps.

On the other hand, Helmholtz's followers certainly constituted a "school" in the looser sense of being a well-defined and self-conscious intellectual alignment. In addition to his particular theories of vision, Helmholtz's commitment to biophysical and mathematical methods (especially of colorimetry) and to the importance of learning and experience, as well as his pragmatic conception of the perceptual processes, appealed to many scientists and provided the methodological core for a "school" of vision studies. Hering himself insisted that Helmholtz's followers constituted a school, and his criticism sufficed, ironically, to endow Helmholtz's principles with an internal coherence they might otherwise not have possessed.

STYLES OF SCIENTIFIC LEADERSHIP: HERING

Styles of scientific leadership strongly influence the success and internal coherence of research schools (Fruton 1990). This applied with special force to Ewald Hering, who was one of the most charismatic research directors of his era. He trained not just students, but disciples. To some of them he passed on his unparalleled talent as a polemicist, his consummate skills as an introspective observer and experimenter, and his militant perception of himself as being an oppressed outsider at war with the physiological establishment. Several factors account for this unlikely charisma of Hering, a man whose writings reveal him as a vicious polemicist, an implacable opponent, and a master of sarcasm.

Part of Hering's charisma arose from the militancy of his scientific stance and from the fact that many of the most famous names in German science feared to cross him in print. His students must have feared and respected him, too. Siegfried Garten, a disciple and junior colleague for over twenty years, recalled Hering as a modest and generous man, who held himself under rigid self-control and yet could explode with primitive rage at a perceived offense and would rarely forgive thereafter (Garten 1918, 522). Helmholtz, one of the few men who ever bested Hering in a public exchange, gossiped to du Bois-Reymond that Hering had been mentally disturbed (Kirsten 1986, 171 [no. 115]).

Fear did not prevent Hering's students from loving him. His fiercely pro-German, anti-Czech political activity at Prague was said to have been crucial to the survival of a German university in the city. This story followed Hering and enhanced his stature among his students as a German nationalist and patriot. Those who left recollections of him—and many of his students did—agree that he lavished attention upon his advanced students, checked and rechecked their publications, and regarded his school as a natural extension of his scientific aspirations (Brücke 1928; Garten 1918; Hillebrand 1918; Hess 1918a, 1918b; Hofmann 1918; Tschermak-Seysenegg 1934). Hering instilled a sense of mission in his students. He offered them, as Tschermak-Seysenegg wrote, not just theories but "a comprehensive conception of nature and of life." He taught them "not to regard life as a physicochemical, machine-like process, but to affirm its intrinsic activity, the autonomous character of its controlling laws, and its goal-directedness, and to search for these characteristics in their particular manifestations." Above all, Tschermak concluded, Hering convinced his students that his ideas "belonged to the future" (Tschermak-Seysenegg 1934, 1232). Through the decade of the 1890s and after his students could undoubtedly sense the master's ideas in the ascendancy.

The writings of Hering's students attest to the emotional tie that bound them to Hering, to his memory, and to one another, and no historical interpretation can do justice to the work of the school that does not take those affective bonds fully into account. In an emotional obituary written a few months after Hering's death, Carl von Hess remembered the old man constantly surrounded by his students, whether in the strawberry patch of the institute garden, in his family parlor, or on a memorable automobile trip through the Tirol. Hess recalled those students as drawing inspiration and brotherhood from Hering's strength, patience, curiosity, and genial humor (Hess 1918a). Some of these recollections must be discounted as the standard fare of obituaries, but Tschermak-Seysenegg was still writing in a similar vein in 1932 near the final dissolution of the school. Tschermak stressed the "close spiritual comradeship" among Hering's disciples, for they had faithfully and systematically "pursued our way" without fear or favor toward anyone and unperturbed by the "ignorant and intemperate criticism" from all sides (Tschermak-Seysenegg 1932, 3).

Franz Hillebrand's memorial tribute to Hering, published in 1918, summarized his teachings and hailed him as the last of the great "psychophysicists" of the nineteenth century, who had built psychology as an autonomous discipline. Otherwise it offered no personal reflections (Hillebrand 1918, 1–5). Some hint of the emotional bond between Hering and Hillebrand, however, is provided by Franziska Hillebrand, Hillebrand's widow and former student. Following her husband's death she published her *Lehre von den Gesichtsempfindungen* in 1929 as a tribute to his memory. It was to survey the field of visual perception and lay out her husband's life's work on the basis of his private papers and notes; in reality it was also to be her own original contribution to the field through her critical commentaries on the literature. The book, however, reveals itself immediately as less a tribute to Hillebrand than to Hering himself. Hering, not Hillebrand, dominates its pages; both scientifically and morally Hillebrand's young widow identified him completely with Hering. In the end the epiphany of her praise for the late Hillebrand was that the virtues "which ought to be attributes of every researcher, and which had developed themselves in Hering to a rare perfection, may also be ascribed to Hillebrand to an extraordinary degree" (Hillebrand 1929, "Vorrede," iv). Ties of loyalty, identification, and love, as well as intellectual commitment, bound Hering's students to their unlikely master.

Hering contributed more to the success of his research school than providing charismatic leadership and instilling a sense of mission. He encouraged his students to publish early and under their own names (although always under his close supervision), and he successfully placed his students in good university positions. Around 1925 Hering's students occupied six of the twenty-seven chairs for physiology in the extended German language university system, and five of the twenty-six chairs of ophthalmology (Eulner 1970, 496, 508). Most of those placements came in Austria, Eastern Europe, and South Germany; only two of the Hering students listed in Table 8.1 saw their careers culminate in Prussian or North German universities, despite Hering's strong ties to Leipzig. Hering also demonstrated an ability to draw recruits from a broader range of disciplines than physiology alone. At Prague Hering was closely associated with ophthalmologist Hubert Sattler, and upon moving to Leipzig he arranged a post for Sattler there as well. Hering counted numerous ophthalmologists as well as physiologists among his students, including Carl Hess, Arthur Brückner, and Alfred Bielschowsky. Similarly, Hering attracted a few experimental psychologists to his views, including Franz Hillebrand, who worked in his institute, and G. E. Müller, who did not. Hering's access to students of psychology weakened after he came to Leipzig in 1895, for psychology there was dominated by Wilhelm Wundt, an old enemy and past victim of Hering's polemical pen.

STYLES OF SCIENTIFIC LEADERSHIP: HELMHOLTZ

Helmholtz, too, exercised great charisma as the most versatile scientist in Europe and later as the acknowledged senior statesman of German science. His institutes, first in physiology at Heidelberg and then in physics at Berlin, produced a modest flow of student research on topics mostly related to his own interests and closely directed by him (Jungnickel and McCormmach 1986, 1:307–10, 2:18–32). In physiology, however, if not also in physics, Helmholtz trained surprisingly few disciples who seized upon and extended the central directions of his work in ways characteristic of the research schools of the period (Cranefield 1966). His personal bearing as an institute leader and research director did not forge the emotional bonds or the sense of mission among his students that Hering's did. Wilhelm Wundt, his assistant at Heidelberg from 1858 to 1863, complained that Helmholtz was so reticent as to be almost unapproachable (Wundt 1920, 155–60; Diamond 1980, 28–31); Ludwig Boltzmann in 1871 found him cold and officious (Mulligan 1989); and Kries encountered similar difficulties during his brief sojourn with Helmholtz (Kries 1925, 130).

Not all his scientific acquaintances found him so remote. Helmholtz's regular correspondents—Brücke, Volkmann, Donders, and others—wrote to him with real affection and found him ready to assist them in numerous ways. Sigmund Exner, a student from the Heidelberg period, congratulated Helmholtz on his seventieth birthday and recollected with unfeigned pleasure "the comfortable hours spent on your veranda" in conversation with "the greatest living scientist" (Exner 1868–91, no. 5 [12.08.1890], no. 6 [15.03.1891]). Physicist Eugen Goldstein recalled the older Helmholtz as reserved and cool, sometimes vague, in his dealings with the laboratory *Praktikanten*, but at the same time patient, generous, tolerant of contradiction, forgiving of student mistakes, and almost excessively modest. Contrary to the stories circulated about him, Goldstein insisted, Helmholtz spent nearly six hours daily in his institute consulting individually with his advanced students, and that despite his heavy administrative duties outside the institute (Goldstein 1921). David Cahan's study accords Helmholtz high marks as a research director in his role as the first president of the Physikalisch-Technische Reichsanstalt, although Helmholtz emerges in that portrait as an Olympian administrator-statesman rather than as an inspirational master (Cahan 1989, 59–125).

Some of the apparent contradictions in the style of Helmholtz's scientific leadership are resolved by considering the character of his science. Much of Helmholtz's achievement resulted from his broad powers of synthesis. His greatest work typically pulled disparate but already existing strands of research and interpretation together into new levels of generalization and theoretical suggestiveness. The character and comprehensiveness of his work, combined with the awe in which he was held, attracted mature and talented researchers to his ideas. That attraction, however, depended little on his personal magnetism, and many who had never worked with the man himself were prepared to build on his ideas. Among those who did work with him he inspired awe, filial trust, and sometimes affection, but rarely the sense of mission and personal devotion that marked Hering's school.

THE NONALIGNED

Table 8.1 also lists thirteen "nonaligned" participants in the controversy. They contributed to the debate not as passive observers, or as a neutral jury waiting to be swayed by the arguments of the warring parties, but as individuals with particular interests, competencies, and goals of their own. Often they urged compromise positions between the two main theories or defended alternatives that allegedly incorporated the advantages of both.

The most important of the nonaligned was Dutch physiologist and ophthalmologist Frans Donders, who after Helmholtz himself was Europe's leading authority on physiological optics. Donders was a close friend and fervent admirer of Helmholtz, yet he was also respected by Hering, and despite the sharp papers they exchanged on occasion, Hering usually spared Donders the worst of his invective. Donders' position on spatial perception shows how very wide was the range of alternatives to the theories of both Helmholtz and Hering. In 1867 Donders warmly defended the theory of projection against Hering's attacks and dismissed the notion of retinal space values as merely a restatement of the facts, not an explanation of depth perception (Donders 1867). At the same time he defended the anatomically innate nature of perceptual mechanisms, and in a private letter of 1868 he cautioned Helmholtz that of all his "magnificent achievements in physiological optics," the only one he could not support was "your *exclusive* empiricist theory" (Donders 1856–88, no. 12 [18.03.1868]).

Other close associates of Helmholtz refused to support his views fully and so are listed among the nonaligned. One was Emil du Bois-Reymond, Helmholtz's close friend and colleague in Berlin. He supported Helmholtz's program of research into color vision, but publicly and privately rebuked his friend for his excessively empiricist theory of spatial perception (Kirsten 1986, 229 [no. 109]; du Bois-Reymond 1870, 1896).

Table 8.1 contains the names of several physiologists (Aubert, du Bois-Reymond, Preyer) and ophthalmologists (Hippel, Javal, Donders). These sorts of specialists tended to gravitate toward the perspective of one school or the other, or to defend compromise positions. The experimental psychologists, on the other hand, usually adopted more independent positions. Wilhelm Wundt, the father of experimental psychology in Germany, wrote extensively on vision from the 1860s on. Wundt, however, always tried to avoid entanglement in the Helmholtz–Hering controversy, and later in his career he proposed an alternative theory of color vision quite different from either of the main theories (Wundt 1888). On spatial perception he espoused a general empiricist line, which nevertheless differed considerably from Helmholtz's theory in the emphasis it placed on eye movements and kinesthetic cues. Wundt consistently refused to compare his own theory with that of Helmholtz, because he regarded the latter as utterly inadequate in its account of psychological processes in vision. Other German psychologists, notably Ebbinghaus, Jaensch, Ladd-Franklin, Lipps, Katz, and Stumpf, increasingly rejected both the alternatives that Helmholtz and Hering offered. As a disciplinary group psychologists more and more came to dominate the ranks of the nonaligned, and after 1900 some brought very different methodological perspectives to the issues in dispute.

CONCLUSION

Rudwick and Collins both insisted on the "private nature" of core sets in their original discussions. Core set members need have no social or institutional ties to one another except for their intense, if differing interests, in the controversy's outcome; hence in many scientific disputes, the relevant networks and their internal negotiations may frequently remain invisible to all but their members. In the Helmholtz–Hering controversy, however, that was emphatically not the case. In this dispute partisan alignments were publicly and starkly drawn, and they were reinforced by powerful emotional ties of personal and institutional loyalty.

This public polarization made the Helmholtz–Hering controversy unique in several respects. On the one hand, polarization obstructed attempts to bring the dispute to closure. The small size of the nonaligned contingent and the marginal status of some of its members thwarted their attempts to mediate in the tacit negotiations between the two warring schools or to impose compromise positions upon the core set as a whole. On the other hand, polarization also contributed to the notoriety of this controversy. Common features of scientific interaction, normally concealed within the core set and its exchanges and forgotten after its dissolution, became increasingly a matter of public record in the Helmholtz–Hering controversy. As the polemics went on, individuals both inside and outside the core set could clearly observe the intense interplay of rhetoric and negotiation, the malleability of concepts, the inadequacy of empirical recourse, and the mutual incommensurability of the competing terminologies. Puzzled and embarrassed outsiders (and some insiders, too) increasingly attributed this apparent anomaly to improper and atypical behavior on the part of participants. In the twentieth century if not before the controversy became a byword for scientific obscurantism and theory spinning run riot. The true anomaly, however, was the unexpected failure of these typical forms of interaction to produce closure, and in producing closure, to obscure the fact that recourse to these forms of interactions had ever been taken.

CHAPTER NINE

The Nativist-Empiricist Debate, 1870–1925

THE MAIN PROTAGONISTS

Helmholtz made his most important contribution to the issue of spatial perception in the third volume of the *Handbuch*, where he delineated the nativist and empiricist positions and mounted a telling criticism of Hering. His own research did not again return to the question of spatiality, but in 1871 he had J. J. Müller investigate the binocular disparity produced by torsional rotation of the eyes and interpret the effect in empiricist terms (Müller 1871; *WAH* 2:947–52, no. 120). More important, Helmholtz continued to develop and regularly reiterate his empiricist position in popular lectures and widely read epistemological discussions down to the year of his death (*VuR* 1:265–328; 2:213–48; *WAH* 3:536–53, no. 215).

Although his epistemological views changed little after 1867, they did not remain entirely static. He struggled with the epistemological status of the principle of causality and retreated from his earlier, quasi-Kantian treatment of the problem (Hatfield 1990, 208–18; Heidelberger 1993). In a series of papers begun in the mid-1860s, Helmholtz defended the possibility of a non-Euclidean geometry. He also attacked Kant's claim for the logical necessity of Euclid's axioms as transcendental forms of intuition, arguing that the claim represented yet another manifestation of the nativist fallacy (Hatfield 1990, 218–26; *VuR* 2:1–33; *WAH* 2:591–662, nos. 103, 104, 112, 144). These issues did not influence the debate over spatial perception directly, but they consolidated a popular image of Helmholtz as an anti-Kantian and spread his version of the empiricist theory to a broader audience of philosophers and mathematicians.

Helmholtz's empiricist account had largely reflected the conventional wisdom of his time about the origin of spatial perception. As such his views commanded widespread assent in popular and textbook accounts. Albrecht von Graefe in 1867 reiterated the important role of inductive inferences in vision; William Preyer delivered a wholly empiricist account of visual, spatial perception in a popular lecture of 1870; and Ernst Brücke's 1873 textbook followed Helmholtz's account of spatial localization to the letter (Graefe 1867; Preyer 1870; Brücke 1873). Through the 1870s and 1880s the subsequent editions of Ludimar Hermann's introductory physiology text presented Helmholtz's terminology and interpretations as the unquestioned consensus of the field and rejected any anatomical explanation of the retinal correspondence out of hand (Hermann 1862–99, eds. 1872, 1882).

Hering, for his part, had responded to key elements of Helmholtz's critique in his *Theory of Binocular Vision* of 1868, but his interest had then shifted in the early 1870s to the perception of light and color and to other kinds of physiological problems. That shift did not imply that Hering had abandoned his running critique of Helmholtz and empiricism or his defense of nativism. As he stated, his aim in *On the Theory of the Light Sense* (1872–75) was to discredit appeals to unconscious inference in explaining simultaneous contrast, and so indirectly to undermine their plausibility in explaining spatial localization as well (Hering 1878/1874, 1).

The *Theory of Binocular Vision* seems to have established Hering as the German authority on eye movements. He was invited to contribute the lengthy section on "The Spatial Sense and the Movements of the Eyes" ("Der Raumsinn und die Bewegungen des Auges") to Ludimar Hermann's *Handbuch der Physiologie der Sinnesorgane* (1879a), where he reviewed in detail the research done in the field over the previous fifteen years. Although he eloquently defended the nativist perspective, that work was, by Hering's standards, almost free of polemic. He wrote of himself in the third person and gave relatively balanced and neutral descriptions of his differences with Helmholtz; his occasional complaints that certain questions "cannot be discussed here" suggest that the editors had insisted on his avoiding excessively controversial issues.

Specialist readers who knew the literature and followed the arguments closely certainly noticed that "The Spatial Sense and the Movements of the Eyes" contained three interesting concessions. First, Hering quietly acknowledged Helmholtz's claim that vertical threads hanging in Müller's horopter circle will not always appear to lie in the plane of the core surface; Hering admitted that their apparent configuration will vary with the distance of the point of fixation, contrary to his own earlier claims. Second, Hering recanted his former insistence that the eyes do not perform so-called cyclofusional movements, even though substantial parts of *The Theory of Binocular Vision* had been devoted to refuting Helmholtz's arguments that under certain conditions movements of that kind can be induced. Hering's third concession was most interesting. He invoked binocular disparity of corresponding retinal images, rather than algebraic summation of innate depth values, as the primary cue to the perception of relief. Without precisely recanting his former theory of depth values, he discussed it so ambiguously as to leave readers in little doubt that he had beaten an orderly retreat from it.

If Hering's nativism found little echo in popular lectures or introductory textbooks during the 1870s, it did receive strong support from several unexpected sources. Emil du Bois-Reymond, in a popular lecture on Leibniz and the problem of the preestablished harmony, argued that Darwinian theory provided a naturalistic and nonmystical explanation of "innate ideas," and a ground on which the "old conflict" between nativism and empiricism could be reconciled. Without mentioning his friend Helmholtz explicitly, he persuasively mobilized developmental evidence against any extreme empiricist theory of vision (du Bois-Reymond 1870). Würzburg psychologist Carl Stumpf, later to be a colleague of Hering's at Prague, announced his conversion from empiricism to a "restricted nativism" that accepted the innate spatiality of local signs while still acknowledging the pervasive role of association (which he distinguished from unconscious inference) in spatial perception (Stumpf 1873). Stumpf added no empirical data to the debate, but Hering nevertheless regarded him as an important and influential convert.

Most important for the nativist cause was the mixed support that Hering received from Frans Donders. To be sure Donders openly criticized many of Hering's views. For example, he dismissed Hering's retinal depth values as a mere transcription of the facts of stereopsis that explained nothing, and he also defended projectionist accounts of localization and the accuracy of convergence as a cue to depth perception (Donders 1867, 1871). But Donders also produced new experimental evidence to demonstrate the remarkable capacity of retinal disparities to trigger accurate, instantaneous perceptions of relief, independent of eye movements or other cues. And as early as 1867 he publicly sided with Hering, against his friends Helmholtz and Volkmann, in declaring that the human capacity for stereopsis is largely inborn. Equally important, he mobilized the clinical data on strabismus patients, on which he was the European authority, to show the existence of anatomically innate associations among some visual functions. Donders refused to be recruited into Hering's camp and always tried to minimize the extent of his disagreement with Helmholtz, but his prestige nevertheless added weight and respectability to the nativist cause. Hermann Aubert, for example, adopted Donders' positions almost slavishly in his influential *Grundzüge der physiologischen Optik* of 1876.

These reactions set the themes of the debate that reverberated through German scientific and philosophical journals during the 1870s and 1880s and which Eduard Raehlmann could refer to as "having split the scientific world into two camps" by 1891 (Raehlmann 1891, 53). Raehlmann's judgment notwithstanding, the nativist-empiricist debate seems to have proceeded rather spasmodically through the 1870s and 1880s, gathered intensity in the early 1890s, and declined considerably after 1915. That debate proceeded on at least two distinguishable levels. The more speculative and philosophical level dealt with the relationship of tactile and visual spatiality, the implications of Kantianism for the question, the plausibility of regarding visual spatiality as an "emergent" capacity, and the very nature of spatiality. At another level the controversy hinged on proximate issues to which experimental results could be more readily brought to bear. The following discussion examines the three most active fronts on which new research influenced the dispute: the issues of development, localization, and the evidence of ophthalmology.[1]

DEVELOPMENTAL ISSUES

From the beginning many felt that the nativist-empiricist debate had been unnecessarily polarized by Helmholtz and Hering, and that a compromise was ready to hand if the issue could be recast into an evolutionary perspective. The empirical acquisition of a spatial sense and its supporting patterns of eye movements and retinal correspondence could then be regarded as having occurred over the evolutionary life of the species rather than as occurring anew during the first months in the life of every individual. Thus, both positions in the controversy could be considered partly correct. Nativists were especially ready to accept the phylogenetic compromise, because it made the mechanisms of perception innate from the standpoint of the individual born with them. Hering explicitly equated individual learning and conscious recollection with acquired characteristics imprinted upon the germ plasm and so driving organic evolution (Hering 1870, 5–32). He wrote that sensory and motor processes must be regarded as the product of a long evolutionary development, so that the infant is born with an immediate and inherited optical awareness of the world (Hering 1906, 133–40). In addition to Hering and his students, du Bois-Reymond, Donders, Herbert Spencer, and many writers after them all offered this mediating position; Ludimar Hermann incorporated it promptly into his textbook series.

Helmholtz and his followers fully accepted the evolution of our sensory mechanisms, but they regarded this fact as beside the point for the nativist-empiricist debate. The phylogenetic compromise said nothing about the degree of residual plasticity left to the individual to be shaped by experience and learning, and this was what Helmholtz and his followers took to be the main issue in dispute (POS 3:535). Johannes von Kries echoed that view in his 1910 discussion of eye movements. Today everyone agrees, he noted, that visual experience and visual mechanisms are largely determined by "laws of development" that have a hereditary and presumably evolutionary basis. But that does not tell us whether what is inherited are fixed behavioral tendencies to move the eyes in certain ways, or patterns of musculature that make certain movements optimally efficient in terms of energy expenditure or maximization of some visual function. If the latter, then every individual must learn anew how to "fit" her eye movements to her inherited anatomical structures in the most efficient way (PO3, 497,516). Taken in itself, Kries believed, an evolutionary perspective did not resolve the nativist-empiricist impasse.

Discussions of the heritable nature of visual behavior usually invoked experiments and observations made on animals. As evidence for an innate spatial sense, nativists commonly pointed to the high degree of spatial coordination evinced among the newly born or newly hatched of many species of animals and birds (Hering 1879a, 564; Tschermak-Seysenegg 1942, 125; Pastore 1973; Hochberg 1962, 318–30). In 1872 Donders cited experiments done by ophthalmologist Emil Adamuk from Kasan showing that electrical stimulation of the brains of experimental animals always produced paired eye movements, as would be expected from Hering's law of equal innervation (Donders 1872, 153–64). Eduard Raehlmann countered with an experiment of Eduard Hitzig claiming to demonstrate a brain site that produced movements of one eye alone, as the views of Helmholtz suggested should be possible (Raehlmann and Witkowski 1877). That kind of recourse to animal experimentation was rare before the twentieth century, however, even though William Preyer, among others, called for more of such investigations to be made.

Observations on human infants played a more important role in the debate than observations on animals, although they offered ambiguous evidence at best. Eduard Raehlmann and Ludwig Witkowski reported their observations on forty infants in 1877. They found that the eye movements of sleeping children depart constantly from Donders' and Listing's laws, that newborns cannot fixate (contrary to a report by Donders), and that they occasionally perform uncoordinated eye movements never seen in adults. The two researchers interpreted those results as strong support for Helmholtz and for empiricism. Hering, however, noted that the infants in the study did mainly perform associated or conjugate eye movements, and they did so immediately after birth; that evidence supported the nativist position (Hering 1879a, 528–30).

Physiologist William Preyer mobilized the ambiguous evidence from infants most effectively. His famous The Mind of the Child (Die Seele des Kindes) reported his detailed observations on the psychological development of his own infant son (Preyer 1884, 4–51; 1895, 1–48). In his first edition (1881) Preyer followed an empiricist line in interpreting his child's sensorimotor development. Although he acknowledged that some infants, including his own, showed conjugate eye movements within minutes after birth, he insisted that random, unassociated ones predominate and that the occasional conjugate turnings may be the result of coincidence. He concluded that there was nothing in vision comparable to the infant's suckling instincts, no trace of any "bilateral-symmetrical nervous mechanism [governing eye movements] which is preformed and ready and capable of functioning even at birth" (Preyer 1895, 24). Newborns cannot control their eye movements, cannot fixate at all before the tenth day, and do not achieve full and regular binocular fixation until the fourth month. In a veiled reference to Hering, he expressed surprise "that representatives of the nativistic conception count the findings on newborns as supporting their position" (p. 25).

But Preyer's widely read study gave some comfort to Hering and his followers. Subsequent editions of *The Mind of the Child*, while not departing from its basically empiricist line, more and more emphasized the role of heredity and evolution. By 1895 Preyer could exclaim about "how false it is, to believe that human beings learn to feel, to desire, and to think only through their senses. Heredity is at least as important to psychogenesis as one's own activity" (p. viii). Readers found in his work demonstrations that sensory capacities develop stepwise in sudden stages, not necessarily as a result of gradual development or learning. As an example, Preyer reported that newborns show a blink reflex upon a flash of light immediately after birth. Only around the sixtieth day do they begin to blink at the approach of a hand or object, even though at that point they have still not developed any conception of a danger to themselves. Preyer concluded that the latter reaction must indeed be regarded as a reflex, not a habit. But unlike the former it must be an "acquired reflex," a reflex suddenly activated when the continued somatic development of the brain and the nervous system after birth had reached a sufficient stage (p. 18).

Du Bois-Reymond had also suggested that the human infant's sensory capacities develop in tandem with its anatomical growth, and with the strong support of Preyer that concept altered the terms of the nativist-empiricist debate. Eduard Raehlmann, in a discussion of 1891, conceded the nativist case for lower animals, but insisted that spatial perception in humans could no longer be regarded as either acquired or innate in the traditional senses of those terms. Instead, he argued, a mass of evidence now suggested that human sensory capacities appear in stages after birth and are correlated with continued anatomical development. In human newborns, as in animals whose sight develops after birth, the "parts of the cortex and the spinal cord which exhibit [ocular] motor sensitivity" are "completely absent," and develop later; in calves and other animals born with full vision they are fully developed at birth (Raehlmann 1891, 58–59).

Raehlmann concluded from this evidence that the nativist-empiricist issue had to be reformulated. At stake was whether the visual stimuli that act on the developing human infant elicit and pattern its perceptions of space, or whether they are "only means for triggering a priori functions which have been activated through the growth of the brain." Of the correct answer to this complex question Raehlmann was in no doubt: "All observations without exception speak for an empirically-acquired conception of space" (pp. 59–60).

As proof of their empiricist position, Raehlmann and Preyer offered their observations on the vision of newborns; both, however, insisted that equally decisive support came from observations on blind adults who had had their sight surgically restored through iridectomies and cataract extractions. That sort of evidence was as old as the nativist-empiricist dispute itself, but the rapid progress of ophthalmological surgery around midcentury, combined with the growing use of general and (after 1884) topical anaesthesia, had multiplied it. Preyer described in detail seven classical cases in the second edition of *The Mind of the Child* (1884); Raehlmann similarly reviewed the evidence and presented two detailed protocols on cases he had examined in 1890 (Raehlmann 1891, 93). Both stressed that despite their full anatomical development, the newly sighted acquire the ability to recognize and localize objects very slowly and in developmental stages that parallel those of the human infant. Franz Hillebrand later subjected these studies to severe methodological criticism, but on the whole the impact of that evidence favored empiricism (Hillebrand 1929, 175–87).

THE STABILITY OF RETINAL DEPTH VALUES

The nativist-empiricist controversy had originated as a dispute about spatial localization, not as a dispute about developmental questions. Even though localization issues had been submerged during the 1880s, Hering's student Franz Hillebrand brought them back to center stage in 1893 with a study entitled "The Stability of the Space Values on the Retina." The very title announced Hillebrand's defiant intention to resume the controversy over depth localization precisely where Hering had left it twenty-five years before (Hillebrand 1893).

Hillebrand began with a clear and concise restatement of Hering's philosophy, methodology, and terminology—the first such restatement to appear since 1879. He reaffirmed what he took to be the key element of Hering's theory: that the depth values associated with retinal points are "stable" and persist unaltered through changes in the point of fixation. Hillebrand explained this in the following way. Suppose the two eyes fixate a point P, and there is in space a small object O near the fixation point that images on two retinal points a and a', which may or may not be corresponding points. Suppose the eyes shift to a new fixation point P', and at the new position there is an object O' that images again on a and a'. If the retinal depth values intrinsic to points a and a' are "stable," then the object O' should have the same apparent spatial relationship to P' as O had to P. This rather abstract formulation expressed Hering's nativist concept of visual depth perception: in the absence of all empirical cues, the visual localization of points in space is solely a localization relative to the core point of visual space; it depends only upon the particular retinal points affected and not upon the convergence of the eyes, the distance of the fixation point, or the configuration of points in physical space.

In defense of this conception, Hillebrand first pointed out that the old projection theory implies the *instability* of retinal depth values. In the thought experiment cited above, suppose the object O lies in the (real) frontal plane of P. Again the point of fixation moves to point P', and another small object O' images on the same retinal points a and a'. Hillebrand offered a geometrical demonstration to show that the projection lines drawn from points a and a' cannot intersect at any point that lies in the frontal plane through P'. If binocular localization is achieved by projection, then the retinal depth values cannot be "stable"; images falling on the same retinal points will alter their apparent spatial relationship to the point of fixation, as the distance of the fixation point changes (p. 13).

These stability relationships are best illustrated experimentally with the three suspended black threads about which Hering and Helmholtz had disputed almost thirty years earlier. We fixate the center thread (which on Hering's scheme then becomes the core point of visual space). The question is, how the two side threads must be arranged in order that all three will seem to lie in the frontal plane (the core plane, or in later terminology, the plane of fixation) through the core point. Hering had originally maintained (although Hillebrand tactfully ignored the point) that the side threads will appear to lie in the core plane of visual space when they are made to hang physically in the so-called longitudinal horopter, the vertical cylinder passing through Müller's horopter circle.[2] Helmholtz had insisted, and Hering by 1879 had come to agree, that in general this is not true. At distances of less than a few meters, the three threads must be arranged along a curvilinear, concave locus (not necessarily a circle) if they are to appear plane. At distances of more than about two meters, the locus must be curvilinear and convex, and at one set distance of the fixation point (varying among individuals) the threads can be arranged in a real plane and also appear to lie in a plane.[3]

Hillebrand's brilliant stroke of 1893 was to show that this set of relationships is, in fact, predicted by Hering's assumption of stable retinal depth values. That demonstration, however, required an unorthodox assumption about how corresponding points are distributed across the retinas. In 1863 physicist August Adolph Kundt had published a note in Poggendorff's *Annalen*, pointing out a curious optical illusion (Kundt 1863). Individuals presented with a horizontal line segment and asked to divide it precisely in the middle can normally do so fairly accurately, if they use both eyes. Asked to do so with one eye closed, however, they almost invariably divide the line segment in such a way that the part of the divided line that images on the nasal half of the retina is too long. Hering had discovered this phenomenon independently of Kundt, and he and Helmholtz had both discussed this systematic error. Hering explained the effect by suggesting that the "breadth values" of the retinal points increased more rapidly on the temporal half of the retinas than on the nasal half (Hering 1865b[32]; 1942/1879, 16). That assumption, however, would invalidate the horopter derivations of both Helmholtz and Hering, for both had assumed a symmetric distribution of breadth values around the apparent retinal meridians.

With Hering's explanation of Kundt's illusion firmly in mind, Hillebrand offered the following demonstration. In Figure 9.1 (I) let km and km_1 be the optical centers of the two eyes, C the location of the center thread in the thread-triple and also the point of fixation, and A and B the side threads. Suppose A, C, and B lie in the real fixation plane and also are *seen* as lying in one plane, and let the distances AC and CB be seen as equal. The direction line Akm will make angle β with the line of sight Ckm; direction line Bkm will make angle α with Ckm; the corresponding angles in the other eye will be the same. If A and B lie symmetric about C, and if the distribution of corresponding points is as Hering had speculated on the basis of Kundt's phenomenon, then angle β must be greater than angle α so that seen binocularly C will appear to partition the distance AB equally.

Let the point C be moved, so that it comes closer to the observer's eyes but still lies in the median plane, as in Figure 9.1 (II). Let the side threads A and B' simultaneously be moved in any such way that angles α and β remain unchanged. To satisfy those conditions A, C, and B must then lie in the general configuration shown in Figure 9.1 (II)—a curvilinear configuration concave to the observer. Now imagine the point C relocated farther from the observer but still in the median plane, and again the angles α and β held unchanged in each eye. The threads A, C, and B must

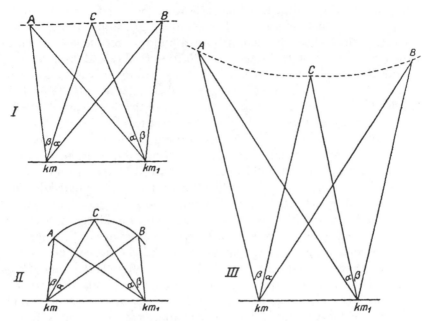

Fig. 9.1 Empirical longitudinal horopter (abathic surface) *ABC* for various distances of the fixation point, as deduced by Hillebrand from the assumption of stable retinal depth values. *Source*: Hillebrand 1929, 120.

then lie as in Figure 9.1 (III)—along a convex curvilinear locus. On the assumption that retinal depth values are stable in Hillebrand's sense, then *A* and *B* will *appear* to lie in a frontal plane with *C* in all three of these positions. More generally, Hillebrand deduced that as long as *C* remains in the median plane and the angles α and β are kept constant but unequal to one another, then the two points of intersection of the direction lines *Akm* and *Akm$_1$* and *Bkm* and *Bkm$_1$* must lie on a conic locus, the form of which will vary with the distance of the fixation point *C* and which, for sufficiently large values, becomes a hyperbola.[4] This prediction from the assumption of stable retinal depth values conforms closely to the empirical result that Helmholtz and Hering had reached years earlier, and which Hillebrand now confirmed through new thread-triple experiments of his own.

As Hillebrand well knew, Helmholtz had offered a different explanation of the thread-triple results. Under real-life viewing conditions, Helmholtz claimed, we unconsciously but quite accurately infer the relative positions of the threads from the retinal disparity of the side threads with the center thread and from the absolute distance of the fixated center thread, and then "see" their spatial configuration accordingly. Under the artificial conditions of the experiment, however, we must judge the absolute distance of the center thread from convergence alone, a notoriously inaccurate cue. When we unconsciously attempt to reconcile these false estimates of the absolute distance with the observed retinal disparities of the side threads, we can do so only by "seeing" the threads as lying in loci that do not correspond to their true physical configuration (*POS* 3:318–22). In short, Helmholtz dismissed the results of the thread-triple experiment as a visual illusion based upon false inferences.

Hillebrand had little difficulty in disposing of Helmholtz's explanation. He agreed with Helmholtz that convergence is a poor cue to absolute localization, and in 1894 produced a shrewd experimental paper showing that Wilhelm Wundt and his students had overestimated the potency of convergence and accommodation as cues to depth perception (Hillebrand 1894). But there is no evidence, Hillebrand insisted, to show that convergence induces a systematic error in estimates of distance, let alone one that varies so as to explain the functional dependence of the horopter deviation on the distance of the fixation point (Hillebrand 1893, 32–36). Hillebrand used prism glasses, stereoscopes, and other experimental arrangements to view a thread-triple at a constant distance while allowing the convergence of his eyes to change; in all those cases, he reported, the initial localization of the threads persisted unaltered (pp. 39–41).

Hillebrand's paper opened up a persistent new focal problem with a literature of its own (Hillebrand 1929, 133–34). The problem attracted Hering's student Tschermak-Seysenegg, who quickly established himself as an authority on the horopter deviation. In 1900 Tschermak demonstrated that the locus of real points in space that will be localized in the plane of fixation differs depending on the nature of the stimulus, yielding, for example, one locus for observations made on hanging threads, another for observations made on falling marbles, and other variations based on the time of exposure. Faced with this array of empirical horopters, Tschermak defined the "true" horopter as the locus of maximum stereoscopic sensitivity, just as Helmholtz had done, and he determined it with three pins stuck erect in a wooden block. He found that empirical horopter to be identical with the loci of hanging black threads that appear to lie in the core plane—further proof of Hering's theory of localization, and derived with the methods of Helmholtz himself (Tschermak-Seysenegg 1900).

Although Hillebrand and Tschermak packaged their results as a strong critique of Helmholtz, their findings challenged empiricism only indirectly, because Helmholtz had never tied localization to the results of projection. Nevertheless, their rhetoric of "stable local depth values" suggested an anatomical innateness calculated to provoke Kries and other

Helmholtz supporters. These supporters, for their part, found Hillebrand's results unimpressive, mainly because they explained Kundt's phenomenon in a very different way. Helmholtz had written in 1866 that when we look at a bisected line, we normally do so with both eyes and we place the midpoint of the line in the median plane of our body, directly before the cyclopean eye. Under those circumstances, the right half appears larger to the right eye, the left half to the left eye. Asked to divide a line segment with only one eye open, we fail to correct for the monocular perspective, try to reproduce the habitual association, and so make the systematic error detected by Kundt (*PO5* 3:204). It follows that Kundt's phenomenon, being merely the result of an erroneous inference, says nothing about the pattern of corresponding retinal points. Kundt's phenomenon may influence how we spatially localize hanging threads, but that is an entirely separate question that has nothing to do with the question of the horopter.

That point of view permeated Kries' querulous discussion of the so-called Hering–Hillebrand horopter deviation, written for the third edition of the *Handbuch* in 1910. Kries complained that all Hering's students, but Tschermak in particular, had begun to *define* the longitudinal or vertical horopter as the physical locus of points that appear to lie in the plane of fixation. But whether the two loci are identical, Kries objected, is just what is at issue. In principle, at least, the empirical horopter can be determined by methods other than depth localization, just as there exist independent methods for determining whether the distribution of corresponding points is asymmetric in the way Hillebrand had inferred from Kundt's phenomenon. Kries regarded Tschermak's result that there can be different horopter loci for different optical stimuli as inconsistent with Hillebrand's insistence on a stable connection of depth localization with binocular disparity (*PO5* 3:488–90).

Paul Liebermann, a student of Kries, certainly spoke for his master in a well-known paper he published in 1910. There Kries and Liebermann moved to block Hering's students from their attempt at terminological cooptation of the whole issue. Liebermann coined the term "abathic surface" for the physical locus of points seen as lying in the plane of fixation, and he refused to equate his abathic surface to the longitudinal horopter. Repeating Hillebrand's experiments he obtained contradictory results: the binocular disparities of the side threads cannot be held constant for all distances of the fixation point, if the threads are also to lie in the abathic surface. In Hering's terminology this meant that stimulating two retinal points will always give rise to the same sensation of visual direction (their "breadth values" are fixed) but not necessarily to the same perception of distance vis-à-vis the core point (their "depth values" are not stable, as Hillebrand had claimed). Liebermann concluded that while the retinal correspondence itself is relatively fixed, depth perception "on the other hand is intricate and variable" and cannot depend on fixed qualities of retinal points (Liebermann 1910, 438). Liebermann suggested that Hillebrand had obtained false results because the artificial conditions of his experiments had deprived the eye of cues necessary to estimate accurately the absolute distance of the fixation point.[5] Thus without explicitly defending Helmholtz's venerable explanation of the horopter deviation, Liebermann and Kries had left the door safely open for it.

THE EVIDENCE OF THE CLINIC:
ANOMALOUS CORRESPONDENCE

By 1900 a third front in the nativist-empiricist debate had eclipsed both developmental questions and depth perception. Patients who suffer from so-called concomitant strabismus are unable to align their eyes in such a way that their primary lines of sight intersect. An object imaging on the fovea of the normal eye will image on a peripheral retinal point of the other eye, and vice versa; the angle of deviation between the two primary lines of sight usually remains constant for all eye positions. These patients ought to see all objects in double images, but they do not. Either they suppress one monocular image altogether, or they display a so-called anomalous correspondence. On the latter condition the eccentric region of the retina of the deviating eye on which the external point of regard habitually images will develop some of the characteristics of a fovea. This so-called vicarious macula may display a heightened acuity and when stimulated evoke directional localizations corresponding to those of the fovea of the normal eye. Patients displaying an anomalous correspondence can be shown to have at least some elements of binocular vision over parts of the visual field and not merely to be suppressing one monocular image. These patients will properly localize at least some of the external points they see binocularly, and always the point of regard.

As surgical intervention to correct strabismus became more frequent in Germany during the 1850s, observations showed that patients who had formerly possessed an abnormal correspondence suffered from double images after the corrective surgery. These double images gradually disappeared as the normal correspondence reestablished itself. Sometimes, however, the patient merely suppressed one set of monocular images and never recovered binocular vision, or in a few extreme cases even regressed to the former squinting position in order to utilize the abnormal correspondence. These facts suggested that retinal correspondence is variable and not anatomically innate; the correspondence between retinal points is acquired (and can be altered and reacquired) in the interests of single vision. Helmholtz in 1866 naturally hailed these facts as strong evidence for the empiricist theory of vision (*PO5* 3:405–7).

But ophthalmological evidence also gave nativists comfort. Donders provided some in criticizing Helmholtz's suggestion that the long-known, involuntary association between convergence and accommodation had been empirically acquired (Donders 1872). Donders pointed out that individuals with hypermetropic (farsighted) eyes need to accommodate in order to see distant objects sharply. That degree of accommodation, however, often forced them to converge their eyes involuntarily to such a degree that only one line of sight can fix the distant object and the other must squint inward. Were the linkage of accommodation and convergence wholly an acquired one, Donders averred, individuals would scarcely habituate themselves to a relationship that forces them to choose between binocular perception and visual acuity. Relationships like that between accommodation and convergence could more accurately be regarded as innate mechanisms designed with a particular "tolerance" that could be adjusted, within certain limits, by the experience of the individual. Hering adopted Donders' antiempiricist argument based upon esophorias induced by hypermetropia, and used it to good effect.

By 1900 the same kinds of ophthalmological evidence that had earlier supported empiricism now seemed ambiguous or even discrediting to that doctrine. This reversal flowed less from particular arguments or discoveries than from a growing consensus, shared by those on both sides of the controversy, that anomalous correspondences were much weaker and more labile than normal ones and that they did not bestow full stereoscopic vision. When the young ophthalmologist Richard Greeff reviewed the question in 1892, he maintained that the acid test of true stereoscopic vision was Ewald Hering's so-called drop test. Never, Greeff insisted, had he observed a squinter who showed binocular depth perception on this test; even squinters whose disorder had been surgically corrected never gained the ability to perform on the test at the level of normal individuals.[6] That applied to squinters who passed other tests of binocularity, such as being able to see stereoscopic pictures in relief, or observing double images when a prism was held before one eye (Greeff 1892). In a major publication on the problem, Ewald Hering admitted that his experience with strabismus sufferers was limited, but insisted that he, too, had never observed a squinter with full binocular vision (Hering 1899c[80]).

But did the limitations of anomalous correspondences support the empiricist or the nativist position? Greeff, working in Arthur König's laboratory in Berlin, drew empiricist conclusions. The inability of strabismus surgery to restore full binocular depth perception suggests that the capacity for binocular depth perception is acquired by the individual, and only during early childhood (Greeff 1892, 45–47). Predictably, Hering and his students drew the opposite conclusion. Moriz Sachs waded into the controversy in 1897 by denying that anomalous correspondences even existed. The usual proof of binocular vision in patients so diagnosed hinged upon the fact that a prism held before one eye of the patient produced double images. Sachs objected that the original single image may actually have been a monocular one with the image from the other eye suppressed; the prism might act merely to bring the suppressed half-image above the viewer's attention threshold (Sachs 1897). Even Hering was not prepared to go quite that far, but he did express his doubts about the many ophthalmological reports of anomalous correspondences. The "binocular" visual field of at least some squinters, he suggested, may really be a mosaic of different monocular regions; that condition could lead ophthalmologists and their patients into the false belief that a limited binocular capacity was present. He and Sachs both stressed that normally sighted individuals all exhibit powerful, largely involuntary compulsions to move the eyes so as to bring about the fusion of images on corresponding points. The vicarious maculas seen in cases of anomalous correspondence seem to unleash no similar compulsion to fusional movements. Anomalous correspondences cannot fully replace the normal correspondence or simulate all its innate functions (Hering 1899c[80]).

Alfred Karl Graefe (1830–99), professor of ophthalmology at Halle and nephew of the famous Albrecht von Graefe, dismissed Hering's argument and found support for empiricism in the same facts. Strabismus, he contended, obliges the eyes to force into correspondence pairs of retinal regions that in normal eyes have very different visual acuities and color sensitivities (Graefe 1897; Hofmann 1925, 2:250). Hence it is not surprising that anomalous correspondences are neither as strong nor as complete as the normal pattern. That they are able to develop at all demonstrates that the normal correspondence must also have been acquired in infancy as our eyes first learned to fixate. In normal eyes the correspondence can then be established most readily between anatomically similar retinal regions; that alone makes possible full binocularity and capacity for stereopsis.

In 1902 the editors of the *Ergebnisse der Physiologie* commissioned Franz B. Hofmann, then an assistant to Hering in Leipzig, to review this vexed question (Hofmann 1902). Hofmann portrayed Alfred Karl Graefe as the leading advocate of empiricism. As the leading advocate of nativism, however, Hofmann cited not Hering, but the famous French ophthalmologist Louis-Emile Javal (1839–1907), even though Javal had earlier been the leading force behind the translation of Helmholtz's *Handbuch* into French (Javal 1867–68). Javal maintained that we are organically compelled to fixate on the two foveas, but that the rest of the correspondence is acquired empirically, built up around the two foveal "zero points." Squinters can acquire an anomalous correspondence only for peripheral regions of the visual field; in the foveal region they see in constant double images or suppress the monocular field of the squinting eye (Javal 1896). In presenting the empiricist case, Graefe conceded that only the normal correspondence allows full and efficient binocular vision, but he insisted that some squinters do acquire an anomalous correspondence that is effective even for the foveal regions, and which confers true, if only partial, binocular vision (Graefe 1897; Hofmann 1902, 807–10).

Advancing Javal as the typical nativist provided Hofmann with an effective rhetorical gambit. It allowed him to criticize Javal without directly offending Hering or his other students, and in doing so to represent himself as seeking a middle ground in the dispute. Hofmann agreed with Graefe that some squinters achieve a true binocular fusion of their monocular fields, even of the point of regard. But he insisted that conceding the evidence of acquired, anomalous correspondence does not oblige us to grant Graefe's claim that the normal pattern of correspondence must be acquired as well. The strength and persistence of the normal correspondence point to its innate quality; among squinters stereopsis is non-existent or extremely rare, and few fusional eye movements occur. At the end Hofmann revealed his true allegiance: "Through these considerations," he summed up, "we arrive yet again at the nativistic conception of the retinal correspondence" (Hofmann 1925, 846).

After 1900 the students of Hering and Sattler played an increasingly prominent role in the study of strabismus in Germany. In 1899 Armin Tschermak began to study his own alternating strabismus by a method of afterimages. Tschermak demonstrated that the anomalous angle of visual direction in the squinting eye did not correspond to the angle of its anatomical deviation (Tschermak 1899). This observation allowed him to interpret the visual anomaly induced by concomitant strabismus as a departure from Hering's law of identical visual direction, and thus to assimilate it to that school's terminology and approach. Alfred Bielschowsky, another of Hering's students, applied Tschermak's method of afterimages in the clinic. He concluded that the many varieties of anomalous correspondence were so variable as to suggest that the stable pattern of normal correspondence must in contrast be inborn and innate.

Despite their nativist commitments, Hering's students did not always agree with one another. For example, the running, minor controversy over whether patients with anomalous correspondence do, in fact, carry out any fusional eye movements, cut across both schools (Hofmann 1925, 2:249). All nativists, however, hailed the demonstration by F. P. Fischer in 1924 that in normal eyes, stereopsis and a common visual direction are possible even on pairs of retinal points for which they could not have been empirically acquired, namely, point pairs on which the image of small external objects is normally blocked by the nose (Fischer 1924). Summarizing all this work in another exhaustive and scrupulous survey of 1925, Hofmann could only repeat the judgment he had offered in 1902, that "all experiences of strabismus-sufferers always lead in every respect back to the assumption that there must be an innate basis for the normal retinal correspondence" (Hofmann 1925, 2:252).

THE ASCENDANCE OF NATIVISM

The 1890s ended with a surge of nativist opinion among members of the German scientific community that continued strongly into the twentieth century. Some of the evidence for that shift of opinion comes from Hermann's *Lehrbuch der Physiologie* and its grudging retreat from Helmholtzian orthodoxy. By the tenth edition of 1892 Hermann had begun to discuss the nativist-empiricist conflict explicitly, to describe the two eyes as parts of Hering's "single apparatus," and to introduce students to Hering's law of visual directions and law of equal innervations. The tendency to move the eyes in accordance with Donders' and Listing's laws is inborn, Hermann affirmed, although subordinated to the purpose of binocular single vision and hence modifiable through empirical factors, as Helmholtz had claimed. In 1892 Hermann cited ophthalmological evidence on acquired correspondence as one of several proofs of the general empiricist position (now defended rather than tacitly assumed), but by the thirteenth edition of 1905 he had quietly dropped this reference.

Other evidence comes from Johannes von Kries and his growing readiness to make concessions to Hering and the nativists. In preparing the appendixes for the third edition of the *Handbuch* in 1910, Kries conceded that innate and hereditary mechanisms underlie visual perception to an extent that Helmholtz "believed to be improbable" (*PO5* 3:533). Kries admitted the anatomical and innate nature of the binocular fusion of the two monocular fields, the innate and qualitatively continuous nature of the retinal local signs (as Helmholtz had), the validity of Hering's law of equal innervations, and the large role played by hereditary mechanisms in ensuring the eyes' conformity to Donders' and Listing's laws (pp. 497–534).

Typically for Kries, however, he was more prepared to make concessions on the form of the debate than on its substance. For example, he was ready in 1910 to consider the *possibility* that sensations of spatial direction may be innately associated with particular retinal points, that is, that the local signs possess intrinsic "height" and "breadth" values, as Hering had put it. But, he insisted, no evidence at all existed to support Hering's retinal *depth* values or to suggest that any innate mechanism is at work in depth localization. He charged that Hering's illusive depth values were suspiciously absent in monocular vision and, if they are somehow activated in the binocular case, they must change their values with the distance of the fixation point (pp. 501–2). Indeed, Kries insisted, it is much more likely that the local signs acquire even their two-dimensional, directional content through a gradual process of association with "psychical phenomena" (p. 504).

As for other elements of the dispute, Kries agreed that innate factors probably influence our adherence to Donders' and Listing's laws. But that adherence can be overridden in the interest of clear vision, he noted, as many experiments show. All eye movements require fine tuning based on visual feedback, and acting on this feedback must be an acquired capacity supplementing the grosser movements derived from equal innervation and other innate mechanisms (pp. 514–16). That the eyes readily compensate for distorted images produced by prism glasses and rotated stereoscopic images demonstrates the large range of free play left by innate mechanisms to be determined by empirical factors. As for studies of strabismus, Kries admitted that they posed the greatest challenge to the empiricist theory of vision, but he testily insisted that their results actually favored empiricism rather than refuting it, as many contemporaries claimed (pp. 526–27).

Eleven years later Kries seemed prepared to carry concessions to nativism much further. In 1921 he admitted that physiologists had come to think of corresponding retinal points as "points of identical [visual] direction" just as Hering had urged (Kries 1921, 681). Much more important, he noted with apparent approval that today "people incline to the assumption" that spatial awareness is given "in the relationships of the nervous substrate," and that they were gradually abandoning Lotze's illusive local signs (p. 684). Studies of strabismus indicate that while an anomalous correspondence can be acquired, the normal one is innately prefigured and developmentally favored. In 1923, in one of his last scientific publications, Kries claimed that even the most extreme empiricists now rejected the view that spatial awareness per se can be understood as emergent from nonspatial sensations (Kries 1923, 216–20). But Kries never retreated from the key empiricist position that the human capacity for binocular depth perception is entirely acquired.

This ascendance of nativism had its basis partly in the specialist debates traced in this chapter, but also in the changing cultural milieu of Central Europe. Helmholtz's empiricist theory of spatial perception had matched the cultural mood of Germany in the 1860s, especially its buoyant materialism and pragmatism and its consciousness of having sloughed off an idealist past (cf. Lenoir 1988, 1992, 1993). No less important to the theory's original appeal had been its obvious debt to British empiricism and its liberal emphasis on individualism, learning, and the flexibility and plasticity of human capacities. Although Helmholtz insisted that our spatial perceptions are indeed inferential constructions of the mind, he also taught confidently that the quasi-scientific procedures that the eye's mind employs in that construction assure maximum congruence between perceptual and real space. But the Germany of 1900 was no longer such congenial ground for Helmholtz's theory of perception. Its period of heroic industrialization and political unification behind it, Germany was struggling with economic recession, urban poverty, a failing liberal tradition, a strong and restless socialist movement, and a national leadership prone to mask fundamental political antagonisms behind appeals to ever-more fervent nationalism. In the rising mood of cultural pessimism that gripped Europe before World War I, German intellectuals increasingly attacked scientific materialism and rationalism and coupled those attacks with calls for a philosophy in closer touch with the imperatives of life, will, and instinct (Forman 1971; Stern 1961, xi–xxx, 122–28; Sheehan 1978, 221–38; Brush 1978, 103–20; Ringer 1969, 253–69, 305–15). In that climate Helmholtz's appeals to experience, utilitarianism, and quasi-rationalistic processes of unconscious inference rang increasingly hollow.

Ostwald Spengler's long discussion of spatial awareness in his widely read *Decline of the West* (1918) epitomized this cultural climate. Spengler argued that every culture possesses a unique consciousness of spatiality that determines that civilization's concepts of time, historicity, and destiny (Spengler 1926, 81–87, 169–74). In mounting this argument, Spengler drew heavily upon Helmholtz's empiricist theory of spatial perception, but in doing so he historicized and radically transvalued that theory. Helmholtz had tacitly regarded the mind's construction of visual space and its approximate conformity to Cartesian relationships as a triumph of the unconscious intellect. Spengler treated that construction as wholly contingent and artificial, a symptom of Western rationalism in the final, decaying stages of Faustian culture. Occasionally he contrasted Cartesian spatial awareness with the instinctual and the phenomenologically primitive. Cartesian awareness of space, he wrote, is but "a mechanical representation" that must be distinguished from the "involuntary and unqualified realization of depth, which dominates the consciousness with the force of an elemental event" (p. 173).

If Spengler reflected deep currents in popular philosophical opinion, developments in academic philosophy also undermined or thoroughly recast empiricist theories of spatial perception. The strong Neo-Kantian movement of the late nineteenth century reasserted the dictum that the categories of space and time are "pure intuitions" imposed by the mind upon experience. Superficially understood, Kantianism seemed to favor

Hering's insistence upon an innate spatial sense, as Helmholtz himself had claimed that it did. That danger sent Helmholtz's disciple Kries, himself an avowed Neo-Kantian, scrambling to reemphasize the Kantian elements in Helmholtz's thought and to relocate Hering into a phenomenological and organismic tradition far removed from Kant (Köhnke 1986; Willey 1978; Kries 1910, 3:640–51; Pastore 1974; Hyslop 1891). The positivism of Ernst Mach stood at the philosophical antipodes of Neo-Kantianism. Nevertheless, Machism's phenomenological approach to knowledge echoed Hering's lifelong insistence that the spatiality of our perceptions is phenomenologically given, and that to try to go beyond that given to hypothetical inferences about its origins or to unconscious experiential deductions is go beyond the realm of legitimate science. Philosophical interest in the positivisms of Mach and Avenarius surged around 1900, and brought Mach's open admiration of Hering to a wider academic audience (Blackmore 1972, 55–63, 180–203; Mach 1959/ 1897, 69, 168).

Neither Spengler, nor positivism, nor fin-de-siècle pessimism spoke directly to the scientific issues of the nativist-empiricist dispute. Still less did the artistic experimentation with superimposed perspectives and the fracturing of visual space that went on in the early twentieth century (Vitz and Glimcher 1984, 108–40). Together, however, these elements testified to a cultural climate in which the correspondence of visual to physical space had become newly problematical. That climate rendered the nativist insistence that our perceptual experience flows from innate predispositions, neural structures, and inherited instincts increasingly acceptable or even obvious.

Hering's supporters greeted these developments enthusiastically. Oscar Zoth, who contributed the review of "Eye Movements and Visual Perceptions" to the *Handbuch der Physiologie des Menschen* in 1905, concluded that the nativist position had already carried the day (Zoth 1905, 325, 396–97). Franziska Hillebrand, writing almost twenty-five years later, claimed triumphantly that over the preceding decades empiricism had "more and more lost ground" (Hillebrand 1929, 198). Citing Kries' concessions, she agreed with Moriz Sachs that the nativist-empiricist question had been decided "in the clinic." Studies of brain localization, the histology of the optical tract, and the pathology of squint, combined with the psychophysical experimentation of Franz Hillebrand and others, had, in her view, brought the nativist position near to a definitive victory (ibid.). Even taking partisanship into account, the confidence of Hering's students suggests that ten years after his death his position on spatial perception had begun to receive extensive support in Germany.

CHAPTER TEN

Color Vision Controversies, 1875–90

FOUNDATIONS

In comparison to the school controversies over spatial perception, those over color vision evinced a sharper sequential development, a more clearly defined cast of characters, much more heated antagonism, and a still less decisive outcome. They unfolded in two phases. The first phase began in 1860, with Helmholtz's paradigmatic reformulation of the study of light perception in the second volume of his *Handbuch*. That synthesis fixed terminological usage and instrumental approaches for decades to come and advanced Young's three-receptor theory as the proper basis for interpreting almost all aspects of light perception. During the 1860s the Young–Helmholtz theory attracted important supporters, generated further research on its core program, and dominated textbooks and popular discussions. But it encountered continuing opposition from ophthalmologists and other specialists for its alleged inability to explain hereditary and acquired color blindness and some of the anomalies of peripheral color vision.

The opposition to the Young–Helmholtz theory did little more than smoulder through the 1860s, mainly because opponents lacked any alternative theory to rally around. But between 1872 and 1875 Ewald Hering provided that alternative in his *Zur Lehre vom Lichtsinne*. That work developed an experimental critique of Helmholtz's psychological theory of simultaneous contrast, and in the final installments set out Hering's radical—although not entirely original—theory of color vision, in which black-white, blue-yellow, and green-red became antagonistic psychophysical processes, capable of combining to produce a neutral gray in the achromatic process, or canceling to produce no sensation at all in the chromatic ones. On that theory, the disorders that Helmholtz called "red blindness" and "green blindness" were explained as the absence of the red-green opponent mechanism and no longer existed as separate classes. Dichromats of this type would see the spectrum in blues and yellows (as they usually reported that they did); their achromatic sensations would be unaffected.

DEBATES OVER COLOR BLINDNESS DURING
THE 1870s

The publication of Hering's theory of color vision coincided with the onset of two decades of intense interest in color perception. Studies of color vision had never exceeded 14 percent of the total literature on physiological optics before the 1870s, but they soared to 28.4 percent in 1875–79 (problem-complex IV in Table 2, Appendix) and color vision quickly replaced binocularity and depth perception as the most active research area in the field. An almost frenzied European concern with color blindness underlay this more general interest in color.

In April 1876 a railroad accident involving great loss of life occurred at Lagerlunda, Sweden. Frithiof Holmgren, professor of physiology at the University of Uppsala, blamed the accident on the color blindness of a railway employee who had misperceived the hue of a signal, and his subsequent investigation of 266 employees turned up nineteen cases of color blindness among them. This well-publicized incident and the reports that Holmgren wrote about it catapulted color blindness into scientific and public attention and generated widespread fear among the traveling public. It also concentrated the research attention of scientists.

Articles on the practical significance and incidence of color blindness (category 20.3h, Table 1, Appendix) jumped from 1 percent of all studies on vision in 1870–74 to 3.3 percent in 1875–79. The literature on instruments and research methods for study and mass screening peaked at 4.3 percent of all publications in 1880–84 (category 20.3e). Holmgren, the central figure in this new mass concern, had studied with Helmholtz at Heidelberg and was uncompromisingly committed to the Young–Helmholtz explanation of color blindness. His writings did much to entrench that theory in the popular European understanding of color perception.

Interest in color vision also burgeoned after 1875 in response to a widely followed popular controversy. Ancient literary evidence suggested to some critics that human color perception capacities had been more limited in the past and had evolved within historical time; some anthropological studies indicated that primitive peoples had different and more limited color vision than Europeans. Others countered that the evidence reflected differences of vocabulary rather than of perception (Segall et al. 1966, 38–47). This controversy was to have a long history continuing to the present, but it peaked in Germany between 1875 and 1885 in the writings of Lazarus Geiger, Hugo Magnus, Rudolf Virchow, Grant Allen, and lesser figures. Category 19.6 (Table 1, Appendix) shows that this literature exploded from insignificance in 1870–74 to 6.3 percent of all publications on vision in 1875–79, only to fall back to relative insignificance in the late 1880s.

Against this background of surging popular interest in color vision, the appearance of Hering's new theory sharpened the theoretical focus and set the stage for a fierce confrontation with Helmholtz's followers. Scientists rapidly chose sides. Almost immediately Hermann Aubert changed allegiance and announced his acceptance of the opponent process theory as the one "founded on the testimony of our sensations, and the one easiest and most conveniently reconciled with the observations" (Aubert 1876, 159). By 1880 figures as prominent as Ludwig Mauthner, Jakob Stilling, Heinrich Schöler, and Eduard Pflüger had publicly announced for Hering or at least conceded that the red blind are invariably green blind, the key prediction of the opponent process theory (Cohn 1879, 12).

Partly as a result of this pressure, the Young–Helmholtz theory received its first major amendment. In 1873 Theodor Leber proposed the so-called displacement hypothesis to explain color blindness. The sight of normal individuals is characterized by the three spectral response curves corresponding to the red, green, and violet (or blue) receptor elements, much as Helmholtz had sketched them heuristically in the *Handbuch*. In the red blind, Leber proposed, we must imagine the response curve of the red mechanism to be displaced toward the green curve and altered in form to coincide with it exactly. Hence the red blind see neither red nor green but always their mixture, yellow; because the red curve has been displaced they see the red end of the normal spectrum dark and foreshortened. The green blind have their green curve shifted to coincide with the red curve; they, too, see the spectrum in violet (or blue) and yellow, but they do not see the long-wavelength end as truncated or darker than do normals (Leber 1873, 470).

Adolf Fick adopted the displacement hypothesis to explain peripheral color vision: at retinal points outside the fovea we must imagine the red and green curves displaced and coinciding so as to make vision dichromatic in blue and yellow, and on the far periphery all three response curves coinciding so that only achromatic sensations are possible (Fick 1873). Fick and Leber both believed that the hypothesis of displaced response curves eliminated every objection currently being voiced against the Young–Helmholtz theory (Leber 1873, 470; Fick 1879, 199).

At the end of the 1870s rivalry between the two camps exploded into polemical exchanges between Holmgren and Hermann Cohn, the latter a junior professor at Breslau, a university already noted as a center of opposition to the Young–Helmholtz theory. The conflict began as a priority dispute and centered on the scientific adequacy of Holmgren's various methods of examination and mass screening of the color blind, but it quickly turned into polemics over competing theories of color vision. Cohn claimed to stand "with the majority of German ophthalmologists on the side of Hering" and blasted Holmgren's critiques of the opponent process theory as puerile and indicative of Holmgren's inability to understand that theory (Cohn 1879, 17–22). Jakob Stilling, a more important player than Cohn, was one of several contemporaries who quickly came to Cohn's defense (Stilling 1879). He showed how simultaneous contrast may be used to diagnose and study color blindness, and he used the results to argue again for a single class of red-green blind and against observers like Holmgren, who argued for separate classes. Throughout the polemics both men confidently portrayed Holmgren as an isolated and anachronistic defender of a discredited theory, the inadequacies of which Hering had demonstrated "in an exhaustive manner" and with "consequent logic" (p. 19).

THE EVIDENCE OF THE UNILATERALS

The only individuals who can directly compare the subjective visual experiences of normals and the color blind are those who have normal color vision in one eye and defective color vision in the other. In 1879 Heidelberg ophthalmologist Otto Becker (1828–90) created a sensation by announcing his discovery of such an individual (Becker 1879). But the vision of Becker's unilateral was so defective that the theoretical clash did not begin until the following year, when Giessen ophthalmologist Arthur von Hippel announced the discovery of a second unilateral. On a battery of tests, Hippel found his unilateral to possess normal color vision in the left eye and to be simultaneously red blind and green blind in the right eye (Hippel 1880).

With Hippel's permission, Holmgren examined the same patient in 1880 and publicly declared him to be "typically red blind." He found the red end of the visible spectrum to be shortened for the color blind eye, and although the patient saw predominantly in blues and yellows, some of the yellow shades were "green-tinged" (Holmgren 1881b). Hippel replied to Holmgren with some asperity, insisting that his patient showed no shortening of the visible spectrum. The report of "green-tinged yellows" had resulted merely from the patient's verbal confusion, before he had learned to appreciate the differences of color perception between his normal and defective eye. Hippel concluded that the evidence could not be brought into agreement with the Young–Helmholtz theory, but that it "fits easily into the framework of the Hering theory, and stands in no contradiction with any aspect of [that theory]" (Hippel 1881, 54).

Conflicting as the evidence from unilaterals may have been, it seems to have produced a consensus that dichromats see only blues and yellows, except for the very rare violet blind (Helmholtz) or blue-yellow blind (Hering). It also seems to have produced a greater willingness among Young–Helmholtz supporters to resort to the displacement hypothesis, despite its undeniably inelegant and ad hoc nature. Holmgren, for example, invoked displacement in 1881 to support his conviction that the predominantly blue and yellow perceptions of Hippel's unilateral were "in perfect accordance with the Young–Helmholtz theory" and did not "shake the basis of that theory" in any way (Holmgren 1881a, 305). Helmholtz himself endorsed the displacement hypothesis in 1889, though without citing Fick or Leber as sources.[1]

THE DEFENSE OF YOUNG, CIRCA 1880

Although Hering's theory gained ground rapidly as a result of the color blindness disputes, Helmholtz's partisans continued to defend their position with aggressive confidence. This tone predominates in the broad survey of physiological optics that Adolph Fick provided for Hermann's *Handbuch der Physiologie* in 1879. There Fick reverently followed Helmholtz's original *Handbuch* treatment of 1860, basing his discussion of Young's theory upon the empirical facts of color mixing and the theory of the barycentric color plane. Fick justified Young's choice of precisely three physiological primaries on grounds of theoretical economy, but he departed from Helmholtzian orthodoxy in urging a blue rather than violet fundamental.[2] Of course, Fick assumed throughout that Young's theory must be amended with the displacement model, and he defended that hypothesis so vigorously that it has subsequently been known as Fick's hypothesis, despite Leber's equal contribution.

As for Hering's theory of color vision, Fick conceded candidly to his readers that although it "appears to find approval in many circles, . . . I cannot understand it" (Fick 1879, 205). This feigned incomprehension did not prevent Fick from criticizing at some length Hering's notion of black as a positive sensation that somehow depended on the action of light. But Fick did not disagree with all of Hering's results. He threw himself squarely behind Hering's contention that simultaneous contrast must depend on some strictly physiological, retinal induction effect. The prestige of Helmholtz notwithstanding, Fick concluded, Hering had demonstrated many contrast experiments "which absolutely cannot be explained through illusions of the judgement" (p. 232).

If Fick's strategy was largely to ignore opponent process mechanisms, another partisan elected frontal attack. In 1882 the young Johannes von Kries published the first comprehensive reply to Hering to come out of the

Helmholtzian camp. Typical of Kries' style, the long discussion in du Bois-Reymond's *Archiv* posed as a neutral comparison of the two theories and called for compromise, but in reality it challenged the very foundations of Hering's theory and framed all the issues that would dominate the debate for the next forty years.

Kries began by pointing out what Hering's and Helmholtz's theories had in common: both are "component" theories, which attempt to explain our manifold visual experiences as compounded of a few simple or primitive kinds of sensations. Hering's theory, to a greater extent than Helmholtz's, relies upon our introspective ability to determine those primitive visual sensations or components, and it assumes that unique physiological processes corresponded to each of those components (Kries 1882, 33). Hering identified black, white, red, yellow, green, and blue as our primitive light sensations, to which corresponded exactly six "terminal" psychophysical processes. Kries conceded that intuition and tradition make that a compelling argument, yet we cannot be sure that our choice of these sensations, or any sensations as particularly simple or fundamental, is not the contingent result of linguistic conventions or cultural influence (p. 45). Hering and his followers ridicule Young's theory for insisting that white is somehow a compound sensation including violet, red, and green, or that yellow is compounded of red and green. But Kries cautioned that even assuming that we can distinguish "simple" and "compound" sensations through introspection alone, that is a dangerously uncertain basis on which to erect a scientific theory of perception.

Kries devoted most of his analysis to effects produced by retinal exhaustion, including (as he claimed) positive and negative afterimages, the Purkinje afterimage, and chromatic fading. He contended that the two theories are nearly equivalent in their ability to explain, or in some cases, not to explain, these phenomena (pp. 113–21). Like Fick, Kries conceded to Hering the existence of retinal induction effects, and acknowledged as "irrefutable" some of Hering's experiments demonstrating inductive effects in simultaneous brightness contrast and some afterimage phenomena (p. 123). But Kries introduced experiments of his own to show that factors of judgment do play *some* role in simultaneous brightness contrast, and he continued to insist that *all* simultaneous color contrast arises through illusions of judgment, as Helmholtz had claimed (pp. 127–28, 132).

On the vexed issue of color blindness, Kries was very decisive. Despite bold claims and fierce debates about what the color blind see, all we know reliably about the condition comes from the methods of colorimetry. We know that most color blind are dichromats—that they can match all colors in the spectrum with mixtures of two colors rather than the three that normals require. This suggests that their color experiences are compounds of two fundamentals only (pp. 132–35). Kries insisted that given our vast ignorance of how the primary visual processes relate to particular sensations even in normals, we need not take recourse to "implausible" hypotheses like Fick's to explain why one of the primary sensations of dichromats seems to be yellow rather than red or green or any other hue. Indeed, Kries claimed, what hues the color blind "really see" is an inherently uncertain matter of little real importance to the scientific study of dichromatism.

What is important to that study, Kries insisted, is whether the great class of "red-green blind" dichromats falls into two distinct subcategories: one with deficient response to wavelengths near the middle of the spectrum, the other with deficient response to long wavelengths. Noting the abysmal absence of hard quantitative studies on this problem, Kries reported tentative results of his own suggesting the existence of clear categories. On eleven dichromats obliged to match a particular sample field, a variability of seventy units between extremes in the group as a whole was reduced to a variability of four when the sample was divided into two subgroups of eight red blinds and three green blinds (p. 146). If sharply separate categories exist, then dichromatism cannot be explained by Hering's theory, which postulates the absence of a single red-green process. It can be explained by the Young–Helmholtz theory, which postulates the absence of one, but not both, processes sensitive to middle or long wavelengths. Needless to say, Kries added, the unfortunate terminology of red and green blindness should not be taken as indicating what particular hues dichromats see or fail to see (pp. 150–58).

Kries appealed for sharper distinctions in contemporary theorizing between peripheral and central mechanisms. The Young–Helmholtz theory, he specified, is one of peripheral, retinal action; only its opponents have suggested that the so-called red, green, and violet responses persist unaltered into the highest cerebral levels (p. 169). Kries was quite prepared to offer Hering a free range for his theory among the central processes, in return for his abandoning all claims for it on the periphery. Probably, Kries suggested, some central process combines the neural input from the Young–Helmholtz receptors into sensory compounds, and this central process may be responsible for the four, apparently simple, chromatic sensations upon which Hering placed such emphasis. But Kries was careful not to concede too much in this tacit negotiation. He thought it unlikely that this central compounding occurred precisely as suggested by Hering (p. 171). Kries also attacked Hering's notorious ambiguity about whether his "visual substance" was located on the periphery or in the center, as well as his insistence on defining "the retina" so broadly as to include the entire optic track. This ambiguity, Kries insisted, blocked any program to distinguish peripheral and central aspects of visual sensation and so to adjudicate clearly between the competing theories.

Frans Donders also defended the Young–Helmholtz theory in his analysis, "Ueber Farbensysteme," of 1881. But he showed himself consistently less partisan than Fick or Kries and consistently more sympathetic to the arguments from intuition and tradition that suggest the existence of four "simple colors" grouped in antagonistic pairs. Nevertheless, he wrote, the colorimetrical research of Maxwell, Helmholtz, and J. J. Müller compels us to accept the existence of three physiological fundamentals from which all our other color sensations are compounded. Donders noted that this apparent contradiction can be resolved by a "zone theory," in which the three "energies" of the "fundamental colors" excite the four "simple colors" in exclusive pairs at some higher neural level. His own proposed model hypothesized a photosensitive molecule, capable of various dissociations and recombinations, each corresponding to particular sensations (Donders 1881, 172–80).

But Donders was not prepared to side with Hering on the crucial issue of color blindness. He admitted that recent evidence from unilaterals had "as good as proved" that both red blind and green blind dichromats see a two-hued spectrum, the "warm" end of which is orangy-yellow, the "cold" end of which is blue or violet (p. 212). That fact reveals just how lamentable is the terminology of "red blindness" and "green blindness", Donders wrote, but it neither refutes Young's theory nor confirms Hering's hypothesis of a single red-green visual substance, despite the "seductiveness" of the latter notion (p. 216).

Fick had tried to deal with the anomaly of yellow-blue vision in dichromats by his displacement hypothesis; Kries had done so by dismissing as insignificant the whole problem of what hues dichromats really see. Donders proposed to deal with the anomaly by abandoning the assumption that color vision is a "reduction form" of normal vision, in which dichromats resemble normals in all respects except that they lack the sensory input from one of the three receptors. The loss of one of the three fundamental processes, Donders hypothesized, also alters the "energies" (the evoked color sensations) of the two remaining processes, and it does so in such a way that the two remaining energies are rendered complementary to one another. Donders introduced several experimental arguments in support of this hypothesis. He noted that the neutral point of the red blind—where they see their dichromatic spectrum as colorless—had long been known to vary quite considerably from one dichromat to another, and this fact suggests that the position on the color plane of the two remaining primaries might vary from patient to patient as well (pp. 211–21).

Donders fully understood just how heretical was his suggestion that dichromatism may not be a simple reduction form of normal vision. Abandoning the reduction-form hypothesis deprived Helmholtz's program of its only effective method of deducing Young's fundamentals (p. 208). That consequence left Donders undaunted. He departed from Maxwell and Helmholtz in arguing that two of Young's fundamentals are probably *spectral* colors—far-spectral violet and far-spectral red— with green as the only physiological primary for which it is necessary to postulate a greater-than-spectral saturation. This choice obliged Donders to criticize and to reject the afterimage experiments of Helmholtz showing the existence of extraspectral red and violet sensations (pp. 170–72).

Decoupling Young's theory from the reduction-form hypothesis did not make the evidence from color blindness irrelevant to the choice between Helmholtz and Hering. On the contrary, Donders agreed squarely with Kries that that choice reduces to a single question: are Hering's so-called red-green blind constituted by two sharply distinguishable groups, deficiently sensitive to middle and long wavelengths respectively? Donders reported studies out of his laboratory on ten dichromats suggesting that this was, in fact, the case. In particular, Donders had measured the spectral brightness (the luminosity curve) for these dichromats. While the green blind had curves almost exactly similar to normals, the red blind showed much greater variability and greatly reduced sensitivity to long wavelengths (pp. 199–213). Hering's theory could not account for the existence of these distinct subclasses, while the Young–Helmholtz theory predicted them.

HERING TAKES THE OFFENSIVE

Although Hering had publicly celebrated the supporting evidence of the unilaterals in a short article in 1880, he remained uncharacteristically quiet on the subject of light sensations during the decade after 1875. Then, spurred by the attacks of Kries, Donders, and others, he plunged into a decade of fierce polemical activity on behalf of his theory. Between 1885 and 1895 he exchanged attacks with at least a half-dozen of Helmholtz's leading defenders. Some of these polemics had little strategic importance. These included his fierce exchanges with Eugene Fick over the role of eye movements in erasing afterimages (Hering 1891b[70], 1892[71], 1893a[72]); his 1885 attack on Arthur König's *ophthalmo-Leukoskop* (Hering 1885a[45], b[46]); and his 1887 refutation of Holmgren's alleged proof of the Young–Helmholtz theory by the illumination of single retinal cones (Hering 1887b[49]; Holmgren 1889). But other fronts in Hering's campaign had great strategic importance for the controversy and for color theory in general.

By 1885 Hering could no longer ignore the growing evidence for distinguishable classes of red and green blind, the groups Kries was soon to rename protanopes and deuteranopes. In a major paper of that year Hering again denied that these groups formed clearly separate classes and attributed their differences to continuous variation among individuals in the coloring of the macula pigmentation and the crystalline lens (Hering 1885a[45]). He introduced experimental data obtained from two assistants in his laboratory to argue that normals also vary widely in this respect, some being "blue-sighted" (if macula absorption is weak) and some being "yellow-sighted" (if the macula and lens strongly absorb long wavelengths) (Sachs 1881). He attributed Rayleigh's discovery of what was later called "anomalous dichromatism" to this effect, through macula absorption of green rays.

Hering's opponents, including Helmholtz himself, later criticized this account as insufficient to explain red and green blindness, particularly as those anomalies manifest themselves on the retinal periphery outside the macula. The account prompted much experimental work on absorption in the lens and macula. Hering stood by his hypothesis, however. In 1893 he counterattacked, arguing that the tendency of the entire Helmholtz school to underestimate macula absorption invalidated nearly all of the color equations on which their theoretical conclusions rested (Hering 1893b[73]). Mixture equations obtained for test fields so small that light falls only on the macula will not match equations obtained for slightly larger test fields where the light falls partly on extramacula regions. These latter fields would be seen to vary slightly in hue across their diameter, except that they induce instant chromatic adaptation.

In 1886 it was Sigmund Exner's turn. Hering attacked a short notice Exner had published on a contrast effect, which he had unfortunately described as an illusion of judgment (Exner 1885). Hering complained that despite capitulation on the point by Aubert and Fick, many writers like Exner clung to Helmholtz's error that simultaneous contrast effects arise through unconscious judgments and mental "illusions" (Hering 1886[47]). Aroused by the ensuing controversy, Hering produced a long string of papers during the following four years, in which he repeated and analyzed the classical experiments Helmholtz had described in the *Handbuch* that allegedly supported his psychological theory (Hering 1887c[50], d[51], f[53], g(54), 1888d[57], 1890a[64], b[65]). In all of these papers Hering tried to show—none too respectfully—that Helmholtz had fundamentally misinterpreted these experiments and had been misled by the presence of afterimages, failure to hold firm fixation, and neglect of proper control experiments. Although brilliant polemical vehicles, these papers did little to elaborate Hering's own theory of contrast or even to demonstrate clearly that it could succeed where Helmholtz's had failed.

Also important were the criticisms that Hering launched against Fick and his displacement hypothesis. From his first reference to the hypothesis in 1880, Hering had treated it as beneath contempt for its viciously ad hoc nature. According to Hering, the hypothesis deprived the Young–Helmholtz theory of all predictive power (Hering 1880[43]). If the response curves were thought capable of continuous variation, then their precise form had to be determined empirically for every individual and, in the study of peripheral color blindness, for every point on the retina. Hering was convinced that the displacement hypothesis implied abandoning the tenet that fixed specific energies, and so fixed color sensations, are associated with each of the three hypothetical fiber-types; this, he wrote, was tantamount to "suicide for the theory" (p. 94). Later, after noting that Helmholtz himself had recently endorsed the displacement hypothesis, Hering cited the growing support of Fick's hypothesis as evidence that the Young–Helmholtz theory was dissolving into a blur of *Hilfshypothesen* and disagreements within the school about the exact nature of the psychological primaries (1889b[62], 73).

In 1889 Hering added an empirical critique to his methodological attacks upon the displacement theory. In the same year Hering's student Carl Hess had carried out a detailed study of peripheral color blindness (Hess 1889). Hess had shown that as monochromatic colored fields are seen at increasing retinal eccentricities, they normally change hue, lose saturation, and eventually appear colorless. But three monochromatic hues and one purplish red (roughly corresponding to the four simple colors of the opponent process theory) undergo no hue changes, although they do lose saturation and eventually fade to white. The two hue pairs also remain complementary, and all other monochromatic colored lights approach these four invariant hues. Hering noted that Hess's results could be visualized in terms of the color plane by imaging a nested set of (roughly triangular) spectral loci curves, all centered on the white point of the color plane; each member of the set will show the spectral locus corresponding to a particular degree of retinal eccentricity of vision.

According to Hering, that geometrical exercise proved the displacement hypothesis to be inconsistent with Hess's findings. Each of the set of nested spectral curves must have the same form as the outermost one obtained for the fovea, otherwise the four constant hues could not remain complementary. But Hering was convinced that on Fick's hypothesis, the successive spectral curves must change their form, as the response curves are altered or shifted with increasing eccentricity. Fick replied that displacement did not necessarily entail such a change of form, although he admitted that Hess's results restricted his hypothesis. The exchange of papers petered out without great acrimony or a definitive solution (Hering 1889b[62], 1890e[68]; Fick 1890). It illustrated, however, Hering's talent for disconcerting his opponents with ingenious and unexpected attacks.

Hering's most important contribution to color theory during this period arose indirectly from his 1882 reply to Frans Donders' long analysis of the state of contemporary color theory (Hering 1882[44], 88). In that rancour-free reply, Hering justified his reluctance to accept a zone theory compromise at that stage of the controversy, and in a clumsy attempt to woo Donders, emphasized to exaggeration the area of agreement between them: the similarity of Donders' photosensitive molecule to his own A- and D-processes; Donders' acceptance of the simple nature of red, green, yellow, and blue; Donders' agreement with him about the nature of black; and much more. Indeed, Hering claimed that the only significant difference between himself and Donders was Donders' conviction that some trichromatic retinal process was necessary to explain the facts of color mixing and the barycentric construction of the color plane. In reality, Hering noted, the opponent process theory could explain these things as well as Young's theory. A demonstration of that fact would destroy the only remaining rationale for believing in Young's theory or advocating compromises between the two theories (Hering 1882[44], 95). Again Hering's attempt to recruit Donders failed, as the latter made clear in a tart reply that emphasized their differences (Donders 1884). Undeterred, however, Hering went on to provide the promised demonstration in one of the most important papers of his career: an abstract, metatheoretical discussion of colorimetrical relationships and color theories (Hering 1887a[48]).

Hering began by insisting that all color theory depended upon "Newton's law of color mixing." Although he never defined this law clearly, it embraced the so-called four laws of Grassmann that guaranteed the barycentric mixing property of colors in color space. Hering complained that this law had never been rigorously confirmed empirically, and some small effects amounting to deviations from it had occasionally been reported. Nevertheless, he assured his readers that it had been approximately confirmed by many experiments and had been assumed or theoretically deduced in some fashion by many theorists including Maxwell, Grassmann, and Helmholtz. After offering experiments of his own in support of Newton's law of mixtures, Hering developed an abstruse geometrical expression of mixture relationships in terms of what he called "mix lines," the "mix plane," and finally the "mix space"—equivalent to the "color space" already deduced by Maxwell and Helmholtz (pp. 206–43).

But what is being mixed in mix space? Hering was adamant that the proper referents were neither physical lights nor light sensations, but rather entities Hering called "optical valences." The optical valence V of any light is its intrinsic potence as a sensory stimulus to produce some particular effect, prior to any considerations of adaptation or individual differences that might alter the actual sensory effect produced by that stimulus. By the mixture law every optical valence is arbitrarily analyzable into n "primitive valences," v_n ($Urvalences$), much as we decompose a force into components. It follows that

$$V = v_1 + v_2 + v_3 + \ldots v_n$$

Two physically different lights that appear to be identical must therefore have equal valences and, pair by pair, equal primitive valences (pp. 208–10). Can we legitimately regard the "optical valence" of a light as constant and possessing a stimulus potency independent of the momentary state of organism it works on? Yes, answered Hering, and he cited in support research by Kries and himself, which showed that a color equation continues as an equation through all changes in adaptation of the eye, as well as through all additions or subtractions of equal-appearing light mixtures. This result Hering dubbed "the law of the constancy of optical valences" and declared it to be the foundation of color vision theory (pp. 210–11).

This tortured discussion had as its purpose the establishment of theoretical entities—the optical valences of lights—to which Newton's law applied. Mix space refers neither to physical lights nor to color sensations, but to optical valences. When we use standard colorimetric methods to locate the spectral locus, or any other colors, on the mix plane, we have not plotted the position of "colors" of particular lights but the positions of optical valences. The color we actually see in the light representing any point in mix space will depend upon our physiological particularities and the state of adaptation (*Umstimmung*) of our sensory apparatus. Hering insisted that failure to note this distinction had led Helmholtz, Maxwell, Grassmann, and all their followers to confuse the objective "valence-table" with a "color-table in the subjective sense," to regard color space as "a tableau of all possible qualities of the light sensation" (pp. 222–32, 226). This error resulted from, and in turn perpetuated, the tendency of Helmholtz's school to assume a one-to-one correlation between hue and wavelength and between brightness and intensity, and to assume that saturation and hue do not vary with intensity.

Hering insisted that the number of primitive valences that constitute an optical valence cannot be determined from the mixture laws themselves, although at least three are required. "It follows from what has been said that the assumption of three components or primitive valences suffices to explain the mix plane. But it in no way follows that lights are in reality mixtures of three primitive valences" (p. 218). This permits a wide range of color theories. They may be classified according to the number of primitive valences they postulate, whether these valences are allowed to take on negative as well as positive values, the relationship between the valences in activating or canceling one another, and their relationship in defining the position of white on the mix plane. Hering went on to analyze the characteristics of four classes of potential color theories (pp. 234–65). He identified the Young–Helmholtz theory as only one of a large class of possible theories that banned negative coefficients and defined the color plane as bounded by an n-gon, where n is the number of primitive valences or fundamentals. His own theory he located in a class defined by paired and geometrically opposite valences that cancel rather than complement each other; the peculiarity of such theories, he noted, is that the white valence, being unpaired, takes on values represented by a plane parallel to the chromatic mix plane. Hering concluded with his central point: the empirical relationships of colorimetry in no way privilege the Young–Helmholtz theory. Many potential color theories (including his own) can fully express the known facts of color mixing (because they all incorporate Newton's law) as well as all relationships of the color plane or mix plane.

HERING VERSUS KRIES

The polemics that Hering exchanged with Johannes von Kries reveal most clearly the conceptual gap that separated the two schools. The exchanges turned on several issues, but primarily upon Kries' assertion, acknowledged and fully shared by Hering, that color equations made by an individual persist through changes of adaptation. Kries repeatedly claimed between 1878 and 1887 that this result, while fully compatible with the Young–Helmholtz hypothesis, absolutely invalidated Hering's theory. Kries advanced several versions of this argument; the first version, presented in 1878, hinged on the following experiment.

We present the subject with a white field, the left half of which has been mixed from monochromatic pure blue and the pure yellow as defined by Hering's opponent process theory. These wavelengths will not activate the red-green process at all. The right half of the field will be mixed from Hering's pure red and pure green, so that it, too, will appear white and there will be no contribution by the blue-yellow process. Now we exhaust the eye by long exposure to pure green light and then restore the original fields. Kries reasoned that since pure green light leaves Hering's yellow-blue process unaffected, exhausting the left half of the retina for green will not change the appearance of the blue-yellow mixture. The mixed white on the left-hand side should undergo no change before and after exhaustion by green. The red-green mix in the right half of the field, however, should now appear no longer white but distinctly reddish, because exhaustion has reduced the retina's sensitivity for green. Against this theoretical prediction, the actual experimental outcome shows that the fields continue to match and to constitute a color equation. Kries concluded that Hering's theory must be false, since it seems to predict that color equations should not persist with adaptation (Kries 1882, 111–13).

In 1887 Hering replied that Kries had simply misunderstood what his theory actually predicted under the experimental situation described. A wavelength that has no effect on the red-green process before adaptation (with the eye in *neutrale Stimmung,* to use Hering's terminology) *will* affect that process after adaptation. In Kries' experiment, both fields will appear slightly redder after adaptation, but they will continue to match (Hering 1887a[48]).[3] Such misunderstandings, Hering mocked, were typical of Helmholtz's supporters.

Kries replied with exasperation that Hering had actually altered his theory in order to deflect criticism; he had earlier written plainly that pure green light did not affect the yellow-blue substance, with no proviso that this applied only in states of neutral adaptation. What Hering now claimed was physiologically possible within the framework of his theory only if monochromatic light of "pure" green *did* act on the blue-yellow process, and in such a way as to stimulate exactly equal levels of assimilative and dissimilative activity. Was it even remotely plausible, Kries asked, that the same light could trigger these equal and opposite photochemical effects in the visual substance (Kries 1887a)?

Now Hering replied in a rage. In suggesting that he had altered his theory, Kries had "slandered his literary character." Hering accused Kries of intentionally misquoting some of his former claims (Kries 1887a; Hering 1887e[52], 30), and he angrily refused to engage in further public exchanges. Hering also rejected Kries' interpretation of his visual substance as being a photochemical substance in the retina, like visual purple, as well as Donders' interpretation of it as a central process that said nothing about the eye per se. In reality, he insisted, "my theory asserts nothing at all about the first, direct effect of light in the peripheral eye" (p. 39).

Kries in return gave Hering a soft answer, denying any intention to insult or misinterpret (Kries 1887b). Retreating slightly from his claims of 1882, he offered a different and more subtle version of the alleged inconsistency between Hering's theory and the persistence of color equations with adaptation. Kries also could not resist attacking what he saw as the fundamental slipperiness of Hering's claims about his visual substance. If, as Hering claims, his theory really applies to psychophysical processes and not to any "intermediate apparatus" that may lie between the physical light stimulus and the site of the psychophysical event, then why does he so strenuously resist any discussion of what that intermediate apparatus might be? Returning to his former attempts at negotiation, Kries appealed directly to Hering to give up his vain attempts to explain color blindness and adaptation in terms of his theory of the visual substance, and to allow these phenomena, at least, to be explained as the results of peripheral, trichromatic processes.

Kries' apology mollified Hering, and he agreed to resume the public discussion. Unmoved by Kries' overtures, however, he did so by responding to Kries' second attempted refutation of the opponent process theory. That attempted refutation had gone as follows. Suppose the eye is presented with two fields, on the left a light L, on the right a light L' that appears identical to L but is physically different. Thanks to Newton's mixture law and the additivity property it confers, we can think of the sensation excited by L as the sum of some number of fundamental sensations A, B, C, ... corresponding to the fundamental physiological processes that mediate color sensation in the eye. Similarly, L' will be the sum of the same number of fundamental sensations A', B', C', ... If these are really the fundamental sensations then we can also know that $A = A'$, $B = B'$, $C = C'$, ... The contributions A, B, A', B', and so on to L and L' must be thought of as products of the particular stimulus value of the total light for the fundamental sensation in question (the "primitive valence" in Hering's terms), times the "receptivity" or "sensitivity" of the retina for that stimulus. If we write $A = \underline{A}a$ to denote this relationship, where $\underline{A}$ is the stimulus value and a is the momentary sensitivity,[4] then equality of L and L' means that

$$
\begin{array}{rcl}
\underline{A}a & = & \underline{A}'a \\
+ \quad \underline{B}b & = & \underline{B}'b \\
+ \quad \underline{C}c & = & \underline{C}'c \\
+ \quad . & = & . \\
+ \quad . & = & . \\
+ \quad . & = & . \\
\hline
L & = & L'
\end{array}
$$

The experimental finding that color equations persist after adaptation expresses the fact, obvious from this theoretical formulation, that L continues to equal L' even if one or all of the sensitivities a, b, c, and so on change (Kries 1882, 110–11; 1887a,b; Hering 1888c[56], 495).

Kries admitted that this derivation does not restrict or specify the number of fundamental sensations, but he went on to argue that additional considerations show that the number must be exactly three, as in the Young–Helmholtz theory. The equality of the two fields implies that they match in brightness, hue, and saturation. These three variables must be three functions of the fundamental sensations. So we can write

$$
\begin{array}{rcl}
F_1\,(\underline{A}a,\ \underline{B}b,\ \underline{C}c,\ \ldots) & = & F_1\,(\underline{A}'a,\ \underline{B}'b,\ \underline{C}'c,\ \ldots) \\
F_2\,(\quad\quad " \quad\quad) & = & F_2\,(\quad\quad " \quad\quad) \\
F_3\,(\quad\quad " \quad\quad) & = & F_3\,(\quad\quad " \quad\quad)
\end{array}
$$

Treating a, b, c ... as constants, it follows immediately that if the number of fundamental components in vision is only three, then $A = A'$, $B = B'$, and $C = C'$. This means that the contributions of the components to the two fields must remain the same for all values of a, b, c; in other words, the equation persists through adaptation. But if the number of components is four or more, then the three equations will not *guarantee* that $A = A'$ and the like. In the absence of further mathematical restrictions, some values of a, b, c . . . might yield A not equal to A' and the equation might not persist through adaptation. But this is contrary to the experimental results achieved by both Kries and Hering. Kries concluded that the trivariance of vision, combined with the constancy of color equations through *Umstimmung*, requires exactly three fundamental sensations.

Hering greeted this demonstration with some perplexity. He did not try to refute the second part of Kries' proof, merely to argue that it was irrelevant to the first part. How the fundamental components of sensation interact to determine brightness, hue, and intensity is an altogether different question from the conditions under which two compound sensations will be seen as equal. The latter condition is satisfied when the separate contributions of the fundamentals are equal, and out of that no limitation on the number of components can be derived, as Kries himself had conceded (Hering 1888c[56], 495–96).

But Kries had also advanced a third, closely related refutation of Hering's theory (Kries 1887b). He noted that Hering's theory specified five fundamental components: blue, yellow, red, green, and white. Hence if two lights L and L' are to appear the same, then where $\underline{B}$ is the total stimulus value of L for the blue component, the condition for the persistence of the colorimetric equation is that $\underline{B} = \underline{B}'$, $\underline{Y} = \underline{Y}'$, $\underline{R} = \underline{R}'$, $\underline{G} = \underline{G}'$, and $\underline{W} = \underline{W}'$. But the opponent process theory also insists that the difference of the two antagonistic components determines the resulting sensation from that process. Hence on Hering's theory a color equation can exist between two lights if

$$\underline{B} - \underline{Y} = \underline{B}' - \underline{Y}'$$
$$\underline{R} - \underline{G} = \underline{R}' - \underline{G}'$$
$$\underline{W} = \underline{W}' \tag{1}$$

To this Kries objected that it is possible that $\underline{B} - \underline{Y} = \underline{B}' - \underline{Y}'$ without it being true that $\underline{B} = \underline{B}'$ or $\underline{Y} = \underline{Y}'$. Only a three-component theory like Young–Helmholtz will eliminate this inconsistency between the two sets of conditions for a color match; it does not suffice to take a five-variable theory and reduce it to three variables through the use of differences between the variables.

This time Hering's reply was devastating. He pointed out that the five components of the opponent process entering into L and L' must not only meet the conditions of the three equations described above in order to guarantee a match between these lights. They must also satisfy the barycentric conditions of mixtures on the color plane. That condition is that

$$\underline{B} - \underline{Y} : \underline{R} - \underline{G} : \underline{W} = \underline{B'} - \underline{Y'} : \underline{R'} - \underline{G'} : \underline{W'}$$

That relationship gives

$$\underline{B} : \underline{Y} : \underline{R} : \underline{G} : \underline{W} = \underline{B'} : \underline{Y'} : \underline{R'} : \underline{G'} : \underline{W'}$$

and that ensures, together with the equalities expressed in Equation (1) above, that $\underline{Gg} = \underline{G'g}$, $\underline{Bb} = \underline{B'b}$, and so on. Hering ridiculed Kries' failure to see the additional constraints that follow from Newton's mixture law; that failure, he claimed, revealed Kries' inability to understand the problems of color theory in a fully general way (Hering 1888c[56], 496–98). Hering averred that this inability followed from Kries' theoretical prejudices on behalf of the Young–Helmholtz theory.

These confrontations resulted in tactical victories for Hering. Kries continued to criticize color theories of more than three fundamentals for overdetermining the three functional relationships for brightness, hue, and saturation (whatever they may be), but he no longer presented this result as demonstratively refuting such theories (Kries 1905, 148; 1910, 427). Kries also abandoned his former attempts to refute the opponent process theory from the fact that color equations persist with adaptation, even though this claim (probably based on Kries' earlier writings) is occasionally met with in later literature. Kries was learning, as Helmholtz had also, that Hering was a shrewd and implacable opponent not to be attacked lightly. Kries' example proved salutary for other partisans. In a major paper of 1886 Arthur König confidently asserted that the sufficiency of three experimental primaries for color mixing proved the existence of precisely three fundamental, physiological primaries as well (König and Dieterici 1886[14], 81). But after following the embarrassment of Kries during the following two years, König quietly withdrew this claim when his original paper was expanded and reprinted in 1892 (König 1892[21], 298).

HELMHOLTZ ON HERING

The exchange may also have been salutary for Helmholtz. In 1889 he published his first public critique of Hering's color theory in the second edition of the *Handbuch der physiologischen Optik* (PO2, 376–82). Avoiding Kries' mistake, Helmholtz conceded that "Herr Hering's theory, if one wants to overlook its physiological liabilities, is able to explain all the facts of color mixing just as well, but also no better, than Thomas Young's theory" (p. 379). Elementary transformations, easily derivable from geometrical considerations, allow us to express the output from three receptors of Young's type in the form expected from Hering's three processes, so that the two theories are mathematically equivalent. Helmholtz left the door open for a zone theory: he did not rule out the possibility that output from Young's three retinal processes is subjected to further processing at higher neural levels. But he evinced skepticism of the possibility, and he reaffirmed his belief that our conscious sensations of color are probably not much different from the red, green, and violet fundamentals excited at the periphery.

Helmholtz's analysis of Hering's theory from 1889 added no new criticisms, but it offered a comprehensive statement of the usual ones. Helmholtz argued (1) that Hering's attempt to identify fundamental or simple colors from intuition alone is methodologically treacherous; after all, Goethe and Sir David Brewster had both insisted that they could "see" blue and yellow in green light. Our conviction that the four pure colors identified by Hering are somehow simple or primitive probably reflects merely the fact that most objects of our experience are of these colors. (2) The fact that Young's fundamental sensations, but not Hering's, can be approximately observed in afterimage experiments, makes Young's theory more susceptible to introspective confirmation (more *anschaulich*) than Hering's. (3) Hering's assertion that achromatic sensations can vary in brightness but pure chromatic ones cannot is counterintuitive and inconsistent with the claims of a theory supposedly built on the evidence of intuition. (4) The physiological mechanisms postulated by Hering are "improbable" and in any case inconsistent with one another; equilibrium in the black-white process produces neutral gray, equilibrium in the chromatic processes produces no sensation at all. (5) Hering's attempt to associate the black sensation with positive physiological processes violates our intuitive appreciation of black as representing the absence of a potential sensation of brightness. (6) Hering's theory cannot explain the existence of the subclasses of red and green blind; absorption in the lens and other media does not suffice to explain why the effect occurs on the retinal periphery, and macula absorption does not completely explain the effect in the center either (pp. 376–82).

While Helmholtz's analysis added little to the debate, it was important for two reasons. First, it demonstrated again his undiminished skill at scientific argumentation. Helmholtz phrased all his objections so as to cast doubt upon Hering's central claim that his theory was more faithful to our intuitive perceptions of color than was Young's. Second, the *Hand-*

buch discussion foreclosed what some had seen as a distinct possibility, namely, that Helmholtz or his school would make major concessions to Hering, or that Helmholtz personally would endorse a zone theory compromise. The foreclosing of that possibility effectively ended the first stage of the color theory debate in Germany.

CHAPTER ELEVEN

Color Vision Controversies, 1890–1915

THE FIRST PHASE of the German debates over color vision ended on an ironic note: both schools had largely established their central claims. Hering's followers had shown that the dichromats whom their opponents called "red blind" and "green blind" almost certainly perceived a spectrum composed of blues and yellows, as predicted by the opponent process theory. Helmholtz's supporters had all but proved the existence of three classes of dichromats: the red blind, the green blind, and the very rare violet-blue blind. The dominant theoretical issue of this phase had been, does the empirical trichromacy and the trivariability of vision necessitate an underlying three-component physiological process? The controversy over that issue had ended with Kries' tacit withdrawal of his claims for the affirmative and Helmholtz's public acknowledgment of the two theories' mathematical equivalency. After fifteen years of intense controversy, the color vision debates in 1890 were stalemated.

Perhaps as a consequence of this perceived stalemate, new color theories began to proliferate in the 1890s. These were mostly hybrids of the two dominant theories, yet they usually resembled one of the two more than the other. The model proposed by American Christine Ladd-Franklin, for example, resembled the Young–Helmholtz theory; that advanced by psychologist G. E. Müller was an elaborate version of Hering's. Except for the singular theory suggested by Wilhelm Wundt in 1888, all were "component" theories, which postulated a small number of fundamental sensations and explained color blindness as reduction forms of normal vision. Most placed high priority upon explaining, as Hering's theory did, the four "simple" chromatic sensations and their exclusive pairings. All postulated mechanisms that would yield separate classes of red blind and green blind, and some insisted with Hering on physiologically separate chromatic and achromatic processes. Nearly all postulated retinal induction effects rather than unconscious inference to explain simultaneous contrast. Several distinguished between peripheral and central processes and so were implicit zone theories.[1] Even as these models proliferated, however, the Helmholtz–Hering confrontation was moving to a new stage.

KÖNIG, RESPONSE CURVES, AND THE FUNDAMENTAL SENSATIONS

The emergence of important new players, above all Arthur König and his collaborators in Berlin, characterized the second stage of the color vision controversies. Between 1885 and 1898 König revolutionized the standards of exact colorimetry in Europe. In 1886 he and Conrad Dieterici announced the results of a new, precision determination of Young's fundamental sensations, and they published the complete data and methodological explanations in 1892 (König and Dieterici 1886[14]; König 1892[21]; König 1886[15]). König based that determination on vast numbers of color matches systematically made between homogeneous spectral lights and mixtures of three experimental primaries that he infelicitously called "elementary sensations." As experimental primaries König employed a far spectral violet, a far spectral red, and (by an indirect method of calculation) an extraspectral green.

König and Dieterici began by measuring the spectral response curves of two red blind and two green blind dichromats for their red and violet experimental primaries or elementary sensations. Using a color-mixing apparatus of Helmholtz's design, they discovered that their dichromats could match homogeneous lights from the outer portions of the spectrum to one or the other of the primaries merely by varying the brightness of the primary. To match lights from the middle of the spectrum, the dichromats required mixtures of the two primaries. In deriving color equations, König actually did not mix primaries at all, but rather had his subjects make equations between the homogeneous test light and mixtures of two similar homogeneous lights of slightly longer and slightly shorter wavelengths. This yielded a sequence of simultaneous color equations. Solving these equations allowed him to express each test light in the sequence in terms of the two experimental primaries at the end of the spectrum (König and Dieterici 1886[14], 63–66; König 1892[21], 231–54).

Using this data König graphed the wavelength of each homogeneous test light in the spectrum against the relative contributions of each experimental primary to the mixture that precisely matched it for the dichromat studied. This yielded two spectral response curves for each dichromat, which König (following the nonprejudicial terminology of Donders) simply called the "warm-color curve" and the "cold-color curve." For a given wavelength on the abscissa, the ordinates to the two curves gave the proportions of the two primaries which, when mixed, were perceived to match the homogeneous light. These curves are shown in Figure 11.1 as König presented them in 1892. By convention König set the areas under these curves equal.

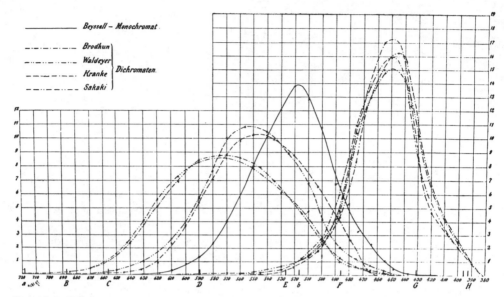

Fig. 11.1 "Elementary sensation" response curves for two red blind and two green blind dichromats and one monochromat, published by Arthur König in 1892. *Source*: König 1892(21), 230.

König found that all four dichromats produced very similar response curves for the cold color (peak at 450 in Fig. 11.1), that the two red blind individuals produced similar warm-color curves (peak about 550), and that the two green blind subjects produced warm-color curves similar to each other's (peak about 575) but quite different from those of the red blind. König took this result as further confirming the existence of discrete classes of red and green blind. Finally, König applied his procedure to one monochromat. Since this individual could match any spectral light with any single primary, the determination amounted merely to an experimental determination of his spectral brightness or luminosity curve. The result, König noted, was striking for showing the monochromat's brightness peak to lie in the green (about 517 nanometers), as Donders and Hering had confirmed on other monochromats (König and Dieterici 1886[14], 61–62; König 1892[21], 226–31). The brightness peak for normals lies in the yellow.

König encountered greater problems in applying this procedure to two normal, trichromatic subjects (himself and Dieterici), because over much of the spectrum they required mixtures of three elementary or primary sensations to match spectral lights. To supplement the procedure he had adopted for dichromats, König resorted to a laborious system of approximation, in which each curve was extended by small steps and the contri-

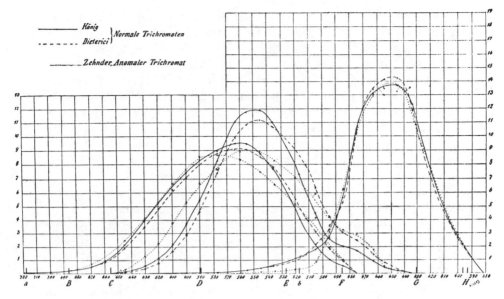

Fig. 11.2 "Elementary sensation" response curves for two normal trichromats and one anomalous trichromat, published by Arthur König in 1892. *Source:* König 1892(21), 288.

bution of the (imaginary) green sensation theoretically calculated at each step (König and Dieterici 1886[14], 73–75; König 1892[21], 268–90). That procedure allowed König to dispense with negative color coefficients, and it yielded the sets of three elementary-sensation response curves shown in Figure 11.2.

König and Dieterici then turned to the theoretical significance of their measurements. If Young's theory and Newton's mixture law are both correct, then each of the three experimental primaries or "elementary sensations" must be a homogeneous, linear function of three unknown "fundamental sensations" that correspond to Young's physiological primaries (p. 298). Deducing the "fundamental sensations" from the "elementary sensations" (the experimental primaries) requires that we determine the nine transformation coefficients that enter into these three simultaneous linear equations. Three of the nine conditions necessary to make this determination are given in the fact that the coefficients in each equation sum to one, that is, their values are only relatively defined. In principle the other conditions can be obtained from studies on dichromats. If the varieties of dichromatism are reduction forms of normal vision, then the same transformation coefficients that apply to trichromats will also express the elementary sensations of dichromats in terms of Young's fundamental sensations. König assured his readers that "a little practice" made it "very easy to find out, by mere inspection, whether relations of this kind exist, at least approximately, among the graphical representations of the curves" (pp. 300, 303–12; König and Dieterici 1886[14], 81–87).

Without showing how he had derived them, König finally produced a set of coefficients that transformed the red, green, and blue elementary sensation curves of Figure 11.2 into the red, green, and blue "fundamental sensation curves" shown in Figure 11.3. For König, the significance of these particular coefficients lay in the fact that they also transformed the cold-color curves of the four dichromats (Fig. 11.1) into a curve identical to the blue fundamental sensation curve of normals, the warm-color curve of the two red blind into a curve identical to the green curve of normals, and the warm-color curve of the two green blind into a curve identical to normals' red curve. The fact that such coefficients can be found, claimed König, showed that both kinds of dichromatism could be represented as straightforward reduction forms, if normal trichromatic vision were based upon the particular fundamental sensations deduced.[2] Significantly, the spectral sensitivity curve of monochromats showed no relationship to any of the normal curves under this transformation (König and Dieterici 1886[14], 81–87; König 1892[21], 310–20). König concluded that monochromatism is not a reduction form of ordinary vision, and he used that conclusion to dismiss Hering's interpretation of monochromatic vision as due to the hypothetical black-white process alone (p. 301).

Using these derived fundamental sensations as the vertices of a color triangle gave a representation of the spectral locus like that shown in Figure 11.4. It made the closest spectral equivalents of the fundamentals to be a bluish-green of approximately 505 nanometers, a purplish extraspectral red, and—within the considerable uncertainty imposed by experimental error and the possibility of macula absorption—a blue of approximately 470 nanometers.[3] That uncertainty about the blue fundamental notwithstanding, König regarded his work as a triumphant confirmation of the Young–Helmholtz theory. He dedicated the work formally to Helmholtz on the occasion of the fiftieth anniversary of Helmholtz's doctoral degree.

The specter of Ewald Hering loomed large over this experimental milestone in the research program Helmholtz had laid down for physiological optics. Swipes at Hering's theory pepper König's footnotes and occasionally erupt into the text, even though between 1886 and 1892 he retreated from his claim that the number of "fundamental sensations" must necessarily equal the number of "elementary sensations"—a claim that would preclude the truth of Hering's theory (König and Dieterici 1886[14], 82; König 1892[21], 298). Boldly bidding to coopt some of Hering's key results, König in 1886 claimed the hues of his fundamental sensations to be

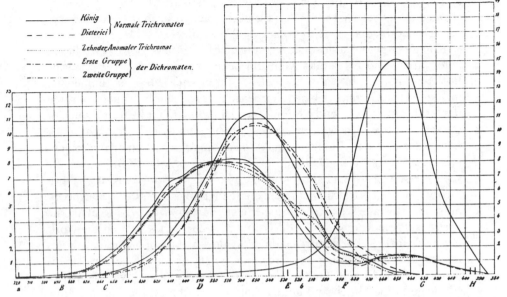

Fig. 11.3 "Fundamental sensation" response curves for two normal trichromats, one anomalous trichromat, two green blind dichromats, and two red blind dichromats, published by Arthur König in 1892. (The "blue" curves of the trichromats and the "cold" sensation curves of the dichromats are averaged to a single curve, peaking at 450 nanometers. The four "warm" sensation curves of the two red blind and two green blind subjects are averaged to two curves.) *Source*: König 1892(21), 310.

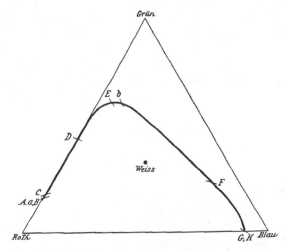

Fig. 11.4 König's color triangle of 1886, showing the spectral locus determined by him and Dieterici and the location of the derived "fundamental sensations" at the vertices. *Source*: König 1886(15), 104.

identical to three of the four "pure colors" postulated by Hering's school (König and Dieterici 1886[14], 86). In the face of protests from Hering, he retreated from this claim, too, in 1892 (König 1892[21], 318).[4]

König's paper became the fountainhead of twentieth-century studies in colorimetry, and his results were still being reproduced in the scientific literature at least into the 1950s (e.g., Le Grand 1968). Its immediate impact on the German debate is harder to assess. Helmholtz incorporated the results into the second edition of the *Handbuch*, but he found some of the data inconsistent with theoretical predictions from his current work on the line element, and he declined to endorse the particular fundamentals deduced by König (*PO2*, 350–72, 439–80; Stiles 1972). The results so impressed Christine Ladd-Franklin, who was working in König's laboratory in 1891, as to lead her to conclude that any successful color theory must incorporate a trichromatic element through which to explain the varieties of dichromatism (Ladd-Franklin 1924). Kries praised the work but made little use of it, and he pointedly declined to incorporate König's results into the third edition of the *Handbuch*, or into the extensive appendixes he provided. One major impact of the paper, however, was to stimulate Franz Hillebrand and Hering to turn their attention to achromatic sensations and the vision of monochromats.

THE SPECIFIC BRIGHTNESS OF COLORS

On Young's theory the sum of the brightnesses of the three fundamental sensations determines the brightness of the composite sensation to which they give rise, and the ratio of those brightnesses determines the hue. Hence brightness and chromaticity are closely related. Hering, however, thought of color sensations as phenomenologically separable into chromatic and achromatic parts, and he associated brightness mainly with the achromatic element. On Hering's system, the brightness of the purely chromatic element in a sensation cannot even be defined apart from the achromatic element that accompanies it. Were it somehow possible to have a sensation with no achromatic element (the sensation that would result from stimulating a chromatic process without simultaneously stimulating the achromatic process), then the brightness of the resulting color would be equivalent to that of neutral gray.[5] All purely chromatic sensations would have this same intrinsic brightness, as would the sum of any purely chromatic sensations (Hering 1874c[41], 1875[42]). Needless to say, Helmholtz and his supporters found much of this incomprehensible.

In 1887 Hering remarked almost in passing that he had changed his mind about chromatic brightness. He had become convinced that some colors (red and yellow) enhance the total brightness of a sensation while others (blue and green) reduce it (Hering 1887b[49], 20). He claimed to have reached this result by 1882, but all the evidence indicates that Hering had been forced to develop and announce the result by the 1886 work of König and Dieterici. They had shown that the spectral sensitivity peak of their monochromat lay in the green, not in the yellow as with normals, and had used the result to challenge Hering's theory. Hering interpreted monochromats as individuals possessing only the black-white process. Although those individuals see the spectrum entirely in shades of gray, they ought to perceive the distribution of brightness across the spectrum the same as normals did, if relative brightness is determined by the achromatic process alone and chromaticity makes little or no contribution.

In 1889 Hering's most gifted student, Franz Hillebrand, published "On the Specific Brightness of Colors," a study that developed and exploited Hering's amendment to his theory (Hillebrand 1889). Although Hering attached a foreword anxiously reaffirming his priority over the central innovation (Hering 1889a[60]), the perspectives developed in the paper flowed from Hillebrand himself. He opened with a defense of Hering's concept of brightness, attacked Johannes von Kries on many fronts, and reaffirmed the major role of contrast and adaptation in color perception. Then Hillebrand turned to the central question. If two sensations have the same achromatic brightness and saturation, but different hues, will the brightness of the sensations as wholes be different? Is there a "specific brightness of colors," variable from hue to hue, which might add to or subtract from the achromatic brightness?

Hillebrand's paper consisted of a series of experiments designed to disentangle the achromatic brightness from the chromatic brightness, if any existed. His techniques were ingenious and in principle easily explained. He dark-adapted his eyes, and then examined various colored fields (rotating color disks, homogeneous lights) under levels of illumination or intensity so low that these fields appeared gray. He made color equations (strictly, luminosity matches) among these gray fields, and so quantitatively determined their relative levels of brightness. Next Hillebrand adapted his eyes to daylight and turned up the level of illumination or intensity so that different hues could be seen. He then redetermined the relative levels of brightness among the fields. Hillebrand found that the brightness ratios were quite different above the chromatic threshold from what they had been below.

Hillebrand reasoned that at low levels of illumination the eye had perceived only achromatic brightness. Those low levels of intensity had not activated the chromatic processes or had left their input below the sensory threshold; only the "white valences" in the light affected the sensation. At higher levels of intensity and illumination the chromatic processes also came into play, and any resulting changes in relative levels of brightness must be due to a variable contribution to brightness associated exclusively with the chromatic processes. The data were such as to suggest that red and yellow enhanced overall brightness and blue and green reduced it. Colors possess a "specific brightness."

Hillebrand also determined what he and Hering called the "white valence curve." This was the luminosity distribution across the so-called dark spectrum—the solar spectrum viewed with dark-adapted eyes and at subchromatic levels of intensity. Hillebrand then graphically compared this "white valence curve" to the luminosity distribution curve of the solar spectrum obtained in daylight viewing. He found the curves to differ, the peak of the former lying in the green, the peak of the latter lying in the yellow. The changes occurred, Hillebrand concluded, because at higher intensities the yellow and red rays of the spectrum evoked a positive specific brightness effect, while the greens and blues evoked a negative one (Hillebrand 1889, 107, 120–22).

All these results, Hillebrand pointed out, spelled trouble for the Young–Helmholtz theory. On Young's theory the dark-adapted eye should become exquisitely sensitive to green light and should see it as green, not as gray; the peak in the spectral brightness curve of the so-called red blind should be shifted toward the green, when in fact it lies in the yellow like that of normals. Hering's theory (with the additional assumption of specific brightnesses) could explain the close similarity Hillebrand discovered between the spectral brightness curve of a red-green blind individual with the white valence curve of a normal individual in the red and green areas of the spectrum. It could explain why two "complementary colors" that "cancel" to give gray always produce a brightness equivalent to the sum of the white valences of the two colors. The Young–Helmholtz theory was powerless to explain these results (pp. 110–19).

A year went by with no public response to Hillebrand's paper, but in 1891, with help from Hering, the uproar began. Early that year Hering announced in Pflüger's *Archiv* that he had experimentally determined the spectral luminosity curve of a twenty-year-old monochromat (Hering 1891a[69]). That curve, he showed, corresponded extremely closely to the "white valence curve" of normal individuals determined by Hillebrand (from the dark spectrum and dark-adapted eye) in 1889. In particular, both curves showed a maximum in the green. Hering pointed out, as Hillebrand also had, that the opponent process theory predicted this close agreement. It interpreted monochromat vision as normal vision reduced to the black-white process; the vision of normals therefore becomes identical to monochromats under conditions of dark adaptation and low illumination, when only the white valences of the light come into play.

No such prediction could be made from the Young–Helmholtz theory. König himself had denied that monochromatism could be a reduction form of normal vision under Young's theory, and Helmholtz had not even mentioned the phenomenon in the second edition of the *Handbuch* (p. 607). In language more confident and triumphant than he had used in decades, Hering reviewed the evidence of monochromat color blindness and concluded that it spelled the demise of the Young–Helmholtz theory.

Within weeks after receiving Hering's paper, König rushed into print, attempting to shore up the considerable damage that had been done to the Young–Helmholtz theory and its program (König 1891a[20]). He reported the results of his collaborator, Carl Ritter, who had repeated the experiments of Hering and Hillebrand and had confirmed "the complete agreement to within expected level of precision" of the spectral brightness curves of monochromats with those of normals obtained from a dark spectrum, just as predicted by Hering's theory. The fact of that agreement, König wrote candidly, left the Young–Helmholtz theory "in a difficult position," and he later admitted that "this fulfillment of Hering's prediction powerfully disconcerted me" (p. 186).

But König reassured his readers that the successful prediction did not guarantee the truth of the opponent process theory from which it had been derived; after all, he wrote, "in the period of the epicyclic theory, solar and lunar eclipses were [also] correctly predicted in advance" (ibid.). All Hering and Hillebrand had really discovered was the long-known Purkinje phenomenon—the effect that reds and yellows lose their color and fade to gray more quickly than violets and greens in gathering twilight. König claimed Young's theory could also explain that phenomenon. We must assume, König conceded, that the coefficients that enter into the linear equation for any fundamental sensation are themselves functions of the intensity. If those functions are properly selected, then Young's theory can be made to explain the shift of brightness in the dark spectrum just as well as Hering's hypothesis about specific brightnesses.[6]

König compensated for this rather ad hoc defense of Young with a vigorous attack. He forcefully restated the traditional objections to Hering's explanation of dichromatism and did his best to contain the damage on the monochromatic front as well.[7] He noted that at least five monochromats reported in the literature had their spectral brightness maximum in the yellow, like normals. He pointed out sardonically that when Hering in 1881 had commented on the first of these cases (Becker's unilateral monochromat), he had cited the yellow peak to support his theory. König's arguments, however, were rhetorical delaying actions; he did not doubt that most cases of inherited monochromatism, including those studied by himself, had their maximum spectral sensitivity in the green. Again in 1892 he conceded as gracefully as he could that Hering had indisputably established a link between normal and monochromatic vision that was not immediately explicable in terms of the Young–Helmholtz theory (König 1892[21], 301).

RODS, CONES, AND VISUAL PURPLE

Events in Berlin continued to unfold quickly. In 1893 Hermann Ebbinghaus, the professor of experimental psychology in Berlin, weighed into the controversy with a color theory of his own and a penetrating criticism of the two major contenders. He not only attacked the Young–Helmholtz theory for its inability to explain the newly established link between monochromatism and normal vision; he even cast doubt upon the theory's greatest triumph, namely, König's alleged proof that dichromatism was a reduction form of normal vision. Ebbinghaus pointed to the large experimental uncertainties that König had encountered in his determination of the blue fundamental response curve in the yellow-green region of the spectrum. These uncertainties were sufficiently large, in his opinion, as to undermine the claim that this curve coincided with the "cold-color" response curve of dichromats (Ebbinghaus 1893, 146–66).

As for Hering's theory, according to Ebbinghaus it failed notoriously to account for red and green color blindness; and the Purkinje effect, although cited by Hering as a support of his theory, actually created major problems for it. Ebbinghaus described the following experiment, which he had conducted in König's laboratory. Let a normal eye look at two matching gray fields, the field on the left formed by a mixture of Hering's pure blue and pure yellow, the field on the right by a mixture of his pure red and pure green. Since the antagonistic chromatic inputs cancel, there can be no contribution from the specific brightnesses and so the luminosity of the two gray fields will be determined entirely by the black-white process. Now reduce the intensity of both fields by the same amount. If Hering's theory is correct and Newton's law also holds, then the fields should become dimmer but continue to match. In fact they do not; the blue-yellow field darkens more quickly than the green-red (pp. 166–86).[8] Ebbinghaus regarded this fact as proving that Hering's antagonistic hues do not cancel but combine to make white; the white contribution of the red-green process acts to desaturate spectral yellow, the very effect which, he asserted, had prevented König and Dieterici from unambiguously determining the form of the violet response curve.

Ebbinghaus's own theory was important mainly for bringing the substance called "visual purple" back to center stage in the color vision debates. In 1876 Franz Boll had announced that the retinal rods contain a reddish pigment that is bleached to yellow by the action of light; further exposure bleaches that "visual yellow" to white. Aside from unlocalized

changes in electrical potential, this was the first purely physiological process discovered to occur in the retina under the stimulus of light. It created
vast excitement and a flood of research. Chemist Wilhelm Kühne at Heidelberg, who led that effort, proposed that visual purple in the rods may
mediate achromatic sensations. But the boom was short-lived. Neither
visual purple nor other photopigments could be detected in the cones,
despite intense research, and comparative studies revealed the existence
of animals whose retinas contained no visual purple at all. The episode
left little trace on the study of visual sensation, although it enriched the
imaginations of color theorists with visions of dissociating photosensitive
molecules and other photochemical processes.

Ebbinghaus in 1893 returned to visual purple by suggesting that it and
visual yellow do exist in the cones, that their decomposition mediates the
sensations of yellow and blue respectively, and that they cannot be observed in the cones because they are intermixed with another photopig-
ment which, with its decomposition product, is of a complementary
color. This suggestion got nowhere, but by one report at least, it stimulated König to reexamine the spectral absorption curve of visual purple.
He assigned that problem to Georg Abelsdorff and Else Köttgen, and
early in 1894 they were able to make the determination on visual purple
extracted from the retina of a freshly enucleated human eye, using a
"spectrophotometer" König had constructed for the purpose. König then
compared the spectral absorption curve for visual purple, the (properly
corrected) luminosity curve of the monochromat studied in his joint research with Dieterici, and the luminosity curve for the dark spectrum and
dark-adapted normal eye, which he and his co-workers redetermined.
The three curves, shown in Figure 11.5 (peaking at 517 nanometers),
resembled each other so precisely as to support powerfully the conclusion
that visual purple is the light-perceiving substance in monochromatic eyes
and in dark-adapted normal eyes (König 1894c[24], 339–49).

Can that fact be reconciled with the absence of visual purple in the
cones of the central fovea? König apparently inclined at first to the view
that the foveal cones do contain visual purple, but in a state so readily
decomposable that it cannot be recovered. Within weeks, however, König
changed his mind, possibly in response to the demonstration by Christine
Ladd-Franklin that a thirteen-year-old local monochromat proved to be
totally blind in the fovea (Ladd-Franklin 1895). After a flurry of laboratory activity through the spring and early summer, König and Köttgen
reported the results of their experimental work to the Berlin Academy in
June, and simultaneously proposed a new and iconoclastic theory of
color vision (König 1894c[24]).

The tenets of that theory are easily stated. König held that the retinal
rods (not the cones) contain visual purple, which under the action of light
is bleached to visual yellow, giving as a psychophysical correlate the sen-

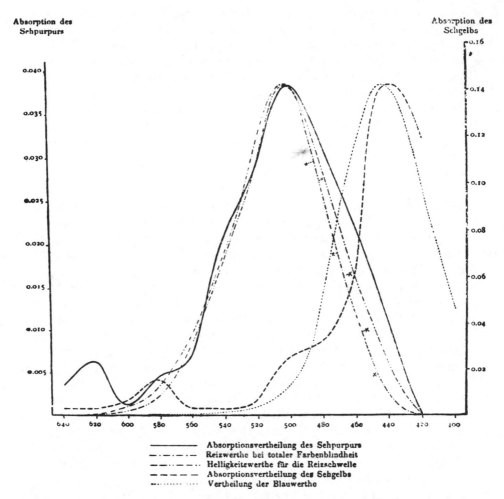

Fig. 11.5 König's determination of the spectral absorption curve of visual purple, the luminosity distribution curve of one monochromat, and the luminosity distribution curve of normal trichromats for the dark spectrum (equivalent to Hering's white valence curve). All peak at 517 nanometers. *Source*: König 1894c(24), 348.

sation of gray such as we perceive at night and under twilight conditions. Under much stronger light, the visual yellow in the rods is bleached to visual white, yielding the sensation of blue. König thus identified visual yellow with the blue receptor material of the Young–Helmholtz theory. König admitted that the fit between the spectral absorption curve for visual yellow and the fundamental-sensation curve for the blue response in normals was much less exact than that between the visual purple absorption curve and the spectral luminosity curve (see Figure 11.5) (p. 351). But the agreement was close enough, he argued, to lend support to the identification of visual yellow with the blue receptor material.

One consequence of this hypothesis is that the fovea, lacking cones and visual purple, must be blue blind! König produced several empirical demonstrations of the truth of this remarkable deduction. If we fixate the center of a row of intense blue dots, then a number of the surrounding dots will disappear, indicating a blue blind region of 55 to 70 minutes of angle at the center of the fovea. Using only this same tiny region, he claimed to be able to match all the spectral colors with binary mixtures of light of 475 and 650 nanometers. In short, the central region of the fovea behaves as if it were dichromatic. One of the resulting response curves allegedly conformed very closely to the green response curve of real dichromats and the other showed some similarity to the red response curve (pp. 355–57).

König had no less radical claims to make about the red- and green-sensitive substances required by the Young–Helmholtz theory. In May 1894 he published the results of research done with Johannes Zumft, in which they had employed Heinrich Müller's venerable (and difficult) method of entoptical retinal shadows to determine the depth within the retinal layer at which light is perceived (König 1894b[23]). Their results suggested that homogeneous blue and violet lights were perceived at a depth that could correspond to the outer members of the cones, but that homogeneous reds and greens were perceived at a deeper level that lay beyond the cones altogether and corresponded to the pigment epithelium. König claimed that this finding refuted all color theories like those of Donders, Wundt, and Ladd-Franklin that traced color perception to modifications of a single substance, and also theories like those of Hering and Ebbinghaus that postulated a single substance for red and green and another for yellow and blue (p. 337). A month later König cited these results in arguing that the cones function only as dioptric apparatus to focus light on the epithelium. Rods, then, with their visual purple mediate gray sensations in dim light and blue sensations in strong light; cones mediate the green and red responses in strong light, although they do not actually contain the photosensitive substances. High-intensity whites arise from the fusion of blue, green, and red sensations as claimed by Young and Helmholtz; those whites are not to be confused with the low-intensity grays produced directly by the bleaching of visual purple in the rods (König 1894c[24], 363).

König advanced this theory very tentatively. Ladd-Franklin, who was in close touch with König at the time of its creation, claimed that he himself did not take it seriously (Ladd-Franklin 1895, 104). Whatever König thought of his creation, the tenets of the theory suggest the constitutive role of the Helmholtz–Hering controversy during this period. The theory explained the Purkinje phenomenon and the peculiarities of monochromatism and its relationship to normal vision within a framework that required only minor modifications of the Young–Helmholtz theory. It eliminated the necessity of postulating spectral response curves for the fundamental sensations that were themselves functions of intensity. This not only avoided introducing an inelegant and arbitrary element into Young's theory; it also ensured the validity of Newton's law at sufficiently high levels of intensity—a methodological stricture essential to the Young–Helmholtz research program. We do not know whether Helmholtz, who died that September, knew and approved of the theory or not, although König indicates that he participated in some of the experimental work during that busy spring.

Whether the theory was a speculative flyer, a final grasp at independence and immortality, or an act of homage to his patron and master, König paid a heavy price for it. His claim for the blue blindness of the fovea, especially, was attacked or ignored in embarrassed silence within the Helmholtzian camp. Ladd-Franklin, who herself attacked the theory in 1895, later claimed that Johannes von Kries and Willibald Nagel pointedly omitted mention of König and much of his work from the third edition of the *Handbuch* because they found the theory such an embarrassment (Ladd-Franklin 1895, 104). Hering, of course, came down upon the theory like a wolf upon a deserted lamb. He observed sarcastically that every daylight visual experience of our lives proves that the fovea is not blue blind. König had been the victim of theoretical preconceptions. His "incoherent" physiological theory required a blue blind fovea and, despite all the uncertainties of accurately determining colors in very small fields, he had convinced himself that he had found it (Hering 1894b[75], 403–5, 411–14).

The more technical arguments that Hering marshaled against König were skillfully designed to undermine confidence in the response curves measured by him and Dieterici. König had supported his claim for the blue blindness of the fovea with a series of dichromat color equations made with binary mixtures of light of 475 and 650 nanometers. Hering pointed out that 475 nanometers is very near the wavelength for which, according to König, the fovea is supposed to be blind! How could it make any contribution to the equations? Hering went on to show that König's own experimental curves of his so-called fundamental sensations place an upper bound on the green-to-red ratio of any light mixed from these particular two wavelengths. But again König's own curves showed that all homogeneous lights from green to cyan-blue have green-to-red ratios that exceed that upper bound; no dichromat lacking the blue fundamental sensation can match those lights with any mixture of these two wavelengths. The fovea may be green blind or red blind or red-green blind, but it cannot be blue blind; König's own data show his claim to be "impossible as well as wrong" (pp. 408–9). König was still obsessed with his curves, Hering charged, even though "scarcely anybody attributes a real significance to them any more except König and his coworkers" (p. 407).

These were criticisms too serious to ignore. König conceded that Hering's charges about the green-red ratio were "formally correct," but that the experimental indeterminacy of the blue fundamental response curve was sufficiently large as to permit adjustments that would accommodate his foveal equations (König 1895a[25]). Hering naturally replied that experimental uncertainties that large inspired no confidence in the theory they were supposed to confirm, and he promptly raised the ante of the controversy (Hering 1895b[77]). Many histologists, Hering charged, described the rod-free area of the fovea as extending over as much as four degrees of arc. If blue blindness extends over that whole rod-free area, as König's hypothesis seemed to require, then every color equation made in Berlin since 1888 had been made in a blue blind area of the retina and their results rendered totally inexplicable![9] König did not reply directly to this gibe. He did, however, retreat somewhat from his original claim that the central fovea does not see blue at all, although he continued to insist that it is dichromatic (König 1897d[31]).

THE DUPLICITY THEORY OF VISION

The uproar that followed König's theory gave way quickly to controversy over another hypothesis, one that Johannes von Kries advanced on the heels of König's notorious article of 1894 (Kries 1894, 1896). Kries proposed that achromatic vision at low light intensities and with dark-adapted eyes is mediated solely by the visual purple in the rods; chromatic vision at higher intensities after adaptation to bright light is mediated by the three processes of the Young–Helmholtz theory located in the cones. Rod vision and cone vision have different sensitivity thresholds for different homogeneous lights, the former being far more sensitive to blue than to yellow and practically insensitive to reds. The Purkinje phenomenon and the shift from the dark- to the bright-spectrum luminosity distribution are caused by the gradual replacement of rod vision by cone vision as intensity increases, as visual purple is bleached out, and as the eye adapts to higher intensities. Kries thus retained all the elements of König's theory that were most dramatically supported by the experimental findings out of Berlin, while jettisoning the most controversial ones, including all

physiological speculation about the blue, green, and red receptor substances, the claim for the blue blindness of the fovea, and the identification of the blue sensation with visual yellow (Kries 1894, 67).

Kries presented his "duplicity theory of vision"—the name he soon
adopted for the hypothesis—as supplementing rather than challenging
any existing theories of vision. He insisted that it should create "no con-
sternation" among those who, like himself, supported the Young–
Helmholtz theory, or who supported zone theories with different color-
coding mechanisms active at the periphery and the center. The duplicity
hypothesis modified the Young–Helmholtz theory only to the extent of
postulating a separate achromatic process responsible for producing low-
intensity grays. Kries even bid for Hering's support. He wrote that the
central assumption of the duplicity theory "is naturally even more compatible" with Hering's theory than with Young's, since Hering had always postulated a separate achromatic process (p. 69). Kries did point
out that his theory required Hering to abandon the specific brightness of
colors, since the effects that Hillebrand sought to explain were better accommodated by the hypothesis of separate rod and cone vision.

Kries' proposal placed Hering and his followers in a strategic quandary
as whether to reject it or claim it as their own. With some justification,
Hering hailed the duplicity theory as a concession wrung from Helmholtz's followers by his own long insistence on an achromatic process
independent of the chromatic ones (Hering 1898[78], 105–7; Hering and
Brückner 1903[82], 535–36). With less plausibility, he even bragged that
Kries and König had borrowed their new account of the Purkinje phenomenon from his idea that colored lights possess particular white valences (Hering 1895a[76], 520). But Hering would not accept one implication of Kries' theory, which according to Hering was the only point
in which Kries had gone beyond what Kühne had proposed long ago.
Hering would not accept Kries' recourse to a "double white"—rod-white
and cone-white. Hering would support only a version of the duplicity
theory in which rods contain the black-white process of the opponent
process theory, while cones contain the blue-yellow and green-red processes, as well as a black-white process identical to that found in the rods.

Over time, that position came to entail severe difficulties for Hering's
school. It obliged them to defend the specific brightness of colors as an
explanation of the Purkinje effect. Specific brightnesses, however, remained as vulnerable as ever to the alleged experimental refutation that
Ebbinghaus had posed in 1891, namely, that brightness equations made
from the four "pure" colors of the opponent process theory do not persist
with changes of intensity. Other problems also emerged. By 1905, for
example, Kries was making much of the finding that the "white valence
curve" obtained by Hillebrand for a dark-adapted eye in the center did

not match the luminosity distribution of the bright spectrum in a bright-adapted eye on the far periphery. Since Hering's theory predicted that in both cases only the white-black process is present and active, the two curves should be the same (Kries 1905, 203). Hering's theory also predicted, in violation of numerous experimental claims, that there should be no sharp distinction between the rod-free foveal region and the rest of the retina for all strictly achromatic phenomena; also, Hering's theory left the relationship of visual purple to the black-white process unexplained.

Despite the vulnerability of Hering's position on these matters, his students rallied to his cause. In a major paper of 1898, Tschermak argued that all color equations persist unaltered with proportional changes in the intensities of the component lights, so long as the adaptation of the eye is held constant. Previous experiments that showed the contrary, including the one performed by Ebbinghaus, had simply failed to control for adaptation. To this Kries countered that adaptation *and* light intensity were crucial to the Purkinje effect and so to the outcome of all experiments like that of Ebbinghaus. Kries introduced experimental data showing that departures from Newton's law were dramatically obvious in the green blind eyes of his collaborator Willibald Nagel, and readily observable in his own normal eyes. Tschermak, Kries alleged, had failed to hold firm fixation during his experiments and had allowed local adaptation to equalize the two adjoining, achromatic fields employed in Ebbinghaus's experiment (Kries 1899; Kries and Nagel 1896, 1900).

Hering's student Carl Hess assumed the burden of arguing that differences between the fovea and the periphery as to adaptation and achromatic vision occur gradually and continuously with increasing eccentricity and cannot be associated strictly with the presence or absence of rods, as Kries' theory required (Hess 1897). In 1897 Hering and Hess reported their investigation of two monochromats, neither of which showed the central scotoma that Ladd-Franklin had found in her monochromat of 1894 and that was predicted by the duplicity theory (Hering 1898[78]). These papers forced minor concessions out of Kries and Nagel. By 1900 they admitted that limited dark adaptation does somehow occur in the central, rod-free area of the fovea, and that a central scotoma was not an invariable concomitant of monochromatism (Tschermak 1902, 790; Kries 1899; Kries and Nagel 1900; Nagel 1909, 379–80). Controversy continued over the so-called Purkinje afterimage and whether it can occur in the fovea, and whether hemeralopia (night-blindness) can be attributed to an absence of visual purple in the rods (Hillebrand 1929, 82–89).

Among these controversies over foveal vision, the most intense concerned the Purkinje phenomenon and whether it can be observed in the rod-free central zone. This debate was complicated by uncertainty about the microscopic anatomy of the central fovea, as well as about exactly what the Purkinje phenomenon was. Hering in 1895 had tried to show that, at least for some intensity ranges, the phenomenon is triggered by changes in the overall adaptation in the eye to the prevailing illumination rather than, as Helmholtz's followers more readily assumed, by the changing intensities of the colored fields themselves (Hering 1895a[76]). Kries, König, Nagel, and Otto Lummer insisted that the Purkinje phenomenon cannot be observed in the central fovea, while Tschermak, Hess, and Felix Koester all insisted that it could be (Hillebrand 1929, 89–97; Nagel 1909, 357–65; Tschermak 1902, 780–800, 790; Kries 1897a). Hering's last scientific paper, appearing in 1915, was an attempt to demonstrate that the phenomenon occurs in the fovea (Hering 1915[84]). Many factors—the rapidity of chromatic adaptation in the region, the necessity of rigid fixation, and the difficulty of color judgments in small fields—made it a difficult phenomenon to investigate and left much room for methodological disagreements.

THE DUPLICITY THEORY AND THE LARGER CONTROVERSY

By 1894 the focus of color vision debates in Germany had begun to shift decisively from color blindness and chromatic perception to adaptation and achromatic vision. The scientific literature on color perception fell from 25.7 percent of the total output on vision studies in 1880–84 to 15.9 percent in 1890–94. The share devoted to adaptation and intensity, however, rose about 2 percent, even though the real burgeoning of this literature occurred after 1896 (categories 21.1 and 23, Table 1, Appendix). König greeted this change as "a new stage in the struggle among color-theories" (König 1896[27]), and Kries was even more explicit. He conceded in 1894 that ignorance of rod function had led him (and by implication many others) to "contradictory and confusing results" in many experiments done in the past, and he called for a new experimental research program designed to isolate and study cone function apart from that of the rods (Kries 1894, 69–70). This program involved much closer attention to intensity levels and states of adaptation, and it involved primarily studying visual sensation in the central fovea. Kries and Nagel pursued that program faithfully at least until the latter's death in 1910, and Hering and his students were drawn relentlessly into it because of their theoretical stake in the outcome.

Now the duplicity theory no more contradicted Hering's theory than Young's, and by the early twentieth century support for the opponent process theory, as a theory of chromatic perception, seems to have been on the rise despite running attacks by Kries (Kries 1899). Ludimar Hermann's 1892 textbook edition had devoted only eleven lines to Hering's theory of color vision, compared to a long and supportive cataloguing of the achievements of the Young–Helmholtz theory. His edition of 1905, however, not only gave equal space to the two theories but seemed to lean distinctly toward Hering. Hermann declared that theory to be "in very good agreement" with the data on color blindness, praised the clean fit of the theory with our color intuitions, accepted Hering's theory of simultaneous contrast over Helmholtz's, and pointed out no specific weaknesses of Hering's theory, even though it mentioned several with respect to Young's.

Those signs of support notwithstanding, Hering's decision to oppose the duplicity theory of vision committed his school to a losing scientific cause. Although Hess, Tschermak, and Hillebrand were able to discomfort Kries and Nagel and wring from them a few minor concessions, those efforts diverted them from elaborating and defending Hering's theory as a model of *chromatic* perception. Despite their efforts, the duplicity theory seems to have been quickly adopted by most physiologists and ophthalmologists in Germany, and by practically all of them abroad (Parsons 1924, 215–25).

Even among themselves Hering's followers never reached consensus about how to deal with the duplicity theory and its challenges. Carl Hess never deviated from Hering's personal line, but Armin Tschermak was much more willing to compromise. In a review of the literature written in 1902, Tschermak declared the duplicity theory "open to discussion" and found the specific brightness of colors inadequate to explain certain phenomena connected with peripheral color vision that he had discovered. While he insisted that the Purkinje phenomenon does occur in the fovea, he admitted that it is much weaker there than outside (Hess 1922; Tschermak 1902, 791–92; 1942, 65–69). Hering's English student, W.H.R. Rivers, reviewed the criticisms of Hering and Hess in 1900 and concluded that they did "not tell seriously against the [duplicity] theory" (Rivers 1900, 1104). Franziska Hillebrand, writing in 1929, admitted that the one weakness of Hering's theory lay in the remaining uncertainty about the relationship of the achromatic to the chromatic processes (Hillebrand 1929, 82–89). Even Hering, in a rare concession to his opponents, confessed that the close similarity of the visual purple absorption curve with the luminosity curve of the total color blind supported Kries' theory, even though he himself did not find that evidence conclusive (Hering 1898[78], 112). As the school's position on achromatic perception became increasingly untenable, its account of the chromatic mechanisms was impugned by implication.

These strategic developments explain why Johannes von Kries was consistently less willing to compromise on the issue of color theory than he had been on the issue of spatial perception. When he reviewed the field in 1910, he conceded that Helmholtz's original theory must be modified by the addition of the duplicity theory, by Fick's displacement hypothesis (which Kries had belatedly come to espouse), and by acceptance of retinal induction effects to explain contrast. With those amendments, he wrote confidently that "even at the present time the theory of Helmholtz is thoroughly justified as to its fundamental conceptions, it is in close agreement with the facts, and as an hypothesis it is qualified to explain a very large mass of actual phenomena" (Kries 1910, 426). He pointed especially to the brilliant success of the theory in explaining dichromatism and in showing it to be a reduction form of normal trichromatic vision, and to the comparable success of the duplicity theory in explaining the characteristics of monochromatism (p. 402). Kries appealed for a return to an aggressive program of color matching and colorimetric analysis such as that begun by König. That data, he claimed, have yielded all our surest knowledge about color vision, and in the absence of reliable physiological and photochemical observations, are likely to continue to do so (pp. 453–54).

Kries still found the opponent process theory hopelessly deficient. Its attempt to explain monochromatism through the hypothesis of the specific brightnesses of colors has been totally discredited, he insisted. It still cannot explain the existence of the red and green blind—classes that Kries had successfully renamed protanopes and deuteranopes in 1897 (Kries 1897b). The attempt of Hess and Tschermak to impugn their existence as distinct classes had foundered on these men's failure to eliminate the effects of rod vision in their experiments. The continued insistence of Hering's school that the distinction between protanopes and deuteranopes is "coincidental and unimportant" has had a deleterious effect upon the entire field, for it has disparaged and discouraged the program of experimental color matching (Kries 1910, 452). As for the widely felt need for a color theory that will affirm the simple and primitive nature of our yellow and white sensations as well as those of green, blue, and red, Kries insisted that such a theory is compatible with and easily derived from the principles of Helmholtz. Kries reminded his readers that he had long ago called for a zone theory, in which a three-variable input from the retinal periphery would be reprocessed centrally to the number of simple sensations dictated by intuition.

The acceptance of Kries' duplicity theory and tacit agreement that separate mechanisms exist for chromatic and (some) achromatic perceptions effectively ended the second stage of the color vision debates in Germany. Despite the continuing controversy about vision in the central fovea, that acceptance seems to have been achieved by 1910 at the latest. By then the controversy had changed in other respects. At least six nonaligned members of the controversy's core set had proposed color theories of their own. The issue was no longer a flat choice between two competing theories, but a choice of the particular characteristics of those theories that should be preserved and incorporated into some final theoretical synthesis. The controversy was also changing in still deeper ways to be examined in the following chapters. By 1915 German research and German theoretical debates no longer monopolized physiological optics; the school debate within Germany was splintering along disciplinary lines; and Ewald Hering's powerful personality no longer dominated the course of the dispute.

CHAPTER TWELVE

The Roots of Incommensurability

THROUGHOUT the course of the Helmholtz–Hering controversy, as previous chapters have shown, the focal problems of the dispute shifted, the relative strength of the schools waxed and waned, and the positions of the antagonists changed in fundamental ways. Nevertheless, after four decades of intense exchange, the dispute remained as far from resolution as it had been at the beginning; neither the ascendance of nativism nor Hering's defeat in his opposition to the duplicity theory remotely constituted a definitive closure. That fact poses a historical problem. Why was one school unable to achieve a decisive victory; or, failing that, why could no acceptable compromise be reached on the central issues? Why, at the very least, could the partisans not agree that the outstanding issues were temporarily beyond empirical resolution and that the dispute should therefore be suspended?

Perceptive contemporaries recognized that the particular intractability of this controversy arose from deep differences of aim and program that separated the protagonists, and perhaps from differences of language and conception that lay deeper still. Franz Hillebrand wrote that beyond all the differences of theory and method that divided Helmholtz and Hering lay a fundamental difference of *Denkrichtung* (Hillebrand 1918; 1929, 189–91, 198–200). Helmholtz, according to Hillebrand, assumed the epistemological primacy of physical space and physical processes and asked how closely our visual images of objects correspond to that reality. Hering, in contrast, attributed epistemological primacy to the phenomenological characteristics of the perception or intuition. He asked, "Why do objects which we see come to be charged with just those locational and other properties with which they appear to us?" (Hillebrand 1918, 87–95).

Christine Ladd-Franklin wrote even more pointedly abut the fundamental incompatibility of the rival theories. "There is no occasion for considering," she wrote in one critique, "all the minor merits and demerits of the Helmholtz and Hering theories. The situation is simply that Hering confutes Helmholtz and Helmholtz confutes Hering" (Ladd-Franklin 1924, 2:465). Elsewhere she wrote that these two theories

> have each its own language, and no one can write, or speak, for five minutes
> on the subject of colour without giving away that he does or does not accept

certain of the fundamental assumptions of one or the other. Thus the view of Hering that the subjective intensity of, say, a whitish bluish green is due solely to the subjective intensity of its whiteness component, either is or is not a part of the speaker's mental furniture. (Ladd-Franklin 1916, 135)

The particular forms of intractability that Hillebrand and Ladd-Franklin emphasized are closely related to the concept that Thomas S. Kuhn introduced in his original treatment of scientific revolutions in 1962: that of incommensurability. Kuhn argued that deep cognitive change in science (like that associated with scientific revolutions) is marked by a clash of competing worldviews in which the protagonists of one view find it impossible to grasp the perspective of their opponents fully and correctly (Kuhn 1962, 110–34). More important, the two sets of antagonists find it difficult to define or to agree upon common, commensurable criteria by which they might measure and compare the relative success or failure of their rival traditions.

In his original formulation Kuhn discussed at least three distinct forms in which the incommensurability of scientific worldviews manifests itself, and as various commentators have noted, his own understanding of incommensurability changed significantly in his subsequent writings. He began to use the term more and more to describe a relationship between rival scientific theories or programs and their vocabularies than a relationship between consecutive normal science traditions per se (Hoyningen-Huene 1990; 1993, 212–18). This shift decoupled the notion of incommensurability from the model of change through sequential revolutions and made it more directly applicable to scientific controversy in general. As such, it has gradually emerged as the most far-reaching and controversial element in Kuhn's legacy to science studies. It also sheds particular light upon the intractability of the Helmholtz–Hering controversy.

INCOMMENSURABILITIES OF PROGRAM

Kuhn's original discussion of the roots of incommensurability emphasized how problems, problem priorities, and solution criteria typically change from one normal science tradition to the next, so that there can be at best only partial agreement between the traditions on what questions are most important or on the evidential value of particular results. The Helmholtz–Hering controversy clearly evinced what might be called programmatic incommensurabilities of this kind. The two sides investigated quite similar problems, but they assigned them radically different priorities. For example, Hering's followers and most unaffiliated members of the core set accorded very high priority to discovering and accounting for the hues that the color blind actually see; Helmholtz's school thought this so uncertain and unimportant as hardly to constitute a scientific problem at all. König and his co-workers emphasized colorimetry and the determination of spectral response curves; Hering and his students took little interest in research of this kind. They did not dismiss it altogether, but they discounted the results as unimportant and potentially fraudulent. Although the schools could agree about many things that a theory of vision should do and show, they could not agree about which of these things was most fundamental and pressing.

This inability to agree about priorities left the schools with no clearly commensurable criteria for judging the comparative success and failure of their research programs or the progressiveness and problem-solving capacity of their traditions. Helmholtz's school, for example, regarded the empirical trichromacy and trivariability of normal vision as the fundamental facts of vision research. They often treated Young's theory as little more than an unproblematic generalization from these indisputable facts of empirical colorimetry. Hering's school accepted the same facts, but discounted their importance because they only weakly constrained the actual range of possible color theories. Conversely, Hering's school always considered the blue and yellow visual perceptions of most dichromats as definitively falsifying the Young–Helmholtz theory, and held that their opponents perversely and illogically refused to acknowledge the refutation. The Helmholtz school responded that Young's theory alone could explain the colorimetric data of color blindness, in particular the classes of protanopes and deuteranopes.

This striking absence of common criteria for theory assessment extended well beyond the circle of partisans. The most casual survey of textbooks from the early twentieth century shows that texts that rejected the Young–Helmholtz theory nearly always did so on the grounds that it could not explain the facts of color blindness, while Hering's theory did so successfully. Ironically, those that rejected Hering's theory did so on exactly the same grounds: that it failed to explain color blindness while Young's theory succeeded in that regard.

THE PROBLEM OF BRIGHTNESS

The failure of mutual understanding between the schools of Helmholtz and Hering showed itself most clearly where the issues were most fundamental, as in the schools' differing appreciation of brightness. As a cornerstone of his approach to physiological optics, Hering had erected the iconoclastic doctrine that black constitutes a variable sensory quality like green or blue. The brightness of an achromatic sensation follows from the ratio of extreme white to extreme black that it contains; the sequence of all possible grays is not to be thought of as an "intensity series," in which some fixed quality called brightness increases steadily with increase of the physical intensity of the stimulus. Hering did not deny that brightness (read whiteness) generally grew with the physical intensity of the stimulating light, but he regarded this as an extremely rough correlation, readily overridden by the eye's state of adaptation and various contrast effects. This understanding carried over into his treatment of all sensations as separable into chromatic and achromatic parts, with the brightness of the total sensation largely governed by the white-black ratio of the achromatic element.[1]

Commentators outside the school did not so much disagree with these claims as fail to comprehend them. Hering's teachings about brightness encountered perplexed opposition in many quarters of the core set. Helmholtz spoke for all his followers in claiming that he could "personally form no conception [*keine Anschauung bilden*] of a color, which could have no degree of greater or lesser brightness at all" (*PO2*, 378). Christine Ladd-Franklin judged that Hering had fallen into "a quite hopeless confusion between our ideas of the *brightness* and the *relative whiteness* of a given sensation" (Ladd-Franklin 1892b, 67). Adolf Fick disclaimed any understanding of Hering, yet still attacked his ideas. He argued that when he looked at a piece of black paper and gradually lowered the illumination until the paper appeared black, he perceived a quantitative change in the sensation but not a qualitative one. All light sensations, not just white ones, pass into black as their intensity is lowered; to Fick this suggested that black stands in no special relationship to white and that brightness is more closely correlated with intensity than with whiteness (Fick 1879, 205–6). Black constitutes a kind of "absolute zero" of vision, much as absolute silence does for the ear (Fick 1900).

This web of disagreements embraced terminology, concepts, and empirical predictions. Kries, seizing upon the remarks of Fick, wrote that introspection simply does not allow us to decide whether the black-white series is a qualitative change of a single sensory modality, with the so-called *Eigengrau* as the midpoint, or a quantitative change in the white sensation, with black as its zero point (Kries 1882, 43). Hillebrand replied to Kries, criticizing his cavalier dismissal of the important and phenomenologically accessible distinction between series marked by changes of quality and those marked by changes of intensity. The brightness of a chromatic sensation may be associated with the physical intensity of the stimulus, but is not determined by it. Using the famous Hering color box, Hillebrand demonstrated that although brown is an orange of low brightness, at least some browns cannot be obtained by adjusting the physical intensity of orange fields. He insisted that these browns arise only through simultaneous contrast effects, in which bright surrounds physiologically reduce the brightness of orange fields (Hillebrand 1889, 73–74, 78–83, 85–87). Hillebrand charged that Kries, by ignoring Hering's distinction between quality and intensity or dismissing it as "merely" semantic, had been led into completely false understandings of sensations and their origins.

These elements of incommensurability can be analyzed readily at the level of semantics, problem priorities, and lexical ostensions—all emphasized by Kuhn. In 1962, however, Kuhn had also emphasized another manifestation of incommensurability. He insisted that before and after the paradigm changes that characterize scientific revolutions, scientists will literally "see the world of their research-engagement differently," and will do so in so fundamental and literal a sense that we may speak of scientists as "responding to a different world" after such a revolution (Kuhn 1962, 110). He portrayed the intellectual conversion that comes with paradigm change as fundamentally perceptual in character and at one point compared it literally to a gestalt shift.

Although Kuhn's subsequent discussions have largely abandoned the search for perceptual roots of incommensurability, his original formulation leaves the interesting question of whether basic differences of perception might have affected the Helmholtz–Hering controversy. Could the followers of Helmholtz and Hering literally have "seen the world differently" through the eye pieces of their colorimeters and on the colored papers of their afterimage experiments? That question cannot be settled, but it deserves consideration. During the period of this study researchers insisted that introspective, visual observations, if they were to have scientific credence, should be carried out by practiced, expert observers. The training and practice that go into the making of expertise, however, imply a process of differential sensitization to particular elements in the sensory compound. The analysis of one's private visual experiences demands first learning, and then applying, expected relationships of similarity and dissimilarity acquired from exemplars of those relationships. Within the work-a-day tradition of a single laboratory, that could plausibly have led adepts to see compounds in particular ways.

Consider the particular kinds of perceptual sensitivity or sensory orientation required to appreciate brightness phenomena as Hering did. One is a strong awareness of a range of black and blacker sensations darker than the *Eigengrau*, and the ability to imagine the occurrence of these sensations. That dark series could then be readily regarded as equally rich and extended as those of our common bright sensations, and so plausibly juxtaposed to them as an opponent visual process. Normal visual experience rarely makes this range of dark sensations available, however; they are obtained mainly through afterimage and contrast experiments. Hering and his school specialized in the study of exactly these phenomena. Hering began his study of visual sensation with them, and his students Carl Hess, Moriz Sachs, and Hugo Pretori pioneered the quantitative study of color and brightness contrast in a series of classic papers of the 1890s (Hess and Pretori 1894; Pretori and Sachs 1895). These circumstances cannot prove, but do plausibly suggest, that a conflation of theoretical structures, perceptual sensitivities, and experimental programmatics induced Hering and his students literally to see and hence to think of black sensations in ways not shared by others.

Hering's conception of sensory compounds also promoted a perceptual awareness of gray independent of intensity. In ordinary life, gray sensations often serve as signs of the intensity of the prevailing illumination and the circumstances accompanying it. The grayness of dawn, for example, offers an implicit comparison with daylight illumination and predicts the time before sunrise. We carry this implicit and functional association of grayness with intensity into artificial experiments on vision and into our theorizing about the gray series. Conceptually dissociating grayness from stimulus intensity first required perceptually decoupling them. In various writings Hering presented experiments designed to allow the subject to perceive the same gray under many different levels of illumination. These experiments not only demonstrated Hering's theoretical point; they also sensitized the observer to perceive gray as a sensory compound in a way naive observers normally could not do.

Hering's concepts also put a premium upon the ability to "see" how chromatic sensations are "veiled" by a particular gray. Hering wrote of this that "practice is important here; but even the most practiced observer, who can easily say which of two adjacent colors is the clearer when they have the same hue and the same *kind* of veiling, often finds it impossible to do so for colors of different hues or when they are veiled by different kinds of black-white colors" (Hering 1964/1905, 53). The problem, Hering went on, is particularly acute for the bright spectral aperture colors used in physiological experimentation. While we can readily see an admixture of white in such lights, they do not appear to naive observers to have a dark component at all, and hence these observers usually fail to see a veiling if it has been done with gray or black. Observers usually attribute differences in the sensation that arise from this kind of veiling to differences in the intensity of the chromatic part, and hence fall into error. Hering insisted that the ability to see the gray nuancing or veiling in a chromatic sensation is similar to the ability to "hear out" the separate notes in a chord or the overtones in a compound tone: it could be acquired through training and attention (pp. 56–65). Hering thus claimed explicitly that he and his students had sensitized themselves to perceive a gray nuancing in chromatic sensations whereas others saw only differences of brightness.

These tentative arguments suggest that the failure of the two schools to fully understand one another flowed plausibly from basic differences in sensory content. The key partisans may not have been "responding to different worlds," as Kuhn suggested, but to very different perceptual sensitivities. That suggestion does not imply that Hering's school tapped into some deep ground of phenomenological reality unavailable to its opponents, or that these sensitivites expressed themselves in particular experimental outcomes that its opponents could not accept or replicate. It does not imply that possessing these special perceptual sensitivities was a necessary condition for accepting Hering's theories and his program. It does imply that perceptual incommensurability in the original Kuhnian sense may partly explain why Hering's school clung so long and tenaciously to a theoretical concept of brightness so far outside the scientific mainstream.

Suggestions about what partisans "saw" cannot go beyond speculation. Nevertheless, it is significant that Hering's laboratory students—Hillebrand, Hess, Tschermak, Garten, Sachs—accepted his claims about the nature of black and of brightness, while others in the core set who were generally sympathetic to Hering's program and his phenomenological approach did not necessarily do so. Among the rash of color theories that proliferated at the turn of the century, many adopted key elements of Hering's system, including the existence of four simple chromatic colors, their antagonistic action, his explanation of simultaneous contrast, and some elements of his account of color blindness. Yet for all that, not one preserved and adopted the full equivalence and antagonism of black and white, which was the cornerstone of Hering's theory and the key to his unique understanding of brightness.[2] This curious fact suggests that the ability to understand Hering's claims and to find them compelling rested upon a sort of tacit knowledge, closely related to perceptual sensitivities, which was elaborated and transmitted only within Hering's institute and as part of its experimental program. This aspect of incommensurability divided Hering's students not only from the opposing set of partisans, but also from other members of the core set who lacked access to these forms of tacit knowledge.

SEMANTICS AND INCOMMENSURABILITY

Kuhn's original discussion of incommensurability had emphasized the importance of semantic differences. The operative concepts in two successive normal science traditions typically change significantly, either by ostension (when an object or phenomenon shifts into a different conceptual category) or by intension, if a concept's meaning per se changes (Kuhn 1962, 110–34; Hoyningen-Huene 1990; 1993, 206–12). Nevertheless, the semantic roots of incommensurability had taken second place to perceptual ones in his earliest formulations.

In his later writings Kuhn largely ceased to describe incommensurability in psychological-perceptual terms and emphasized semantic elements instead, particularly conflicting ostensions. Kuhn held that the tacit knowledge that constitutes the scientist's world and underlies his practice is embodied in perceived relationships of similarity and dissimilarity among objects, phenomena, and problems. These relationships are not learned through definitions, but through supervised exposure to "exemplars" of these relationships. For this reason, they often cannot be conceptually formulated, and they come to embody chains of implicit expectations and associations that have been tacitly acquired (Kuhn 1970, 191–207; 1974; 1979, esp. 417).

By the end of the 1970s Kuhn's conception of incommensurability had completed its linguistic turn. His formulations attributed incommensurability more and more to the impossibility of fully translating all the terms and statements in the "lexical structure" characterizing one paradigm into that of its successor. Kuhn held that theoretical languages constitute linguistic grids as do natural languages, grids that express the complex network of ostensions and similarity relationships available to a native speaker of that language. This formulation also admitted degrees of incommensurability. If not all statements can be translated from one language into that of an incommensurable successor or rival, many can be. And Kuhn held out the possibility that even when actual translation was impossible, an individual might become "bilingual," by learning the series of ostensions in the other language, just as he had learned those of his own as a native (Kuhn 1970, 198–204; 1979; 1983; Hoyningen-Huene 1990, 487–88).

The Helmholtz–Hering controversy evinced with special clarity the role of semantic incommensurability and its consequences. Basic disagreements about lexical ostensions pervaded the controversy and prevented efficient communication between the schools. One school grouped yellow with the mixed sensations, the other with simple ones; one grouped simultaneous contrast with the class of optical illusions, the other with the class of pure sensations. Most important, however, was the similarity relationship on which the nativist-empiricist controversy turned. Is the "spatiality" that accompanies a visual point-image to be grouped with the class of sensations, so that depth, for example, becomes like a color or like a degree of brightness? Or is the spatiality to be classed with the perceptions, so that it becomes analogous to the recognition of a familiar object or a pattern we have encountered before?

Semantic incommensurability expressed itself in other ways. While Helmholtz's language mostly incorporated traditional terminology, plus a few innovations by Fechner and Brücke, Hering created a broad and innovative body of new terms that quickly came to define and characterize his school and differentiate it from its opponents. Terms like *Sehraum, Sehding, Kernflache, Raumwert, Umstimmung, Gegenfarben*, and the *Reinheit, Nuancierung*, or *Verhüllung* of colors do not all translate easily into English, and not all found ready equivalents in the alternate German terminology used by Helmholtz's students. Hering never chose terms lightly and never without polemical awareness. His refusal to employ the almost universal term "saturation" (*Sättigung*) to describe chromatic sensations typified his approach. He insisted that "saturation" had been corrupted by Helmholtz's use of the word to describe both the whiteness adhering in sensations due to homogeneous light and the whiteness arising from broad-band illumination; this conflation allegedly imposed physicalist connotations upon all talk about desaturated sensations. Worst of all, according to Hering, "saturation" as used by Helmholtz's school always denoted the ratio of chromatic content to white, whereas colors could potentially be mixed with any gray or even black (Hering 1964/1905, 41–44). Hering originally spoke of the "purity" of a color in this regard, but he increasingly moved toward a description of colors as "nuanced" or "veiled." This preferred terminology semantically required that the sensation by which colors were veiled be specified.

The preceding chapters have offered many examples of the critical struggle for semantic control in the Helmholtz–Hering controversy, especially in Hering's polemical strategy. At the beginning of his career, for example, Hering campaigned to redefine the idea of retinal correspondence so that it denoted the pairing of points with the same visual direction. He knew that this redefinition would bring with it tacit acceptance of much of his theory of spatiality. In the same spirit his student Tschermak sought to redefine the notion of the vertical horopter in order to link it to Hering's concept of the core plane—or so Kries and his students charged in their attempts to head off this strategy. Hering made every effort to exploit the semantic weaknesses of his opponents. As long as they insisted upon describing dichromatism as red blindness and green blindness, Hering's school held them to the literal meaning of these phrases, namely, the absence respectively of normal red and normal green sensations. He finally compelled Helmholtz's school to retreat to the more sanitized terminology of protanopia and deuteranopia. But Hering's boldest bid for semantic control came in his popular lecture of 1870, "On Memory as a General Function of Organized Matter." There, as previously noted, he sought conceptually and terminologically to conflate the "memory" of the individual with the "memory" of the species derived from its phylogenetic heritage. This metaphoric strategy, if successful, would have collapsed the nativist-empiricist controversy in a manner wholly favorable to Hering.

Hering's students carried on this semantic strategy in fully conscious fashion. Franz Hillebrand defended the importance of classification and of proper terminology. Naming is never arbitrary, he insisted, since assigning a thing to a class tacitly endows it in common usage with all the properties of that class. It followed that denoting brightness an intensity rather than a quality as Kries did imposed upon it characteristics of other intensities that contradict our phenomenological experience (Hillebrand 1889, 78–83). All Hering's supporters furthered the school's cause by unfailing recourse to Hering's language and terminology. One Helmholtz sympathizer complained that the famous research of Pretori and Sachs (1895) on the quantitative relationships of color contrast were "scarcely comprehensible except in terms of . . . [Hering's] theory" (Parsons 1924, 279). When Franz Hofmann surveyed the literature on squint in 1902, he introduced his long discussion with the claim that "it is only possible to describe binocular vision fully and correctly through use of the terminology created by Hering" (Hofmann 1902, 803–4). There as throughout his writings Hofmann rarely indulged in direct polemics, but he promoted Hering's cause through constant and self-conscious use of Hering's language and terminology.

The supporters of Helmholtz, who occupied the dominant position in the controversy and employed a more traditional terminology, found this semantic strategy frustrating and difficult to counter. To attack Hering on his own ground required that they laboriously translate their own concepts and empirical findings into the language of Hering's school, yet their attacks were commonly answered with the charge that they had not adequately understood Hering's real meaning (Hering 1887e[52], 1888c[56], 1888f[59], 1891a[69]).

Hering often attacked the Helmholtzian school for its adherence to terminology that in his opinion blurred the physical and the sensory aspects of perception and was implicitly theory-laden. He objected to terms like the "projection" of sensations, retinal fatigue, and "red" light waves. Typical of these attacks was his reply in 1887 to Sigmund Exner, who had reported a new contrast effect and had unfortunately referred to it as an "illusion of judgment" (*Urteilstäuschung*) (Exner 1885, 1887; Hering 1886[47]). Under Hering's attack, Exner replied that he had used this expression only because it "prejudiced the issue as little as possible" and that he had meant to imply nothing about the underlying causal mechanisms. Hering answered indignantly that in ordinary language an illusion of judgment implies that we take as objectively true what is actually of subjective origin. If we look at a gray spot on a red ground and see it as green, that might possibly be an illusion of judgment. But once we realize that the spot appears green because of simultaneous contrast, *and it still appears green*, then the effect is not longer a judgment and no longer an illusion but a valid sensation. It was disingenuous of Exner, Hering complained, to believe that he could use such a theory-laden term as *Urteilstäuschung* and have it not be interpreted as an espousal of the Helmholtzian theory of contrast (Hering 1887f[53]).

The Helmholtz school in turn resented tirades of this kind as fussy, pedantic, and expressly polemical in intent. Hering charged that his opponents' very terminology presupposed a perfect correspondence between wavelength and hue, intensity and brightness, saturation and colormetric purity (Hering 1887a[48]). Kries retorted that this was blatantly incorrect. Everyone understands, Kries wrote, that the correspondence between physical stimulus and sensory response is inexact. Those who use the designations interchangeably, or who speak of "red" points on the color plane, or who speak of the "brightness" of a light rather than of a light sensation, do so only to avoid circumlocutions. The correct meaning follows from the context in nearly all cases. Physiologists might disagree about whether current terminology, especially as it relates to colorimetry and the color table, requires reform, but Kries insisted that no real theoretical issue was involved. This aspect at least of his controversy with Hering "concerns nothing other than a question of more or less appropriate nomenclature" (Kries 1887b, 117).

Sometimes partisans and the nonaligned disagreed among themselves about what Hering meant. Donders dismissed Hering's theory of depth values as tautological: "Insofar as the theory is correct, it is only a descriptive paraphrase of the facts, not an explanation" (Donders 1867, 42). Aubert agreed with Donders, and Ladd-Franklin later expressed the same sentiment about Hering's theory of contrast (Aubert 1876, 616; Ladd-Franklin 1893, 83). Helmholtz and Kries, on the other hand, read strong theoretical claims into the theory of retinal space values; so did Hillebrand, who defended it as the basis of Hering's theory of spatial perception.

The Helmholtz school only occasionally criticized Hering's semantic practices, beyond their frequent use of sneer-quotes about his specialized terms. When they did it was always on the grounds of the inherent vagueness of Hering's language. In the course of a polemical exchange with Hillebrand during the early 1920s, Franz Exner praised the concepts of the Young–Helmholtz color theory—hue, saturation, and brightness—as clear and susceptible to exact mathematical and quantitative description and measurement. Exner charged that Hering's approach, in contrast, expressly rejected quantitative expressions and measurements. The heuristic formulas advanced by Hering contained variables that could not be operationalized, and his recourse to vagaries like the "clarity" or "weight" or "veiling" of sensations only made the situation worse. Exner concluded that the differences between approaches were so deep as to preclude further discussion (Exner 1921).

This semantic incommensurability between the schools explains in part why compromise proved so difficult. The proposed compromises were usually advanced by partisans of Helmholtz or by neutral members of the core set like Donders, and they were invariably rejected by Hering. He did so because the compromises proffered to him, as he saw them, were always cast in the language of his opponents. They threatened semantic and hence conceptual cooptation in return for modest theoretical concessions.

Two examples illustrate the point at issue for Hering's school. Donders, Kries, and many other theorists after them called for a zone theory compromise that would see a three-component response on the periphery providing input to sets of antagonistic responses at a higher neural level that would function somewhat like Hering's opponent mechanisms. Hering and his school consistently rejected these compromises. Hering wrote that a zone theory is possible only if the three specific energies of Young's theory are interpreted not as sensations but as "three physiological processes associated with various fibres connecting the eye and the brain" (Hering 1882[44], 88). Kries responded that that is precisely how he *did* understand them (Kries 1905, 129–32; 1910, 431; Hillebrand 1929, 96). But Hering refused this reassurance. He wrote that Helmholtz and "the scientific world" understand those specific energies not just as *Erregungsvorgänge* but also as *Empfindungsvorgänge*, that is, as being at the same time the "fundamental qualities of the sensations." After all, he noted, even Kries invariably described them as red, green, and violet sensations and treated all visual sensations as compounds of them. A zone theory understood in this way would still identify the psychophysical event yielding color sensations with mechanisms of the Young–Helmholtz type; that kind of compromise would mean the semantic and conceptual cooptation of Hering's program (Hillebrand 1929, 96; Hess 1922, 65).

Hering's school also rejected another tentative compromise sponsored by Kries. On several occasions Kries proposed in effect that empiricists acknowledge the existence of an innate and primitive spatial awareness that accompanies our earliest visual perceptions. Nativists in return would acknowledge that localization within this innate, primitive space is largely an acquired capacity, learned in the process of becoming aware of our bodies as the point of reference of our visual perceptions. Kries advocated this position as nothing more than a return to the views of Hermann Lotze and as fully consonant with Kant's original insistence on the synthetic a priori status of spatial perception. Kries even insisted that Helmholtz himself had held this position, even though he had not always recognized or publicly acknowledged it. Kries realized that this compromise would settle few of the specific issues in dispute, but he hoped that it would create common philosophical ground from which inquiry could begin (Kries 1910, 520–34).

Both Hering and Hillebrand rejected this proposal as resting on an alleged conceptual confusion they found inimical to their own program. Hillebrand wrote that the proposal assumed the existence of a "collective space" (*Gesamtraum*), a space without qualities and of which we are born with an innate awareness. It presupposed the idea of space as a "receptaculum," a propertyless container within which experience will teach us to arrange our perceptions. But, Hillebrand insisted, there can be no perception of space without the simultaneous perception of other visual qualities; where there are no qualities, there is no "place." Hering's "visual space," unlike physical space or the Kantian space of synthetic a priori perception, is not a "receptaculum" (Hillebrand 1929, 169–71). Hillebrand found the compromise proffered by Kries to be no compromise at all, since it treacherously imposed upon Hering's concepts semantic connotations alien to those of Hering's school.

The elements of semantic incommensurability that pervaded the Helmholtz–Hering controversy left the two schools in the position of separate linguistic communities. The communities found themselves forced to communicate in dissimilar dialects that left residual mistrust and uncertainty hovering about every exchange. Prestige and authority also hinged on this struggle to communicate. At stake was the monopolization of what Pierre Bourdieu called "symbolic capital"; the issue was, which dialect would establish itself as the standard or normalized language (Bourdieu 1991, 37–42, esp. 51). According to Bourdieu, cultural fields like natural science constitute special, "high-tension," linguistic markets, because they require such great investments of symbolic capital. Failure in those markets means not only marginalization, but destruction; hence the confrontations between scientific communities are typically tense and protracted.

The linguistic dynamics of the Helmholtz–Hering controversy reflected the high-stakes nature of the struggle. Terms such as "brightness," "spatiality," "local sign," and "to project" assumed incompatible, even contradictory meanings for the two schools. In Bourdieu's phrase, there were "no longer any innocent words" that could moderate the struggle for symbolic power (pp. 37–40). Nonaligned members of the core set like

Donders and Aubert advocated terminological innovations in the interest of a "neutralized language," but in general they could not escape the web of contradictory meanings that beset the controversy. Not until the late stages of the dispute did the so-called new psychologists, led by Erich Jaensch and David Katz, obtain limited success in transcending the linguistic impasse. They did so, not by reconciliation or effective translation, but by positing a new semantics that claimed to transcend both the old dialects and render them simultaneously unintelligible.

SCHOOLS AS LINGUISTIC COMMUNITIES

The incommensurability that allegedly accompanies deep cognitive change in science has not only been the most influential of Kuhn's ideas, but also one of the most controversial. He considered the incommensurability between competing paradigms to be often so fundamental that no logic of verification, no neutral observation language, no calculus of progressivity could exist that would definitively resolve the problem of theory choice. Neither for the practicing scientist, nor for the philosopher or historian of science, could there be any appeal of theory choice beyond the consensual judgment of the local scientific community as committed experts, or more specifically, to its relevant core set.

This Kuhnian shift to the community contributed to the unfolding of a rich literature on the dynamics of communities and core sets: their negotiations, rhetoric, exercise of power and control, professional investments and interests, and, sometimes, the intersection of these with larger, macrosociological interests and ideologies. In that sociological extrapolation, however, the problem of cognitive incommensurability itself was often lost. Writers simply presupposed it, or dismissed it as epiphenmenal to the social and structural dynamics of core sets. While those dynamics promised insight into the root causes of scientific change, manifestations of incommensurability promised only to show further why change was so difficult and unpredictable.

More recently Mario Biagioli has suggested that some manifestations of incommensurability may be closely tied to the sociodisciplinary interests of the scientific groups involved, and both may be central to the process of scientific change. He notes that the inability of one party in a controversy to understand or to communicate with the other—whether that inability be feigned or real—might under certain circumstances further the sociodisciplinary status of the group. Incommensurability might then function like a sterility barrier in speciation events; it can constitute an antiswamping device that allows a new tradition to establish itself and compete effectively. In periods of theory choice, rival scientific traditions "do not need to talk to one another" and the occurrence of deep change may depend upon their not doing so (Biagioli 1990, 184–85).

This perspective captures an element fundamental to the Helmholtz–Hering controversy. The Helmholtz school, as the dominant tradition, had little to gain from legitimizing Hering through direct confrontation. In the 1870s and early 1880s they pursued a "strategy of noncommunication," during which—with some notable exceptions—they largely ignored Hering or professed an inability to understand him. They left critical comparison of the two theories largely to figures like Donders, du Bois-Reymond, Stumpf, and Classen, all of whom stood outside the immediate circle of partisans. By the late 1880s this strategy had shown itself to be no longer feasible. Under the provocation of Hering's criticisms the Helmholtz school moved to the attack. Even then Fick, Kries, and König occasionally employed a "strategy of condescension" in dealing with Hering (Bourdieu 1992, 68). Without directly attacking him, they would sometimes try to employ his language and terminology in brief and well-bracketed analyses of the point in question. This rhetorical technique reassured their readers that they were cognizant and wary of Hering, and it acknowledged his existence while reaffirming his status as an outsider and an inferior.

Hering, as an outsider-opponent of the alleged orthodoxy represented by the Helmholtz school, naturally found it in his interests to pose as totally bilingual between the two theories. His constant attacks upon his opponents, in addition to their obvious polemical function, played the larger role of demonstrating to the nonaligned that Hering could speak the language of his opponents with a fluency they could not manage for his. This was an accurate self-representation in large part; bilingualism was functional for Hering and his students in a way it was not for their opponents. In one other sense, as well, Hering's writing aimed at more—or less—than real communication with his opponents. From the early 1890s, when Hering's students began to publish in significant amounts, their writings took on a epideictic function. They wrote in part for one another, deepening and nuancing the common language that defined them, buttressing each other's results, defining their common boundaries, and publicly reinforcing the shared values of their research school.

That fact points to a larger consideration of how school formations influence scientific debates. In order to survive, a language or a dialect requires a linguistic community, one large enough and cohesive enough that its members' speech-acts become mutually reinforcing and—at least temporarily—insulated from outside corrupting influences (Petyt 1980, 13–31; Wardhaugh 1986, 22–53, 113–26; 1987, 1–38). Indeed, these may be necessary conditions for the "speciation" of a new scientific tradition (Biagioli 1990). However, the conditions of modern scientific communications, especially in an age of international journals, militate against the existence of such linguistic pockets. Whether from the perspective of exchange theory or constructivism, science as collective practice pushes toward normalized languages and linguistic uniformity. In that kind of communications environment, research schools—institutionally localized, inward-looking, internally reinforcing, militant toward external rivals—offer the only settings in which linguistic or dialect pockets can establish themselves even temporarily. Research schools may be the only real nuclei of deep scientific change under modern conditions, because they are the only adequate loci of semantic innovation.

THE LIMITS OF INCOMMENSURABILITY

At the same time that semantic incommensurability promotes cognitive innovation, it can also perpetuate controversy, and in doing so it delayed or prevented closure of the Helmholtz–Hering dispute. While incommensurability limited the mutual understanding between the schools, however, it did not foreclose it altogether. Despite being widely misunderstood on the point, Kuhn always insisted that the incommensurability of scientific worldviews was a matter of degree. Not all statements formulated in one natural language can be translated adequately into another, but many can be.

Throughout the period of the controversy, the schools of Helmholtz and Hering shared fundamental assumptions about human vision and how it should be explained. Perhaps the most important of these areas of consensus were their abandonment of projection, their emphasis on retinal local signs, their deemphasis of kinesthetic visual cues, their common commitment to "component" theories of visual sensation, and their full acceptance of experimental colorimetry and the empirical trivariability of the eye. At a deeper level the schools shared a tacit commitment to punctiform analysis of the visual image and to the distinction between sensation and perception. These common elements distinguished the schools of Helmholtz and Hering from several approaches to vision studies current before and after them.

Incommensurabilities of method and program certainly did not mean that the protagonists remained inflexible in the face of opposition, or even that they failed to achieve agreement on some disputed questions. For example, the schools achieved rough agreement concerning the nature of the horopter deviation (although not its causes) after much dispute and shifting of ground. Hering's school almost completely abandoned its original insistence that protanopes and deuteranopes do not constitute distinguishable classes of color blind; in the face of Hering's critique, Helmholtz's followers retreated en masse from his psychological interpretation of contrast. Nativists and empiricists both accommodated their programs to the emerging evidence for organically programmed developmental stages. The displacement hypothesis, the duplicity theory, and the specific brightness of colors all repesented major theoretical amendments adopted by one school in response to the attacks of the other.

Incommensurability also did not prevent the schools from mounting effective appeals to nature, nor did the controversy differ significantly from other scientific controversies simply because the issues often hinged upon subjective, introspective observations. In general each side was consistently able to invoke experimental outcomes that its opponents successfully replicated or at least left unchallenged, even when the outcome of the experiment told against the opponent. That was not universally the case, as the previous chapters have made clear. At the beginning of the dispute the disagreement between Helmholtz and Hering on the spatial localization of monocular half-images deteriorated to experimental impasse; they and their students long disagreed on the outcome of experiments on the empirical horopter and on measurements of the significance of macula coloring; and at the end of the controversy the schools diverged sharply about their observations on small-field, visual effects in the central fovea.

On the other hand, the schools showed remarkable agreement about other experimental results, and these included some of the experimental outcomes that were most central to the controversy. Helmholtz's students, for example, rarely challenged Hering's experiments done to criticize psychological theories of contrast; König replicated and accepted Hering's demonstration that the monochromat luminosity distribution closely resembles the dark spectrum of normals, even though the fact embarrassed the Young–Helmholtz theory. Hering accepted Helmholtz's experiments on the horopter deviation even though they told against his theory of the core plane; he did not dispute König's results about the absorption spectrum of visual purple; and he reluctantly conceded the existence of separate classes of red and green blind. Of course, the schools disagreed violently about what this empirical evidence meant, but they shared a broad if far from total agreement on what that empirical evidence was. Elements of Kuhnian incommensurability pervaded and prolonged the dispute; nevertheless, they never stifled effective experimental dialogue between the schools or precluded a constitutive role for controversy.

CHAPTER THIRTEEN

Controversy and Disciplinary Structure

THE HELMHOLTZ–HERING CONTROVERSY unfolded at a period when the formation in Germany of new, autonomous scientific disciplines was proceeding most intensely and most turbulently. The founding histories of at least four scientific disciplines impinged upon the controversy, and the imperatives of disciplinary consciousness and disciplinary interests powerfully influenced its progress and eventual stalemate (Stichweh 1984, 1–94; Guntau and Laitko 1987b; Turner 1986).

Those disciplinary interests ought not to be narrowly interpreted as only the drive for careers and status. Scientists make investments in particular resources necessary to their practice: instruments, skills, alliances, bodies of expertise. Individuals or groups advance, embrace, or reject new claims by calculating whether those claims promise to enhance or restrict the return on their particular investment (Pickering 1984, 3–21, 403–15; Pickering 1990). So all-inclusive are "resources" in this sense that they collectively specify how individuals see and talk about the world they investigate. They merge seamlessly into the kinds of "cognitive interests" that some theorists have preferred to the invocation of "social interests" as determinants of scientific choice (Roth and Barrett 1990).

To these sorts of disciplinary interests might be added the role of "affective investment": the emotional reward and protection of shared endeavor and identity. As an element in scientific consciousness affective interests assumed particular importance in nineteenth-century Germany. There the scientific career imposed severe material, social, and psychological risk upon its followers, and, as its apologists stressed throughout the century, demanded a life of unstinting renunciation. Allegiance to a research school offered affective compensation for that sacrifice and reduced the individual's risk by linking one's personal interests to those of the group. Hering's circle in particular showed how powerfully those bonds of allegiance could knit together a research school.

THE DISCIPLINARY BASIS OF VISION STUDIES

Vision studies per se never constituted a real scientific discipline during the period examined here. The field (except for ophthalmology) did not achieve institutional recognition in European universities, never possessed a journal addressed exclusively to its concerns, and never generated arguments for its methodological or philosophical autonomy vis-à-vis other branches of science. Virtually no contributors to the field pursued vision studies to the exclusion of all other research problems. Instead, the field cut broadly across at least four recognized disciplines: physics, physiology, ophthalmology, and experimental psychology. Philosophers, biochemists, and comparative anatomists also wrote on vision problems.

This heterogeneous list might suggest that research on vision was fragmented and compartmentalized among its participating disciplinary groups, but at least until the very late nineteenth century this was not the case. As early chapters have demonstrated, physicists, physiologists, ophthalmologists, and psychologists worked on similar outstanding problems and contributed collectively to most of the research lines shown in Table 1 in the Appendix. They did so within a broadly shared context of theories, methods, and relevant controversies, and they published their results in the same, or at least broadly overlapping, groups of journals. Several factors contributed to the openness and high integration of the field. One was that sensory physiologists in Germany dominated the other groups numerically, and with their methodological eclecticism they long provided a center of gravity. Another was the Helmholtz–Hering controversy itself. Each school enrolled at least a few supporters of every disciplinary persuasion, and each school advanced integrating methods and theories relevant to the practice of every discipline. The school alignments obliged participants in the controversy to engage with a range of disciplinary perspectives, and so counteracted tendencies to disciplinary fragmentation and compartmentalization.

A third integrating factor was that sensory studies in general made a significant bid to become an autonomous and unified discipline. Hering himself led the call, asserting in 1885 that "the study of sensory perception may truly claim to be designated as a special discipline." It demands special and well-defined experimental skills and an awareness of the sources of error that enter into that kind of experimentation. As part of his polemical tactics, Hering regularly denounced neophytes who published *Anfängerarbeit* in ignorance of those special skills (Hering 1885a[45], 143). When the *Zeitschrift für Psychologie und Physiologie der Sinnesorgane* was founded in 1890, its editors praised the emergence of "a single, great twin-science," neither of whose branches could be successfully advanced independently of the other.[1] Ultimately, however, the bid for disciplinary status failed. Sensory studies did attain division status in a few German physiology institutes, but the broadscale institutional basis for even subdisciplinary autonomy was not forthcoming in the nineteenth century. By 1900 the search for deep commonalities among the various sensory modes lost its urgency, and existing disciplines partitioned the study of sensation among themselves.

THE PHYSICS OF SENSATION

At midcentury physicists pursued the experimental study of vision at least as ardently as physiologists. One in every twenty papers published in Poggendorff's *Annalen der Physik und Chemie* during the 1850s dealt with topics in visual perception. Physicists like Wheatstone, Maxwell, Helmholtz, Listing, and Fechner had been mainly responsible for the revolution in vision studies that had occurred around midcentury, and their achievements had been based on the heavy importation of physical and mathematical methods. By 1900, however, physicists had lost their numerical prominence in the field. Their contributions were increasingly limited to mathematical forays into what has been called "higher colormetrics" (Trendelenburg 1961, 96). Physical methods, however, remained very important in vision studies.

As Hering never tired of complaining, the theories of Helmholtz appealed especially to physicists. They made up a high proportion of Helmholtz's partisans in the nineteenth century (see Table 8.1), whereas Ernst Mach was the only major physicist openly allied with Hering. Helmholtz's theories appealed to physicists because they maximized the importance of resources that physicists normally possessed and minimized those that they did not. Much more than Hering's program, Helmholtz's emphasized precision colorimetry, elaborate instrumentation, mathematical and error analysis, and data interpolation and graphical methods. These were resource skills that physicists normally possessed, but other scientists had to acquire. On the other hand, empiricism's tendency to explain visual perception in terms of individual learning and experience minimized expected returns from developmental studies, comparative anatomy, and neurological research—territory relatively unfamiliar to physicists.

The skills of the mathematical physicist reigned especially preeminent in a new research line that Helmholtz himself created late in his career. In the 1890s Helmholtz resumed his earlier attempts to generalize Fechner's psychophysical law, $dE = A(dH/H)$, so as to extend its validity at high and low values of the physical intensity H (*WAH* 3:392–406, no. 199). In 1892 he boldly extended the generalized Fechner formula beyond brightness to hue as well (*WAH* 3:407–38, no. 203). He wrote the differential element of sensation dE as the sum of three primary hue sensations dE_1, dE_2, dE_3 corresponding to the three physiological primaries of Young's theory (*WAH* 3:438–75, no. 204, 205), and expressed each E_n by his generalized Fechner formula as a function of H_n alone. This made E_n a line element in a three-dimensional color space with a Riemannian metric given by

$$dE^2 = dE_1{}^2 + dE_2{}^2 + dE_3{}^2$$

From his line-element formula Helmholtz could predict the variation of the eye's sensitivity to small changes of hue across the visible spectrum. The close agreement of these predictions with data derived from König was taken as strong support of Young's hypothesis (*WAH* 3:438–75, no. 204; Parsons 1924, 243).[2] Other mathematical physicists developed line-element theory further, and it came to constitute a branch of color theory relatively inaccessible to other kinds of specialists in the field.

Instrumental as well as mathematical resources could preempt areas of vision research for the attention of physicists and those who commanded their methods. By 1890 spectral colorimetry based on the mixing of homogeneous lights had become the research standard in Germany, and resort to the rotating color wheel, formerly the most ubiquitous instrument in vision research, was becoming rare. Arthur König and his collaborators set that new standard; to compete with them researchers henceforth had to possess colorimeters at least as sophisticated as that available in Helmholtz's laboratory. They had to command the physical optics necessary to understand and calibrate the instrument, possess the mathematical techniques necessary to interconvert spectra, and understand the elaborate interpolation and approximation techniques König routinely used. These were not trivial demands on physiologists and psychologists.

Some of Hering's supporters resented this instrumental preemption of the field. Jakob Stilling attacked spectral colorimeters as lending nothing more than "a veneer of mathematics" to vision research, and as being too complicated, costly, and implicitly physicalist in orientation (Stilling 1910, esp. 395). Hering and his students remained more circumspect, in order to avoid attacking the ideal of precision measurement. Against König they pursued a strategy of criticizing his alleged obsession with curves and overly elaborate instruments and of ridiculing the alleged lack of physiological understanding that went with them (Hering 1885a[45], 1887b[49]; König 1885a[8]). Hering designed and used a very sophisticated spectral colorimeter himself (see the following section), but he chose to publicize only his simple and inexpensive ones, like his so-called color box and his color-mixing apparatus of 1888. These devices adjusted brightness by angle of reflection and produced colors by the use of stained glass or pigment reflection (Hering 1888b[55]; Hillebrand 1889).

Hering's experimental style has sometimes been characterized as qualitative, introspective, and phenomenological, and so contrasted invidiously to that of Helmholtz (e.g., Schrödinger 1926; Boring 1942, 28–34). Physicist Franz Exner, for example, made that charge in 1921, when he accused Hering's basic concepts about color phenomena of being insusceptible in principle to quantification or measurement (Exner 1921). In reality, Hering's methods are better described as a striving for *Anschau-*

lichkeit, an experimental-explanatory orientation that Kenneth Caneva found widespread in the physical sciences in Germany before the 1840s (Caneva 1978). According to this orientation, every natural phenomenon reveals itself in a great diversity and complexity of forms, which are as variable as the enormous range of possible experimental circumstances in which the phenomenon can be elicited. Some experimental manifestations, however, reveal the essence of the phenomenon with particular simplicity, clarity, and naturalness; through these particular demonstrations the phenomenon becomes *anschaulich*—vivid, intuitive, plain, essential. Experimental science does not strive to capture some essence of the phenomenon that lies behind the experiments, or to explore the phenomenon through hypothetico-deductive testing, but to discover and display the exact circumstances in which the phenomenon reveals itself with particular *Anschaulichkeit*.

Hering's experimental style looked back to this older German tradition more than it looked forward to the later, self-consciously phenomenological methodologies that he influenced. His earlier writings, in particular, abound with the striving for *Anschaulichkeit*, and the approach coexisted, sometimes uneasily, with his penchant for physiological models and exact psychophysical measurement. That style, however, isolated Hering from physicists and the methodologies they espoused. By the 1840s German physicists were turning to hypothetico-deductive methodologies and new understandings about the relationship between theory and measurement (Caneva 1978, 95–122; Olesko 1991, 266–317).

Hering's students—Hillebrand, Hess, Pretori, Sachs—emphasized graphical techniques and exact measurement much more than Hering had done. They never regarded this as a departure from his precepts, however, and they vociferously disputed characterizations that Hering's methods were qualitative and phenomenological, like those that Exner advanced. Armin Tschermak-Seysenegg formally named Hering's methodology *der exakte Subjektivismus*, a methodology applicable to all aspects of the study of life (Tschermak 1932, 1942). According to Tschermak, exact subjectivism recognized that physiological optics was more than "mere applied physics"; it rejected attempts to isomorphically map sensory response onto physical stimulus; and it took the sensory contents of consciousness as its primary data. Tschermak emphasized, however, that exact subjectivism treated sensory content as fully susceptible to exact measurement and mathematical description and fully subject to rigorous causation; indeed, it drew no distinction in these regards between "subjective" and "objective" realms of experience (Tschermak 1942, 156). Arguments like these self-consciously attempted to answer the appeal of the Helmholtzian tradition in physiological optics to physicists and those who placed a premium upon the physicist's tools and predilections.

COLORIMETERS AND EXPERIMENTAL PRACTICE

Even their most sophisticated instruments subtly expressed the two schools' different orientations toward the physicists' methods. In 1920, two years after Hering's death, his student Siegfried Garten published a detailed description of a spectral colorimeter that Hering had designed and used in his institute since 1884 but never described in print (Garten 1920). The comparable instruments in the laboratories of Helmholtz, König, and Kries—the latter two variations of the first—had already been described frequently. Spectral colorimeters enjoyed almost iconic status in vision research at the end of the century and reflected much about the consciousness of those who used them.

The colorimeter König and Dieterici used in their classic research of the 1880s and 1890s was based upon an apparatus that Helmholtz had designed early in his career for mixing spectral colors.[3] König noted rather pointedly that Helmholtz's original instrument had never been used for exact measurements and had had to be modified for that purpose (König and Dieterici 1884[6], 217). König's instrument, shown in his sketch of 1892 (Figure 13.1), consisted of two collimator tubes C_1 and C_2 that could pivot about a fixed axis through P. Light passing down the two tubes would be refracted in the large prism at P and thrown into the telescope barrel B. The ocular of the telescope was replaced with a plate carrying a narrow slit. Looking through the slit, the observer would see a luminous field, the left half of which would consist of light from the right-hand collimator, the right half from the left-hand collimator. Light entering the tubes from the sources G_1 and G_2 would pass through adjustable Nicol prisms N_1 and N_2, through the adjustable bilateral slits S_1 and S_2, and finally through the moveable, double-refracting prisms K_1 and K_2. For a setting like that shown for K_2, the prisms will produce two overlapping spectra, so that each half-field seen through the slit at S will be a mixture of two homogeneous lights. The wavelength of those two components can adjusted by pivoting the collimator tubes with the adjustments at R_1 and R_2 and by moving the prisms K_1 and K_2. The overall brightness of each half-field can be adjusted by the micrometer screw at the slits S_1 and S_2, and the relative brightness of the two components in each field can be altered by rotating the Nicol prisms with the scales D_1 and D_2.

Perhaps by more than coincidence, Hering had his original colorimeter built in 1884, the year in which König and Dieterici first published the spectral response curves they had obtained with Helmholtz's modified instrument. How Hering's original device differed from Helmholtz's is

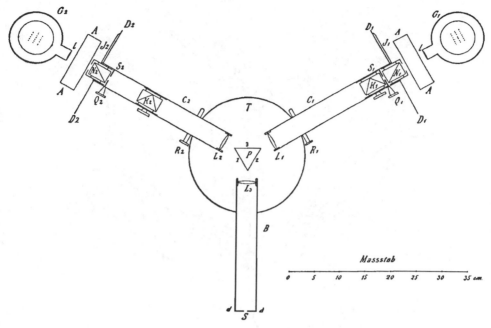

Fig. 13.1 The König–Helmholtz spectral colorimeter, as depicted by König in 1892. *Source*: König 1892(21), 218.

unclear, but the final version described by Garten in 1920 is quite distinct. As Garten's diagram (Figure 13.2) shows, Hering's developed instrument used three collimator tubes C, C_1, and C_2 and a central prism equipped with a small mirror, so that light from C_1 illuminated the left half of the observed field, and light from C_2 and C the right half. In order to superimpose two homogeneous lights in a single collimator tube, Hering used an ingenious double-slit apparatus at the positions S_1, S_2, and S_3, by which any two homogeneous colors could be chosen and their relative brightnesses regulated. His apparatus, then, employed no Nicol prisms, double refraction, and polarization. Hering's instrument differed from the Helmholtz–König device in substituting mechanical for physical-optical sophistication. The lenses L_1, L_2, and L_3 in the viewing tube enlarged the image of the two half-fields, so that Hering could obtain a uniform image subtending twenty degrees (Garten 1920).

Garten's published account of this instrument in 1920 aimed at countering the popular prejudice that Hering dispensed with precision instrumentation, and even at showing the superiority of Hering's instrument. In respects not emphasized by Garten, the colorimeters of König and Hering

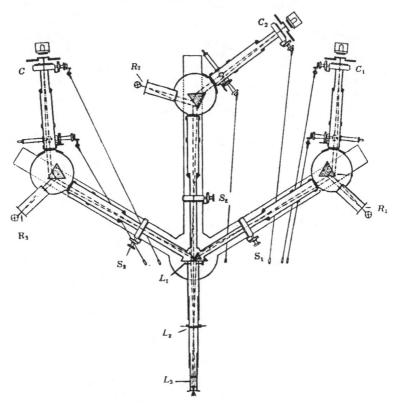

Fig. 13.2 The Hering spectral colorimeter, as depicted by Siegfried Garten in 1920. *Source*: Garten 1920, 92.

reflected theoretical differences and differences of experimental style. While Helmholtz and König could mix only two lights in each field (and in practice König made metameric matches with only three homogeneous lights), Hering in principle could mix four homogeneous lights in one half-field and two in the other. In a manner no less significant for being heuristic, this feature operationally freed Hering and his school from what Tschermak mockingly called "the impoverished three-light economy" behind the Young–Helmholtz theory (Tschermak 1942, 63–69). Equally significant, the devices R_1, R_2, and R_3 allowed Hering to superimpose standard white light onto the homogeneous rays in each of the collimator tubes. The instrument could therefore systematically model the separate chromatic and achromatic components of vision that were central to Hering's understanding of sensation. König's apparatus served for derivation of spectral response curves; Hering's could produce a greater diversity of stimulus conditions but was only occasionally used to gather data systematically for curve plotting. Both schools seamlessly conflated theory, experimentation, and instrument design in their laboratory practice.

The conflation of instruments and ideas showed itself in one other respect. Hering equipped his colorimeter with adjusting rods so that the controls for altering the fields were within easy reach. This allowed an observer to proceed without looking away from the eyepiece, to work conveniently under a dark hood when the experiment required it, and in general to control more precisely for adaptation. König's instrument, on the other hand, seems to have lacked similar devices. It required the experimenter to reach up to sixty centimeters to make fine adjustments of the fields under observation in the telescope barrel. If König asked his observers to make their own adjustments, they would have experienced eventual strain and the temptation to shift momentarily away from the eyepiece in uncontrolled ways. That would have made it more difficult for König to control for adaptation and perhaps tempted him to use low-intensity fields in order to equalize the level of illumination between the field and the room.

Now Hering frequently criticized König for ignoring the effects of adaptation, and Kries after 1894 also criticized König for regularly obtaining color equations under conditions of adaptation and field intensity too low to guarantee photopic vision (Kries and Nagel 1896). During this period König was almost alone in regularly reporting deviations from Newton's law; those results may have resulted from the circumstances of instrument design and experimental procedure cited above. They may also have grown out of theory-induced expectations about sources of error. Hering's hypothetical visual mechanism made adaptation one of the central phenomena of vision; the Young–Helmholtz theory, at least before the duplicity amendment, conceived adaptation as a different kind of effect and gave it less theoretical attention. The colorimeters designed by König and Hering reflected these different levels of consciousness about the phenomenon and its importance. They demonstrate the close integration of instrument design, experimental procedure, and theoretical expectations in the practice of the two rival schools.

GERMAN PHYSIOLOGISTS AND THE VISION DEBATES

The disciplinary investments of German physiologists led them to no clear-cut preference between Helmholtz and Hering as did those of physicists. Nevertheless, Table 8.1 shows that they dominated the core set of the Helmholtz–Hering controversy numerically. Physiology long provided the disciplinary center of gravity for the vision debates. Vision studies was called "physiological optics," even when the real issues were psychological in nature, and the school controversy was fought out mainly in journals of physiology and the great physiological *Handbücher* of the period.

Several factors allowed physiology to play a mediating role among the various disciplinary perspectives. German physiologists had always concentrated heavily upon sensory research, and by 1870 their field enjoyed the largest and firmest institutional base of all the disciplines involved with vision. Where there had been nine autonomous chairs of physiology in 1850, there were twenty in 1870. By 1880 chairs of physiology, usually with associated institutes for laboratory training and research, had been established in twenty-six of the twenty-seven universities of the German-language university system in Europe (Eulner 1970, 46–65, 508).

The methodological eclecticism of German physiology also favored its mediating role. At midcentury physiologists routinely employed the psychophysical, introspective observational techniques later associated with psychology. The field also absorbed the biophysical program as an important current in its drive for disciplinary differentiation from anatomy and more traditional morphological approaches. Physiologists associated Helmholtz's achievements in sensory physiology with that program and readily enrolled them to support their disciplinary aspirations. By the 1870s, however, the enthusiasm of German physiologists for biophysics and reductionism in general was waning, and the field simultaneously retreated from its earlier methodological eclecticism (Cranefield 1966, 36; Kries 1892). New subspecialties like physiological chemistry found their opportunities for institutional autonomy more limited, and psychophysical experimentation was becoming more commonly associated with psychology than physiology.

In vision studies, physiology's retreat from psychophysical experimentation was accompanied by a turn to "pure physiological" research methods based on animal experimentation, comparative and microscopic anatomy, and electrophysiological and biochemical studies. Problem complex II (Table 2 in the Appendix) shows the relative levels of literature output from research of this kind, that is, research on vision not based on reports by an experimental subject. Table 1 in the Appendix indicates the individual research lines that accounted for this expansion: research on brain localization and the optic track, comparative visual anatomy and embryological development, studies of the retina and optic nerve, and investigation into retinal photopigments. Research of this kind showed a dramatic trend of secular growth.

But research on animal systems, despite its growing centrality to physiological practice, simply could not be brought to bear upon the issues of the Helmholtz–Hering controversy. Comparative physiology and microscopic anatomy did support the duplicity theory, but they scarcely touched the debates over color vision. Neither Hering's nor Helmholtz's theory received any significant anatomical or chemical instantiation, and the hope that some would come, first out of the work of Heinrich Schultze and then out of the discovery of visual purple, was disappointed. The controversies over spatial perception showed the same pattern. By 1900 more and more research on vision was being done that had no immediate significance for the Helmholtz–Hering controversy. Conversely, the issues of the controversy were proving impervious to the methodological resources in which most physiologists were investing.

Physiologists received Hering's theory of vision, at his own insistence, as one instantiation of a much more general conception of organic function. From the beginning he had offered his theory of antagonistic assimilative and dissimilative activities in the visual substance as a model for all neural and regulative processes in the body. In 1877 he had applied that model to the temperature sense (Hering 1877[24], 1879b). Then, in a series of popular lectures beginning in the 1880s, Hering emerged as one of the foremost representatives of a philosophy of the organism that made "self-regulation"—what would later be called "homeostatic feedback"— the central feature of living systems.[4] He taught that in the absence of external stimuli, life is a dynamic equilibrium of antagonistic processes that he conceived as biochemical and metabolic. External stimuli can disturb this "autonomous" equilibrium, but the processes themselves contain self-regulating mechanisms that act even in the presence of a constant stimulus to restore it to "allonomous" equilibrium (Hering 1888a). Organic response therefore depends as much upon the state of the organism itself as upon the nature and intensity of the stimulus.

Hering also stood out among German critics of the reductionist program, the pernicious influence of which he found still alive and strong in the 1890s. Where that program had erred, Hering wrote, was not in introducing physical and chemical methods to the study of life, but in assuming that life can be wholly explained in terms of the non-living. In reality, "life can only be understood in its entirety out of itself" ("aus sich selbst *ganz*"; Hering 1899a, 107). Both vitalism and reductionism are scientifically dangerous dogmas, he wrote in 1899, but today reductionism has replaced vitalism as the more dangerous of the two.

If physiologists found these views congenial, they must have found others of Hering's mildly heretical. He continued to attack what he called the "homogeneity theory" of nerve conduction, the view held by all the "masters of physiology" that the nerves, like telegraph wires, transmit only one kind of action at varying levels of intensity ranging down to zero. This conception, Hering believed, could accommodate neither his own doctrine of antagonistic responses nor the complexity of real organic function. It violated the real meaning of Johannes Müller in his specific law of nerve energies, and it promoted a vision of the organism as a passive physicochemical machine, inhabited at its center by a ghost called the consciousness, the mind, or the sensorium (ibid.).

Physiologists evaluated Hering's theory not only for its predictions about sensory response, but also for the physicochemical plausibility of the mechanisms he postulated to mediate vision. Hering's theory made stronger and more specific claims about those mechanisms than Young's did, and by 1900 those claims had come under attack. Donders and Kries opened this line of criticism in the 1880s (Donders 1884; Kries 1887a). Hering's theory, Kries charged, assumes "that certain lights cause a dissociation, others a corresponding synthesis, for which as far as I know, photochemistry offers no example" (Kries 1887a, 118). By contrast the Young–Helmholtz theory "conceives the effect of light as we in fact know it to be from photochemistry," in that the effect increases with the intensity and varies with the wavelength. Christine Ladd-Franklin noted that the "physiological economy" offered no example of the "purposes of life" being served directly by anabolic activity, as on Hering's theory. Complex substances are synthesized only in order that they might be later destroyed, to release energy for the organism's purposes. That Hering's theory rejected this physiological principle was to her a "fatal objection" to that model (Ladd-Franklin 1893, 80).

Psychologist G. E. Müller delivered the most thorough indictment of the plausibility of Hering's mechanism, even though he was convinced that minor changes could fully vindicate the theory. Hering's model, he charged, violated the fundamental principle of psychophysical explanation because it did not isomorphically map sensations onto specific physiological states. Instead of correlating particular sensations with the absolute levels of A- and D-actions in the visual substance, it correlates them with the *ratios* of those actions, an altogether different principle (Müller 1896–97, 1–6). Furthermore, Müller went on, suppose Hering were right in his claim that antagonistic A- and D-actions analogous to those supposed to occur in the visual substance underlie all organic functions in the body. Then responses like afterimages and fatigue, which arise from these antagonistic actions in the visual substance, ought to be much more general and to occur in all sensory and organic function. In fact, they are restricted entirely to vision, Müller observed, despite misleading analogies such as muscular fatigue.

Müller found the energetics of Hering's model highly implausible. If the D-process releases energy, then the A-process must consume it, or vice versa, so that one of the processes cannot release potential energy to the nerves and so be responsible for sensation (pp. 64–74). English psychologist William McDougall made the same charge. Hering's theory does not explain the source of the energy necessary to drive the endothermic reactions involved in assimilation, nor (if the source is assumed to be simultaneous dissimilation) how the assimilation-response can ever exceed its antagonist. At the very least, he claimed, the model cannot be generalized to all inhibitory responses, including muscular ones, as Hering tried to do (McDougall 1903).

Hering had defenders. The influential physiologist Max Verworn (the student of Hering's student Wilhelm Biedermann) made Hering's model the basis of his widely known and controversial "biogen" hypothesis of neural action (Verworn 1915, 591–616; Peritz 1909). Emil Brunner attempted to reformulate the underlying chemistry of the model as a reversible chemical reaction, the rate and direction of which governed the sensory response (Brunner 1908). As expected, Kries declared that these attempts created more new problems for the theory than they solved (Kries 1910, 2:452). Hering and his immediate students stayed aloof from this discussion. The charge that Hering's model lacked physiological and chemical plausibility, whatever its merits in explaining the psychophysics of vision, surfaced frequently in the literature of the early twentieth century (Ladd-Franklin 1924, 80; Parsons 1924, 275).

THE INSTITUTIONALIZATION OF OPHTHALMOLOGY

Ophthalmology achieved institutional autonomy among the disciplines of the German medical faculties by differentiating itself from general surgery. Its institutionalization occurred later and more rapidly than that of physiology, with most new chairs and ophthalmological clinics being founded between 1870 and 1880.[5] As is common in such formations, proponents invoked heroes and heroic achievements to justify their appeal for autonomy and disciplinary status. Helmholtz took his place alongside Albrecht von Graefe and Donders in ophthalmology's triad of hero-founders. His invention of the ophthalmoscope endowed the new speciality with a vital diagnostic tool, and his enshrinement linked the ambitious young specialty to the growing prestige of scientific physiology and exact instrumentation (Tuchman 1993a; Leber 1884). This was very important to a field that at midcentury was little more than an accretionary set of surgical techniques, rooted in very traditional therapies and still too readily associated with low-status groups like spectacle-makers (Hirschberg 1986, 7:266–68; 8A:91–93).

The patterns of literature output shown in Tables 1 and 2 (Appendix) demonstrate the real, if tenuous, relationship between scientific research and practical ophthalmological concerns. Most of the relevant literature is catalogued in problem complex III (Table 2 in the Appendix), which includes research lines 9.1 through 14.4, all related to the dioptric functioning of the eye. After the 1860s relative literature output in the more theoretical research lines (categories 13, 12.2, 11.1, 11.2, 10.2, 10.1) declined quite sharply, as Donders, Meissner, Listing, Henson, Helmholtz, and others clarified and consolidated the outstanding issues in the field. Literature production then shifted toward research lines with more direct diagnostic and therapeutic significance, including those on refractive errors, spectacles, and diagnostic techniques and instruments (categories 11.5, 11.6, 11.7, 11.8). By 1885–94 these chiefly medical research lines accounted for about 34 percent of the literature in the problem complex, and as much as half if the literature on astigmatism is also characterized as chiefly medical.

As for the Helmholtz–Hering controversy, the issues that divided the two schools usually did not bear on practice and so did not enlist the disciplinary interests of ophthalmologists in direct or obvious ways. Despite Helmholtz's enormous prestige among ophthalmologists, Hering had closer ties to the German ophthalmological community than did Helmholtz or his main students. Table 8.1 shows roughly equal numbers of ophthalmologists among each group of partisans. Nevertheless, around 1920 Hering's students or close associates held five of the twenty-six chairs of ophthalmology in the extended German university system, while Helmholtz's direct supporters who had held chairs had long since died or retired. At Leipzig the elderly Hering recruited research assistants primarily from among the specialists in ophthalmology trained by his colleague Herbert Sattler.

Hering valued his association with the ophthalmological community and played to it. He addressed his article of 1899 on the impossibility of an anomalous retinal correspondence to "Ophthalmologen vom Fach." In questions like that one, he concluded, "the judgement of experienced ophthalmologists, not that of physiologists, is decisive" (Hering 1899c[80], 16). On accepting the Graefe Medal of the German Ophthalmological Society in 1908, he praised practicing physicians as alone capable of deciding among the conflicting opinions of physiologists, as they are closest to full complexity and mystery of life and death. In the same speech he warned contemporary physiology in Germany against the temptation to dissolve itself into a "comprehensive biology" and so lose its historical link to medical practice (Hering 1921, 140). In general ophthalmological evidence served Hering well in his scientific polemics. Pathological cases of acquired color blindness had furnished the main support for his theory of that phenomenon, and his more optimistic supporters regarded the nativist-empiricist question as having been settled decisively in Hering's favor by medical evidence.

The issues of the Helmholtz–Hering controversy did touch one important area of ophthalmological practice. Heterophoria, common among children, is the condition of latent squint that manifests itself only when the eyes are tired, are turned in certain peripheral directions, or when one eye is suddenly covered so that binocular vision is no longer possible (Miller 1984, 293–304). Except in these circumstances, the "fusion mechanism"—the compulsion to image an object simultaneously on both foveas in the interest of clear vision—overrides the tendency to squint. If uncorrected, heterophoria can lead to loss of vision in the squinting eye.

At midcentury most German physicians regarded heterophoria and other forms of fixed-angle strabismus as a mechanical anomaly arising from abnormal form or place of insertion on the eyeball of one or more of the ocular muscles. They corrected the condition by various surgical procedures including myotomy, in which the overactive muscle was partially severed in order to weaken it (Hirschberg 1985–88, 5.3:330–31; cf. Graefe 1935; Fahrenbach 1983, 113–16). Partly in reaction to what a later critic described as "indiscriminate muscle-cutting," Frans Donders in 1863 proposed a new theory of strabismus. He argued that hyperopia in the squinting eye commonly caused esotropia (convergent strabismus) by forcing a dissociation between accommodation and convergence that became habitual (Donders 1863). Donders thus drastically deemphasized surgery and made correcting the refraction the critical step in treating heterophoria. Unfortunately strabismus is not invariably associated with refractive anomalies, and there were running disagreements about the etiology and treatment of the condition.

Controversy centered on the recourse to surgery, and this important question also fueled the later debates over retinal correspondence. If the anomalous correspondence that some squinters acquire provides a good approximation to binocular vision, or if surgical intervention cannot restore full binocularity, then surgery provides at best a cosmetic correction. If, on the other hand, the normal correspondence is natural, innate, and easily restored, then surgery is strongly indicated (Sachs 1897; Tschermak 1899; Bielschowsky 1900).

By the end of the nineteenth century European ophthalmologists divided along national lines over the etiology of heterophoria. On the whole, German ophthalmologists regarded the condition as muscular-mechanical in origin (Graefe 1897). French and English ophthalmologists more frequently regarded it as a disorder in the cortical nervous centers (Bielschowsky 1907, 321; 1945, 32–34). Claud Alley Worth, surgeon at the Royal London Ophthalmic Hospital, represented the latter view. His very influential theory held that convergent squint arose from a congenital defect that prevented the fusion mechanism from developing strongly or early enough (Worth 1915, 53–55; Hofmann 1925, 2:249). This left the eyes in unstable equilibrium, so that any provocation—hypermetropia, anisometropia, motor anomalies—would induce them to squint. Suppression of the visual field would then ensue within a few weeks or months, frequently leading to amaurosis. The only effective treatment, Worth taught, was fusion training with various stereoscopic devices applied at critical stages of the child's development; such training alone could awaken the latent "desire for binocular vision." Worth regarded surgical intervention with skepticism, since it did not address the real cause of the disorder (Worth 1915, 132).

Worth's theory showed the clear influence of empiricist theories of vision, probably derived from William Preyer's writings on visual development in the child. Worth regarded the fusion mechanism as a habit or association that can be shaped by experience and training. His theory incorporated the notion of developmental "windows," organic stages at which new visual capacities are cued by interactions with the environment and fail to develop properly without them. He assumed in empiricist fashion that congenital abnormalities, although responsible for visual impairment, may be compensated in part by training and the formation of new associations.

Hering's student Alfred Bielschowsky emerged as Worth's main critic, although his own position in the strabismus debates tended to moderate eclecticism. At Leipzig he had collaborated with Franz Hofmann in experiments designed to support Hering's position in the nativist-empiricist dispute (Hofmann and Bielschowsky 1900). They had shown that fusional movements are neither voluntary nor involuntary in the usual sense of the terms, that the capacity for fusional movements varies widely among individuals, and that although exercise can increase the amplitude of possible fusional movements there exists an upper limit beyond which training produces no further improvement.

In his later medical writings on strabismus, Bielschowsky acknowledged the "momentous role" that the fusion mechanism plays in the etiology of squint. Nevertheless, he argued that Worth had exaggerated the improvements to be expected from fusion exercises and been too pessimistic about the chances of successfully treating heterophoria outside the narrow developmental windows he had defined. Echoing Hering's philosophy, Bielschowsky insisted that the physician's primary responsibility is carefully to separate anatomical-mechanical contributions to heterophoria from neural-behavioral ones instilled by habit. Acknowledging the role of innate anatomical-mechanical factors gives greater warrant for ophthalmological intervention. Bielschowsky supported quicker recourse to surgical correction than had Worth, and he defended muscle-weakening operations against Worth's criticisms. Always, he insisted, selecting the proper therapy depends crucially on distinguishing between various levels of organic control over ocular motility (Bielschowsky 1900; 1945, 32–55). The nativist-empiricist controversy over the nature of stereopsis and retinal correspondence therefore impinged directly on the ongoing dispute over the etiology and treatment of heterophoria.

VISUAL PERCEPTION AND THE NEW PSYCHOLOGY

More than physiology or ophthalmology, experimental psychology inherited the dilemmas of the Helmholtz–Hering controversy. Psychology had traditionally been taught as a branch of philosophy in the German universities, and this association continued after 1870, even as psychologists reoriented their field toward experimental methods and the natural sciences. In larger universities, one of the several chairs for philosophy might be tacitly reserved for experimental psychology; in smaller ones an associate professorship might be created. Eleven laboratories or institutes for experimental psychology had been founded by 1900, and by then the field possessed the disciplinary trappings of distinguishable research schools, specialized journals, and authoritative texts. This institutional arrangement occasioned tension and sometimes open conflict between philosophers and psychologists, but it sustained a uniquely German integration of the two fields that lasted well into the twentieth century (Ash 1980).

The impetus behind the new experimental psychology had come partly from Gustav Fechner and psychophysics, but even more out of the agendas and research methods of sensory physiology (Ben-David and Collins 1966). Until late in the century German psychologists concentrated heavily on the experimental analysis of sensation and perception, often to the exclusion of other forms of mental function. The common participation of Germany's leading psychologists and physiologists on the editorial board of the *Zeitschrift für Psychologie und Physiologie der Sinnesorgane* attests to the close intellectual integration of the two fields. By the 1890s psychologists were contributing heavily to the research literature on vision, especially research lines involving contrast, geometrical illusions, and depth perception. This led them irresistibly into the issues of the Helmholtz–Hering dispute. Psychologists predominated among the nonaligned members of the core set shown in Table 8.1. They mostly tried to mediate the controversy and lead it in new directions. On the other hand, psychologists were infrequent among the two groups of partisans. Hering's supporters included psychologists Franz Hillebrand and

G. E. Müller; Helmholtz had no comparable defenders among the new psychologists, although Theodor Lipps espoused a general empiricism on the origins of depth perception (Lipps 1885, 1892).

The new psychologists wanted above all to establish the autonomy of psychological phenomena and the legitimacy and necessity of purely psychological modes of investigation. Helmholtz's empiricism, despite its congenial emphasis on mind, learning, and experience, did not meet this need particularly well. It portrayed the mental processes that mediated perception as inferential in nature, and explanations of that kind harked back dangerously to the tradition of philosophical psychology from which the experimentalists were trying to distance themselves. Psychologists therefore led the attack on unconscious inference, usually favoring a stricter associationist interpretation of apperceptive processes than Helmholtz had offered (Brentano 1924, 155–56; G. E. Müller 1873; Stumpf 1873, 313–14).

Neither did Hering's philosophy fully meet the disciplinary needs of the new psychology. Its biological-reductionist overtones threatened to dissolve psychology back into physiology. What did appeal to psychologists in Hering's writings was the primacy he gave to phenomenological experience. Hering insisted (although he did not always observe the precept) that the primitive sensory capacities have to be studied as we find them and not reduced to rationalistic inferences or (at least in the first instance) physicochemical mechanisms. Most psychologists regarded Hering's theory of color vision as psychologically natural in a way that Young's was not, and most (although not Wundt or Brentano) agreed that a sensation so apparently primitive as that of space could not be an emergent quality or a psychic synthesis of other sensory elements. By 1900 many experimental psychologists, including Carl Stumpf, Hermann Ebbinghaus, and Ostwald Külpe, had formally taken positions much more compatible with Hering's than with Helmholtz's (Stumpf 1873, 97–103; Ebbinghaus 1919, 490–94; Külpe 1893, 385–87).

German psychologists never abandoned their intense concern with the issues that had divided Helmholtz and Hering, but in the early twentieth century those issues began to lose their relevance for the immediate research agenda of that field. Psychologists were turning to the study of thought, feeling, and volition; sensation and perception no longer monopolized the attention of the field as before. In 1906 the famous *Zeitschrift für Psychologie und Physiologie der Sinnesorgane* split without editorial comment into two independent series, the *Zeitschrift für Sinnesphysiologie* and the *Zeitschrift für Psychologie*, the latter without pretence of specialization on the senses. Psychologists who studied sensation and perception retreated from associationist theory and from the attempt to analyze sensory content into hypothetical elements.

Especially important for the psychology of vision were Erich Jaensch (1883–1940) and David Katz (1884–1953), both students of G. E. Müller. Each adopted Hering's careful phenomenological approach and praised it as Hering's greatest contribution to psychological method. But each came to reject Hering's further tendency to analyze experience into sensory elements, and each broke with Hering and Müller over their penchant for strong physiological models of events at the psychophysical interface (Katz 1952; Jaensch 1920, 258; 1909, 380–88).

Katz claimed that he explicitly set out to "psychologize" psychology (Katz 1952). In 1911 he insisted that color sensations are powerfully influenced by our perception of the spatial characteristics of the colored fields, and he analyzed the differences among what he called "surface colors," "film colors," and "volumetric colors" (Katz 1911, 1935). In doing so, Katz was developing the insight that had led Carl Stumpf to deny any basic distinction between spatiality and other sensory qualities and so to espouse a moderate nativism (Stumpf 1873, 109). Katz also adopted Hering's physiological explanation of simultaneous color contrast, but he explained color constancy and Hering's "memory colors" much as Helmholtz had done (Kroh 1921, 183–85). Katz criticized Hering and Helmholtz alike for seeking to reduce sensory experience to sensory elements, whether simple colors or the contribution of isolated retinal points to the visual field (Katz 1911, 4).

Jaensch began his career with the same sorts of questions. Even while building explicitly on the work of Hering's students Hess and Pretori, he challenged Hering's physiological theory of contrast, contending that it would not explain a larger class of color-shift experiences (some involving memory colors) to which he gave the name "transformations." Jaensch insisted that contrast and color constancy are both central effects and that both are influenced by experience and association, but he denied any wish to go back to the unconscious inferences of Helmholtz (Jaensch 1920, 269–72). He believed that the new concepts and terminology of "transformation theory" would make possible a new psychological theory of contrast, and so reconcile or transcend the old dispute between Helmholtz and Hering.

Jaensch and his students carried this independent orientation into their study of spatial perception as well. Jaensch repeatedly criticized the experimental evidence from which Hillebrand had deduced the stability of retinal depth values. He argued that visual depth perception is not associated directly with retinal disparity, but with shifts of attention that are evoked by those disparities, and he was prepared to grant a role to experience and association in shaping the concentration of visual attention (Jaensch 1911, 123–29). In the 1920s he and his students repeated the classic thread-triple experiments of Helmholtz, Hering, and Hillebrand, using up to seven hanging threads rather than three. Their findings suggested that the spatial localization of the threads depended upon the subject's collective conception of the threads, and that it could not be reduced to a simple distribution of space values across the retina (Kröncke 1921; Jaensch and Reich 1921).

Jaensch discussed the theoretical significance of this research in an important note of 1921. He claimed that the old "anatomical nativism" of Müller, Panum, and Hering had been undermined by the new psychology, which had shown that there could be no "isomorphic ordering of sensations and the anatomical substrate." We are witnessing, he claimed, the metamorphosis of anatomical nativism into a "new nativism" that was abandoning insistence on anatomical and physiological substrates and substituting for these "a system of [psychological] functions which condition sensory experience and first make it possible." The functions themselves were to be recognized as "flexible, variable, and highly adaptable to environmental circumstances" (Jaensch 1921, 234).

The Gestalt movement, which broke upon German psychology around 1920, extended and formalized some of the principles implicit in phenomenological psychology. By stressing the holistic nature of sensory experience and searching for "laws of form," Gestalt theorists further abandoned the punctiform mapping of elemental sensations onto retinal elements that had characterized the schools of both Helmholtz and Hering. Much more important, Gestalt theorists rejected the basic distinction between sensation and perception that had been at the heart of the Helmholtz–Hering controversy. Kurt Koffka made both these principles clear in his 1919 essay "On the Influence of Experience on Perception."

In that essay Koffka discussed the visual perceptions associated with stroboscopic movement, the so-called Phi phenomenon, introduced by Max Wertheimer in 1912. Experiment, Koffka argued, shows that those perceptions cannot be explained as inferences from our past experience in viewing objects, yet experiment also shows that observing particular stroboscopic movements creates dispositions to see some patterns of movement rather than others. Gestalt theory transcends this dilemma by rejecting the idea that perceptions are the sum of particular associations or individual sensations. That standpoint, however, requires abandoning the nativism's old program to understand spatial perceptions as raw sensation. It also makes untenable the distinction between inherited and experientially acquired determinants of perception. Perception no longer has "elements," the different origins of which might be consigned to one or the other of these two disputed categories (Ash 1982, forthcoming; Boring 1942, 246–56). From Koffka's point of view German psychology had no need to choose between Helmholtz and Hering; by 1920 it had bypassed both alternatives.

These developments in psychology challenged and frustrated partisans on both sides of the Helmholtz–Hering controversy. Each recognized the new psychologists as a crucial scientific public whose allegiance needed to be captured. Hering appealed to psychologists in some of his earliest writings, claiming that his approach to the study of sensation was tantamount to a "physiological psychology" or even to a "physiology of consciousness" (Hering 1878/1874, 4–5). In his later writings he was ever ready to drop the names of prominent psychologists such as Ebbinghaus and Brentano, who had supported or corresponded with him (Hering 1890a[64], 1893b[73]).

Kries, who was all too aware that he had been forced onto the defensive in many areas, drew much aid and comfort from the phenomenological movement. In 1923 he hailed the transformation theory of Jaensch as signifying a return to a psychological theory of contrast along Helmholtzian lines. Kries also waxed enthusiastic about Jaensch's rejection of stable retinal depth values and his openness to empirical determinants of the psychological "functions" that condition perception. Kries boasted that the "new nativism" that Jaensch had announced in 1921 could equally be taken as a "new empiricism" (Kries 1923, 218–19, 284). The new psychology obliged Helmholtz's supporters to "translate the Helmholtzian view into a different terminology," but on the whole, Kries asserted, it was bringing about a gradual compromise between nativist and empiricist approaches (Kries 1921, 684).

Kries correctly sensed that the phenomenological and Gestalt movements challenged the very tenets of explanation that Hering's school espoused. That challenge became clear in the controversy over the Phi phenomenon. In his famous paper of 1912, Wertheimer had developed an elaborate physiological model of the Phi phenomenon, based upon the assumption that two separate points in the brain are alternately excited again and again. At each excitation, waves of stimulus-energy spread out from the excited point and eventually encompass the other point. If the phase relationship of the two impinging waves is correct, the waves can produce a "short circuit" in the excitation sequence at one brain point or the other. Wertheimer believed that the many resulting possibilities could adequately model the perceptual phenomena of stroboscopic motion (Wertheimer 1912; Koffka 1919).

In 1922 Hillebrand offered a rival interpretation framed in the language of Hering's theory. For Hillebrand, the stroboscopic stimulus necessitated rapid shifts of visual attention; each shift triggered compensations in the space values of the retinal local signs in ways that Hering had discussed on several occasions. Hillebrand hypothesized that because the compensations were less than instantaneous, an apparent perception of movement resulted. Equally important, Hillebrand bitterly attacked

Wertheimer's own explanatory model as pseudophysiological at best. Indeed, he claimed, it was no explanation at all. It did not build on previously known facts about the spatial sense, whether physiological or psychological, but strained after complete novelty. It merely translated psychological facts into physiological language (Hillebrand 1922, esp. 36–41).

Wertheimer offered in reply a sequence of experiments designed to refute Hillebrand's own theory. He bitterly denied that the Phi phenomenon could be explained by elementist appeals to retinal depth values or absolute localization. He countered that what Hillebrand attacked in his model were in fact its greatest virtues: its radically new analysis of the spatial sense and its striving for new analogies through which to imagine how explanatory physiological models might be brought into closer conformity with psychological facts (Wertheimer 1923, 122).

Franz Hofmann also sensed that the principles of Gestalt psychology challenged the basic explanatory tenets of Hering's school. Although he defended Hillebrand against Wertheimer, he was fully prepared to accept apparent motion as a Gestalt effect and argued that it led to "a new form of nativism" similar to that which Jaensch had announced. But as a student of Hering, Hofmann remained ambivalent about what he clearly saw as the Gestalt school's abandonment of practical attempts at physiological reductionism. He insisted that Gestalt formation should be explained in terms of simpler, "physiologically grounded" perceptual patterns such as those elaborated earlier by G. E. Müller (Hofmann 1925, 591). At the end of the Helmholtz–Hering controversy, German psychology was offering both schools ambiguous support at best.

CONCLUSION: THE FRAGMENTATION OF VISION STUDIES

These accounts of the disciplines involved with vision studies show the fate of the Helmholtz–Hering controversy in the twentieth century. Fragmentation of vision studies along disciplinary lines tended more and more to override the more pervasive but essentially interdisciplinary breach represented by the competing perspectives of Helmholtz and Hering. The issues of the controversy were too fundamental to disappear: they were reviewed and reformulated in textbook accounts deep into the twentieth century. But a resolution or compromise was no longer pressing to the separate disciplinary interests involved; the dispute seemed intangible and irrelevant, and it no longer represented the burning division of the field it had been for the scientific generation of the 1890s.

One contemporary acknowledged the acute disciplinary fragmentation of vision studies. American psychologist Leonard Thompson Troland complained in 1922 that the 180 articles on vision published in 1920 had been scattered in fifty-eight different periodicals and reflected eleven separate disciplines or fields. Even the literature reviews were discipline-specific, so that none captured more than a small portion of the total literature. "The diffuseness of the literature," Troland went on, "is reflected by the methods and conceptions employed by investigators publishing in the several fields, each showing a lack of acquaintance with the problems and results of the other" (Troland 1922, 10).

The twentieth-century breakdown of communication among the disciplines that studied vision suggests an irony about the historical role played by the schools of Helmholtz and Hering. Research schools have been described as the primary vehicles of scientific change and specialization. In this particular case the schools played the opposite role. While they flourished as transdisciplinary constellations, they encouraged the collation of many diverse results into a theoretical and methodological whole that could be brought to bear for or against the perspective of one school or the other. They integrated vision studies on the Continent and slowed, although they did not ultimately prevent, the onset of disciplinary fragmentation and specialization.

Part Four

CONCLUSION

CHAPTER FOURTEEN

In Search of Denouement:
The Twentieth Century

HISTORIANS offer narrative reconstructions of the past that are essentially stories, and stories nonetheless when they deal, as this one does, with the arcane disputes of scientific specialists. As narrators, historians choose the points at which their stories begin and end, and that choice inevitably influences both the form of emplotment and the dramatic significance that the narrative as a whole will evince. This account of the Helmholtz–Hering controversy has already been deeply shaped by narrative choices of this kind. For example, it opens abruptly with the initial confrontations of the two chief protagonists and largely disclaims historical continuities extending back before the 1840s. In doing so it eschews other narrative possibilities that might employ longer prologues or earlier beginnings set in the more distant history of speculation about vision. Versions of that latter type more readily seek the story's narrative significance in a historical recurrence of a deep and transcendent conflict of ideas surpassing individual personalities and historical contexts. The narration employed here seeks the significance of the controversy in the local and contextual ironies of the exchange itself.

But if this particular narration postulates a clear beginning for the Helmholtz–Hering controversy, it can unfortunately offer no equally decisive denouement. The great methodological issues that divided the two schools in the nineteenth century, and to a surprising extent many of the specific and empirical questions that they debated, are still alive and controversial in the sensory physiology and psychology of the present. From the standpoint of the storyteller, the controversy threatens to display no ending at all, or rather to offer several possible endings, any one of which would impose a subtly different significance on the narrative as a whole.

THE INTERNATIONALIZATION OF VISION STUDIES

Whatever ending might be found for a narrative account of the Helmholtz–Hering controversy, the plot of that story undergoes a basic twist in the 1920s. Sometimes during that decade the dispute lost the character of a school controversy. Disciplinary fragmentation contributed to that loss, but so did changes in the cast of characters. Hering's school was devastated by its leader's death in 1918, and his most formidable disciples outlived him by only a few years. Siegfried Garten died in 1923 at fifty-two; Carl von Hess in 1923 at sixty; and Franz Hofmann in 1926 at fifty-seven. There were other students, to be sure, but by 1930 only Armin Tschermak-Seysenegg was still polemicizing on Hering's behalf, and Tschermak never attained a full professorship, the sine qua non of academic influence in Central Europe. Franz Hillebrand, the most adroit of Hering's disciples, published little and spent his career at the small Austrian University of Innsbruck, where he lacked research facilities and sympathetic colleagues (Stumpf and Rupp 1927). He died there in 1926 at sixty-three, after having been incapacitated for years by a lingering illness.

Death also took its toll on Helmholtz's key supporters. J. J. Müller had died at age twenty-nine, and Kries' student and collaborator Willibald Nagel died in 1911 at forty-one. Neither loss was as damaging as that of Arthur König in 1901 at age forty-nine, for his death ended the flourishing research school he had developed at Berlin. The survival of Helmholtz's doctrines, however, never depended upon personal discipleship to the extent that Hering's had. In general, Hering's students did not train prominent schools of their own and did not inspire their students with their own scientific militancy. Hering's ideas survived, but after 1930 they were no longer coupled to the affective and institutional interests of disciples who had staked their careers upon them.

From the 1920s the issues of the former Helmholtz–Hering controversy were to be debated on a larger and more international stage. American L. T. Troland remarked with satisfaction in 1922 that vision research had by then "ceased to be a predominantly Teutonic endeavour" (Troland 1922, 4–5), and bibliographical evidence confirms his judgment. Analysis and comparison of the great bibliographies on vision studies compiled by Arthur König in the 1890s and Franz Hofmann in the 1920s show that the proportion of scientific literature written in German had declined substantially in most research areas over the period. Germany's long dominance over physiological optics was being slowly eroded in the early twentieth century.

This "internationalization" of vision research enhanced the relative influence of the Helmholtzian positions and weakened those of Hering and his school. England, for example, provided stony ground for Hering's ideas. In philosophy and psychology, England's venerable associationist tradition undergirded an empiricist approach to spatial perception more similar to Wundt's theory than to Helmholtz's, in the heavy stress that it laid upon eye movements and other muscular and motor phenomena

(Hyslop 1888, 1891; Sully 1878, 1886, 1886; McDougall 1912; Stout 1929). As to the study of color vision, physicalist approaches predominated in England. Sir William Abney, photographic chemist and educational official, succeeded König as the leading international pioneer in precision colorimetry, and Abney took the Young–Helmholtz theory virtually for granted (Abney 1914). British ophthalmologist John Herbert Parsons published perhaps the single most influential text on color theory of the twentieth century, his *An Introduction to the Study of Colour Vision* (2d ed., 1924). Parsons showed sympathy and understanding in his discussion of Hering's theory and the researches it had inspired, but he devoted almost three times as much space to the Young–Helmholtz theory and left his readers in little doubt as to which was to be preferred.

The tradition of experimental physiology that developed at Cambridge University proved somewhat more hospitable to Hering's ideas. C. S. Sherrington, who studied there in Michael Foster's laboratory, collaborated with Hering's son, published studies on flicker fusion that supported the physiological basis of simultaneous contrast, and developed influential theories of inhibition and neural integration that closely paralleled Hering's in their basic philosophy (Eccles 1979; Swazey 1975). W. H. Rivers, who also taught at Cambridge, had studied with Hering at Prague (Geison 1978, 304, *passim*). His advanced textbook of 1900 provided what was by far the most knowledgeable and sympathetic account of Hering's work to appear in English (Rivers 1900). Sympathy, however, did not translate into advancement of Hering's theories. Rivers' professional interests shifted to anthropology, and Sherrington published little on vision at the height of his career. William McDougall openly opposed Hering's theory in his *Physiological Psychology* of 1908 (McDougall 1908, 1912).

In the United States sympathy for Hering's positions on spatial perception was not entirely lacking. Joseph Le Conte's study of binocular vision (1881) tried to hold a middle ground between nativism and empiricism, but it leaned implicitly toward the former (Le Conte 1881, 104, 151). William James espoused an abstract nativism that relied heavily on Hering, and he vigorously attacked the "anti-sensationalists" Helmholtz, Wundt, and Lipps; his position influenced Josiah Royce and others (James 1890, 2:900–912; Royce 1911). On the whole, however, experimental psychology in America was empiricist in temper, partly because of Wundt's strong personal influence upon its founders (Boring 1950, 517–24; Titchener 1902, 169–71; Dunlap 1922, 275–76). Leonard T. Troland in the Harvard Psychology Department was the leading American authority on vision through the early twentieth century. Troland tried to maintain an atheoretical stance on the origins of the spatial sense, but he drew his accounts of the horopter and stereopsis as well as his terminology directly from Helmholtz with little reference to Hering or his students (Troland 1922a,b, 1929).

American scientists also showed mixed attitudes toward the conflicting accounts of color perception. Columbia physicist Ogden Rood proselytized vigorously for the Young–Helmholtz theory in his influential *Modern Chromatics* (Rood 1879; Homer 1964; Vitz and Glimcher 1984, 83). American psychologists, however, more frequently criticized Helmholtz for the psychological inadequacies of his color theory. J. McKeen Cattell reviewed the second edition of the *Handbuch* in 1898 and denounced the work as obsolete and a barrier to further progress in the field. Despite the fact that the Young–Helmholtz theory is "imposed annually as ascertained truth on thousands of students in their introductory courses of physics and physiology," Cattell wrote that it would find "not a single adherent" if introduced anew today by an unknown scientist (Cattell 1898, 796).

Suspicion of Young's theory did not translate into support for Hering, or (usually) for any other specific color theory. During the first half of the twentieth century American psychology texts and handbooks usually included a short description of Hering's theory as "another point of view." These descriptions, however, nearly always stressed the four-color characteristic of his theory over the element of opponency, rarely dealt with his theory of brightness, and almost never gave a clear sense of the large role that contrast and adaptation played in his thinking. The judgments offered on Hering's theory ranged from outright dismissal, to theoretical agnosticism, to calls for a zone theory compromise (cf. Troland 1922a,b, 1929; Judd 1951; Graham 1951). By the 1930s American scientists acknowledged that the study of "color" was badly polarized between "physicalist" and "psychological" approaches (Jones 1953; Optical Society of America 1966). Those psychological approaches, however, drew mainly upon David Katz and not upon Hering or his immediate students.

The English-speaking world knew Helmholtz's ideas far better than Hering's. In 1926 the Optical Society of America sponsored an English translation of the third German edition of Helmholtz's *Handbuch* in an attempt to bring American vision research thoroughly up to date with the best German work. The translation also included updates of the extensive appendixes and commentaries that Johannes von Kries and his collaborators had prepared for the third German edition. English and American readers, who had long had access to Helmholtz's popular lectures in English, now had readily available not only the *Handbuch* but also Kries' adroit defenses of Helmholtz's views against those of Hering. By comparison, none of Hering's scientific work was translated before 1942, and his long and diffuse German writings were not widely available. For all these reasons, English and American scientists who were quite familiar with Helmholtz's original writings and those of his defenders knew Hering mostly through hostile secondary accounts.

In Germany, by contrast, Hering's ideas continued to be treated with respect and in detail, even after the collapse of his school (e.g., Trendelenburg 1943, 1961). Hering's ideas seem to have had few direct supporters in Germany after 1930, but his surviving influence on color theory there could be seen in the proliferation of zone theories. Erwin Schrödinger demonstrated again in 1926 that the Helmholtz–König results could be expressed in terms of Hering's theory by simple mathematical transformations, and he hypothesized that neural interactions at a zone interface might carry out the physiological equivalent of those transformations (Schrödinger 1926). G. E. Müller's complex, three-zone theory continued to attract interest, and at least three additional zone models were proposed in Germany in the 1940s. All assumed three types of primary cone receptors and drew on the latest neurological research in postulating complex lateral wiring between ganglion cells to render plausible opponency effects at that level (Richter 1951). In comparison, these models found little echo in the English literature, and much less work was done on zone theories outside Germany. Both developments point to the relative decline of Hering's influence as a result of the internationalization of vision studies.

ZONE THEORY ESTABLISHED

For all these reasons, 1930 offers a feasible point at which to conclude the story of the Helmholtz–Hering controversy. By then the historical continuity of the dispute had been broken by disciplinary fragmentation, the passing of the schools, and the internationalization of the field. How stories end, however, dictates what they have been about, and the choice of 1930 imposes an ironical, even satirical cast upon the narrative. By then the alternatives that Helmholtz and Hering had offered were no longer instantiated in clearly defined schools or—except vaguely in the trichromatic theory of vision—in active research programs. Scientists regarded the controversy as an unfortunate and anachronistic lapse, and most believed that they had transcended the terms of the dispute. From the standpoint of Hering's school, a denouement in 1930 imposes a tragic cast upon the story. Outside Germany, and perhaps within it as well, the 1930s and 1940s marked the nadir of Hering's historical influence on the study of vision.

A different date yields a dramatically different ending to the story. During the 1950s and 1960s physiology and psychology turned sharply and unexpectedly toward theories of light perception ostensibly very similar to those Hering and Ernst Mach had advocated long before. This theoretical turn occurred on a wide front, but most dramatically in studies of color vision. By the 1970s a zone-theory mechanism of color vision similar to that advocated by Kries and Donders almost a century earlier had been so broadly accepted as to be dubbed the "textbook model" of color vision (Hood and Finkelstein 1983; Hardin 1988; Hurvich 1981). This development has a complex and still unexplored history, but its outlines, at least, can be sketched.

Until the 1950s most twentieth-century research on color vision had pursued and extended the basic trichromatic theory. Physicists and psychologists mobilized psychophysical data from color mixing, threshold measurements, hue discrimination, adaptation, and color blindness in repeated efforts to derive the spectral response curves of the fundamental sensations and to deduce from them the nature of the retinal color-coding mechanisms (Le Grand 1968, 429–53). What characterized this tradition was less its tacit assumption of trichromatism than its confidence—also an element of the Young–Helmholtz theory—that any neural processing that might occur between the retinal receptors and the sensorium would not invalidate those deductions about receptor physiology. These efforts required ever-greater precision in the difficult psychophysical measurements required for the program, and so were closely associated with the attempt to define universal colorimetric standards, as in the establishment of the C.I.E. Standard Colorimetric Observer in 1931. The approach was highly physicalist in orientation. One of its major representatives was Selig Hecht (1892–1947), professor of biophysics at Columbia University (Hecht 1930). Another was physicist Walter. S. Stiles (1901–85) of the British Physical Laboratory. Stiles ingeniously combined chromatic adaptation techniques with threshold determinations to produce an entirely new method for detecting and measuring mechanisms of color perceptions at work in the visual system (Stiles 1978).

For all its sophistication, this research tradition made little progress toward a unified theory of vision. Hecht's work raised fears that no set of fundamental response curves could simultaneously satisfy all the data constraints (Vries 1946; Le Grand 1968, 433; Jameson 1981, 9; Granit 1947, 330); Stiles' methods detected as many as seven mechanisms of vision, the relationship of which to the three hypothetical ones of Young's theory remained unclear (Le Grand 1968, 449–53; Marriott 1976, 509–32; Stiles 1978, 28–29). By the 1930s, however, important breakthroughs in the study of vision had begun to come from an entirely different research tradition.

By the 1930s physiologists had learned to measure the electrical response to stimuli of individual fibers of the optic nerve, and eventually to make direct microelectrode measurements in the retinal layers themselves (Le Grand 1968, 429–53). Regnar Granit at the University of Stockholm pioneered research of this kind; in 1939 for the first time he inserted microelectrodes into the ganglion cell layer of the retinas of frogs and measured spectral response curves at these sites (Granit 1947). Granit developed his own "dominator-modulator" theory, which he presented as a neurophysiological specification of Young's (pp. 316–44). Nevertheless, his specific findings proved difficult to reconcile with psychophysical data from humans or with the assumption of three fundamental response mechanisms. Granit insisted that he had confirmed one prediction of Hering's theory, namely, the existence of a photopic brightness mechanism independent of chromatic responses (p. 320). Equally important, his own influential theory presupposed lateral interconnections in the retina, and so tacitly abandoned Helmholtz's assumption that every cone possessed a "private line" to the brain.

Granit had developed his microelectrode techniques in collaboration with his student Gunnar Svaetichin, who in 1953 claimed to have obtained the first results from microelectrode studies of individual cone responses. Working with the large double cones of fish retinas, Svaetichin discovered that most positions of the electrode yielded broad and positive electrical responses. These he compared to Granit's dominators, which were hypothesized to mediate achromatic vision. By 1956, however, he had found the property of chromatic opponency in some cells. Long wavelength stimuli produced positive local potential responses, short wavelength stimuli produced negative responses (Svaetichin 1956). He also discovered two classes of cells with different sets of maxima. Svaetichin promptly labeled these "R-G" and "B-Y," and in his first paper he pointed explicitly to the conformity of these responses with the behavior predicted by Hering's opponent process theory of color vision (Figure 14.1).

Svaetichin's work attracted much attention, as well as skepticism that his local potential readings had been taken from individual cone cells, or from single cells at all. Despite that skepticism, his results opened a floodgate of research on the chromatic response of individual cells in the visual system. By 1970 chromatic opponency had been discovered all along the visual path. Research on the lateral geniculate nucleus of monkeys confirmed two classes of chromatic opponent cells with the specific spectral sensitivities roughly similar to those required by Hering's theory (Wiesel and Hubel 1966; De Valois 1965; De Valois and De Valois 1975).

In the late 1950s methods of foveal reflectometry allowed researchers to detect and measure the absorption spectrum of two cone photopigments, even though these could not be extracted and isolated. In the 1960s the microspectrophotometer began to yield difference spectra from

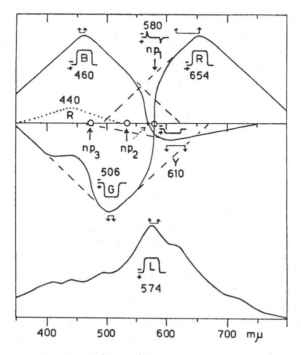

Fig. 14.1 Svaetichin's schematic representation of
spectral response curves obtained from fish cones.
Source: Svaetichin 1956, 41. Reproduced with the
permission of the *Acta Physiologica Scandinavica*.

individual cones. Data from humans and monkeys indicated the existence
of three pigments peaking at 445, 535, and 570 nanometers (Marks et al.
1864; Brown and Wald 1964; De Valois and De Valois 1975, 121–23).
Single-cell response studies seemed to confirm the existence of three
Young-type mechanisms in the retinal cones and opponent-processing
mechanisms at higher neural levels, just as predicted by the classical zone
theory hypotheses on the basis of totally different kinds of evidence.

Neurophysiology and psychophysics converged on a common zone
theory from opposite directions. American psychologists Leo Hurvich
and Dorothea Jameson emerged in the 1950s as the foremost architects of
that theory. Hurvich had studied at Harvard, where he encountered the
work of Ewald Hering in a graduate seminar on the history of psychology
conducted by E. G. Boring.[1] Dorothea Jameson studied psychology at
Wellesley, and their common interest in vision was reinforced when they
took research positions in the Eastman Kodak Laboratory in Rochester,
New York, in 1947. Their work returned squarely to Hering's program
of research on color vision, and to the question of how to develop it on a

zone-theoretical basis (cf. Hurvich and Jameson 1951). In both respects their work was radically discontinuous with the then-dominant traditions in American psychology and vision research.

During the mid-1950s Jameson and Hurvich developed a quantitative model of how inputs from the three retinal photopigments are recoded at the opponent process level to produce our observed sensory responses. They employed a hue cancelation technique in which the subject was presented with, say, a blue-green monochromatic light and instructed to add yellow (most conveniently, the unique or pure yellow) until the test field was left with no tinge of yellow or blue. This technique allowed them to determine the relative levels of red-green, blue-yellow response present in every hue of the spectrum, and therefore to represent the two opponent mechanisms graphically as spectral response curves, positive abscissas representing red or yellow, negative abscissas green or blue (Hurvich and Jameson 1957; Hardin 1988, 39). They equated the response curve of the achromatic mechanism to the photopic luminosity function (see Figure 14.2). Further, this data allowed Hurvich and Jameson to calculate the tristimulus values of any monochromatic light for any set of experimental primaries, or conversely to calculate their response curves from color-mixture data. They could thus display graphically both levels of the zone theory and demonstrate their quantitative relationship.[2]

The work of Jameson and Hurvich suggests again Hering's remarkable ability to inspire disciples. In their later careers they continuously presented themselves as followers of Hering, despite the obvious differences between their zone model and the original opponent process theory. They translated Hering's most comprehensive presentation of his theory into English and wrote valuable historical accounts of his work. Hurvich, especially, resisted designation of his model as a zone theory. The three retinal photopigments may provide neural inputs to the opponent process mechanisms, Hurvich wrote, but those inputs cannot be associated with color sensations. In that most crucial sense, Hering was right and Helmholtz was wrong in their controversy, just as Hering had always insisted (Hurvich 1969).

Like Hering and his school, Hurvich and Jameson waxed sarcastic about what they perceived to be the tendency of many scientists, and physicists in particular, to describe as "red," "green," or "blue" everything from light waves and photopigments to electroneural excitations and human genes. Their reminiscences of their early work refer to the trichromatic theory as a pervasive but illusive dogma in the field, just as Hering and his students had done (Hurvich and Jameson 1989, 182–95). Like Hering, they offered the principle of opponency as a blueprint for understanding all neural action and stimulus-response effects (Hurvich and Jameson 1974). Their work, together with the supporting evidence

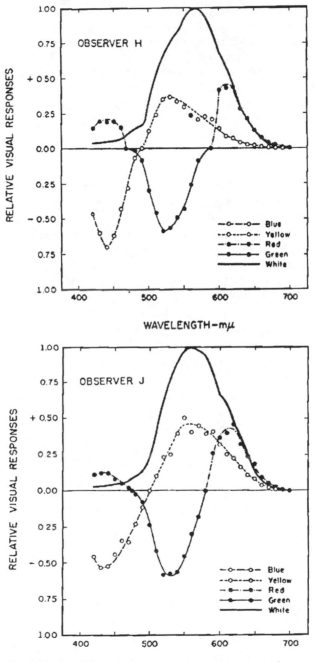

Fig. 14.2 The Hurvich–Jameson opponent process chromatic response curves derived from hue cancelation studies, with the achromatic spectral function. (Two observers, equal energy spectrum.) *Source*: Hurvich and Jameson 1957, 389. Reproduced with the permission of the American Psychological Association.

from neurophysiology, was primarily responsible for the new "textbook model" of visual perception and for the revival of widespread scientific interest in Hering's ideas.

The narrative drama of this decisive reversal of fortune would not have been lost on the rhetorically conscious Hering. An account of the color vision controversies that ends in 1970 necessarily introduces a comedic element: the conflicting views of Helmholtz and Hering emerge as suddenly and unexpectedly susceptible to harmonious integration. Extending the story further, however, introduces other narrative complications.

Despite its success at the level of advanced textbooks, the two-stage zone model never lacked for critics (Brindley 1970, 209; Marriott 1976). They pointed out that the fit between physiological and psychophysical data was approximate at best. Some cells in the visual track showed the opponency characteristic required by the two-stage theory, but many others did not. A greater difficulty came with closer investigation of opponent properties themselves. In the early 1980s psychophysical methods based on adaptation techniques allowed researchers to demonstrate the existence of second-stage mechanisms that showed clear color opponency. While the red-green opponency axis measured in this way was found to correspond to the "pure red" and "pure green" of the Hering-type mechanisms postulated by Hurvich and Jameson, the yellow-blue opponency axis failed to do so (Krauskopf et al. 1982). A similar discrepancy was detected neurophysiologically, in certain cells of the lateral geniculate nucleus in macaques that in other respects showed the blue-yellow opponency required by Hering-type mechanisms (Derrington et al. 1984). The results cast doubt on the assumption that sensory response could be associated directly with the output of second-stage opponency mechanisms, and they raised the possibility that more than two zones were required to model chromatic processes adequately.

CONTRAST AND STEREOPSIS

By the 1950s the same kinds of electrophysiological research that supported the zone theory of color vision had led to a reinterpretation of contrast phenomena in terms of neural interactions in the retina. This was indeed a reinterpretation. E. G. Boring, reviewing twentieth-century research on simultaneous contrast in 1942, claimed flatly that nothing had been added to the classic studies done by the students of Wundt and Hering at the end of the nineteenth century. The one exception to this generalization, Wundt noted, was that the Gestalt school had demonstrated how contrast effects were related to perceptual wholes. Contrast therefore arose in the center, not in the retina, and this suggested to Boring a return to a quasi-Helmholtzian view of the phenomenon (Boring 1942, 170–71).

Even as Boring wrote, however, electrophysiological studies had begun to yield different results. In 1938 H. K. Hartline detected three classes of fibers in the optic nerves of frogs, one class of which showed an inhibitory "off" response at cessation of stimulus (Hartline 1938). Granit and his students quickly confirmed this result using their own methods, and noted that it resembled the neural response required for successive contrast. As early as 1935 electroretinogram readings had shown evidence of lateral interaction between stimulated retinal points suggestive of simultaneous contrast. Hartline and others measured the receptive fields of individual fibers of the optic nerve, and in the 1950s directly observed lateral inhibition among neighboring retinal elements in the eye of *Limulus*, the horse shoe crab (Hartline and Ratliff 1957–58). The receptive fields of visual cells were found to contain concentric zones, some zones responding to stimulation with inhibitory effects, some with exhibitory, and with complex averaging when the whole receptive field was illuminated (De Valois and De Valois 1975, 128–39). Color contrast and the uniformity of contrast across large fields continued to present problems to neurophysiological accounts, and much evidence showed that higher perceptual and psychological effects enter into contrast phenomena. Nevertheless, by the early 1960s direct physiological action was widely held to be responsible for contrast, afterimages, and contour enhancement, just as Mach and Hering had claimed (De Valois and De Valois 1975, 151–62; Dodwell 1975, 57–77).[3]

The nativist-empiricist controversy had turned primarily on the issue of binocular depth perception. Twentieth-century studies of stereopsis scarcely moved the issue from where it had stood at the end of the nineteenth century. In 1962, however, Bela Julesz of Bell Laboratories introduced random-dot stereograms, in which a portion of the random pattern is displaced in one monocular presentation. The fact that these stereograms nevertheless give rise to binocular relief was taken to refute the empiricist view that we infer the spatial meaning of binocular disparities on the basis of past visual experience of objects in space (Julesz 1962, 1964, 1971). Equally important was the discovery in the 1960s of single cells in the visual system that respond to specific degrees of retinal disparity (Barlow et al. 1967). This evidence encouraged psychologists to regard stereopsis responses to disparity as anatomically innate, however experiential cues might supplement the effect, or whatever visual experience might be necessary to trigger the proper developmental sequences (Hochberg 1988, 226–28; Dodwell 1975, 65). Here, as in studies of contrast, Hering's position had become the consensus view, although not a view universally accepted.

PERCEPTION THEORY IN THE TWENTIETH CENTURY

The most pervasive theme in the long story of the Helmholtz–Hering controversy is the fundamental differences between the protagonists concerning the nature of human perception. Helmholtz represented what was by far the dominant point of view. Although many psychologists and philosophers rebelled against his terminology of unconscious inference, few departed from the pervasive belief that mental processes must somehow bring the evidence of past sensory experience to bear upon proximal stimuli, in order to complete or supplement them and so give rise to perception. Psychologist Julian Hochberg identified empiricism and its inferential understanding of perception as the "classical" theory of perception. Only since the late 1940s, he argued, has that classical theory been challenged by three new research directions that reject or attempt in significant ways to alter that theory (Hochberg 1988, 228–33).

One was the neurophysiological direction, in which David H. Hubel and Torsten Wiesel at Harvard Medical School played major roles. During the 1960s they investigated cells in the striate cortex of cats and mapped receptive fields using patterned retinal stimulation. They discovered arrays of cells that show particular responsiveness to set stimulus patterns (bars or edges), particular spatial orientations of these patterns, or particular directions of motion (Hubel and Wiesel 1965, 1968). This receptor specialization in adult animals could, of course, be assumed to have been built up through visual experience, and other experiments showed that raising animals in darkness, or otherwise depriving them of normal visual experience, could retard or permanently prevent the development of visual ability. In a much-cited paper of 1963, however, Hubel and Wiesel announced that very young kittens raised without visual exposure possessed the same specialized receptor cells in the cortex as adult, visually experienced cats. They speculated that visual deprivation did not prevent development, but "led to the disruption of connections that were there from the start" (Hubel and Wiesel 1963, 1001). Skeptics objected that neurophysiology made little headway in showing how output from a mass of specialized receptors is integrated into object perception or whole-field effects. Nevertheless, neurophysiological findings and other methodological approaches that supplemented them persuaded many scientists that the mammalian visual system and its capacities are more extensively innate and hard-wired than previously believed (Dodwell 1975, 65; Gardner 1985, 260–90, esp. 273–74).

Another current in postwar American psychology counterbalanced the reductionist and arguably nativist impact of neurophysiology. The so-called new look in perception studies after World War II emphasized the role of past experience and motivation in perception. Then in the 1970s what has been called the "cognitive revolution" threw off the last remnants of behaviorism and turned to a search for deep analogies between perception and information processing and how the former might be simulated in computers (Gardner 1985, esp. 138–81; Gilgen 1982, 74, 111–38). The new "cognitive science" was programmatically oblivious to cultural or affective determinants of consciousness, but at the same time was suspicious of neurological reductionism. It was also resolutely interdisciplinary, and drew heavily, not only upon computer science and artificial intelligence, but also upon linguistics, philosophy, and anthropology (Gardner 1985, 38–45). Technological needs reinforced the drive of cognitive scientists to develop boundary-sensing computer programs, form analyzers, and mathematical models of binocular stereopsis and motion perception.

The information-processing models of perception developed as part of the cognitive movement implicitly restored scientific respectability to talk of mental structures and representations. They suggested that such structures stand to brains as programs stand to computer hardware, and they provided methods for simulating models of mental structures and testing them quantitatively (Hochberg 1988, 248–49). In their approach and assumptions, information-processing models of perception also displayed clear continuity with classical empiricism. Some of the pioneers of cognitive psychology expressly noted the similarity of their approach with the empiricism of Helmholtz and compared their own works to the famous *Handbuch* (Ash 1985, 334; Gardner 1985, 305–7). A recent historical treatment has portrayed Helmholtz as the founder of the modern, information-processing approach to perception (Meyering 1981, 1989).

The third new direction in perception theory owed a debt to the influence of the Gestalt movement upon American psychology. Koffka, Wertheimer, and Köhler all immigrated to the United States between 1927 and 1934, where their ideas were strongly opposed by the powerful American traditions of operationalism and neobehaviorism. Those traditions discouraged research into sensation and perceptions, or channeled them into behaviorist and quasi-empiricist orientations (eg. Taylor 1962, vii; cf. Dodwell 1975, 65). Nevertheless, Mitchell Ash has shown that Gestalt theorists exercised an indirect impact on the training of certain influential American psychologists as well as upon a few students of their own, and that they preserved an undercurrent of research interest in perception and cognition (Ash 1985, 329–33).

Koffka, especially, influenced psychologist James J. Gibson, considered by some the twentieth century's most original contributor to the problem of spatial perception. He became the foremost advocate of the most radical departure of postwar theorizing on perception, the so-called direct theories of perception (Reed 1988; Hochberg 1988, 240–48). In his 1950 work, *The Perception of the Visual World*, Gibson followed the Gestalt theorists in abandoning the sensation-perception dichotomy and denying that the world as we perceive it is an interpretation or construction out of some more primitive data that are themselves not "thing-like" (Gibson 1950, 187).

In his later writings Gibson went far beyond the Gestalt theorists in spelling out the tenets of the direct theory of perception he called "ecological realism" or "visual realism." He taught that the visual array incorporates and preserves certain invariant relationships in the distal stimuli of the physical world. Under normal viewing conditions our nervous systems respond directly to these invariants, so that the retinal image is "adequate" in and of itself for veridical spatial perception (Gibson 1982, 53–89; 1966, 186–223). Direct theories like Gibson's hinged on the search for such invariants: texture and motion gradients, simplicity principles for the integration of three-dimensional forms, rigidity principles for object perception.

The breakdown since the 1950s of what Hochberg called the "classical theory" of perception offers another feasible note on which to conclude a narrative account of the Helmholtz–Hering controversy. At least a few clear lines of historical continuity seem to run from the school debates of the late nineteenth and early twentieth centuries to the various new approaches to perception that have proliferated since the 1960s. The neurophysiological evidence that response to specific visual stimuli is localized in particular anatomical sites and processes, and that these responses are to a large extent innate, is often taken to confirm the nativist principles that Hering tenaciously defended during his lifetime. Cognitive models of perception based on information processing seem similarly to express in contemporary guise the basic tenets of Helmholtz's empiricism. Told within these limits, the story becomes one of the essential continuity and unity of scientific attempts to treat the problem of perception, and a story tinged by the satirical hint that these warring perspectives cannot readily be transcended.

In the final analysis accounts of postwar theorizing about perception may take story of Helmholtz, Hering, and the historical confrontation of their ideas too far. The lines of historical continuity grow increasingly faint upon close examination, and the apparent similarity between contemporary ideas about perception and those of the early protagonists can be treacherously misleading. Hering's nativism, for example, should not be misread in retrospect as primarily a program of physiological reductionism. To Hering, it was a search for the psychophysical interface, a program to complete the "tunnel" from objective stimulus to subjective experience. Empiricism, for Hering, confused and complicated that program, by imposing "experience" and "inference" in what he regarded as unnecessary ways between nervous stimuli and the phenomenologically given. Helmholtz's talk of unconscious inference translates with deceptive ease into the modern terminology of information processing. In fact, he postulated very different models of the inferential process from most of those current in modern cognitive science. At the core of Helmholtz's thinking was the questing, rational ego. Despite his ambiguities on the subject, Helmholtz conceived the mental processes through which the ego constructs perceptions and the world as constrained not by rules and processing protocols, but by rationality itself.

The discontinuity between ideas about perception from the late nineteenth century to the late twentieth is most marked in Gibson's direct theory of perception. For Gibson the "adequacy" of the retinal image makes inferential processes like those Helmholtz had postulated extraneous and unnecessary. Yet Gibson's notion of learning as an active and exploratory process, in which the perceiver achieves successively finer discrimination of invariants from variants in the optical array, parallels Helmholtz's particular volitional empiricism. Although Gibson was frequently labeled a nativist, his views are subtly incommensurable with those of the Gestalt school or of Hering himself (Gibson 1950, 22–23; 1982, 303–16). The "adequacy" of the retinal image obviates the necessity of postulating, as nineteenth-century nativists did, innate neural structures that act on the proximal stimulation in order to bring it into more direct correspondence with some distal property. In his most mature writings, Gibson insisted on a commonsense, realist view of time and space relationships quite different from those espoused by Helmholtz or by Hering (Gibson 1982, 374–84), and quite alien to the context of German thought about perception at the end of the nineteenth century. With respect to the Helmholtz–Hering controversy, contemporary debates about perception are another story.

CONCLUSION: CONSENSUS AND CONTROVERSY

In 1982 philosopher Larry Laudan asked what it was about the practice of natural science that *most* requires explanation. Is it that scientists *agree* so extensively? That they achieve and maintain intense levels of internal consensus over the fundamentals of their practice, even as that consensus itself undergoes startlingly rapid and continuous change? Or is it that despite the powerful social and methodological mechanisms that compel scientific fields toward theoretical consensus, they nevertheless are and have been rife with chronic disputes, rival research programs, and incommensurable knowledge claims?

No historical case study resolves questions like these. But case studies—and particularly the unique case study examined here—shed intense light on the mechanisms of consensus and controversy in science. The Helmholtz-Hering dispute exhibited, for example, the intimate entanglement of consensus and controversy. The core set controversy fought among Helmholtz, Hering, and their students presupposed the far-reaching integration of the formerly inchoate field of vision studies that occurred in Europe at the middle of the nineteenth century. The controversy was possible not only because Helmholtz and Hering disagreed so fundamentally, but also because, in relationship to other competitors and to the recent past of their field, they shared such extensive common ground. The early chapters of this study have stressed the extent of that agreement. As late as 1866 Helmholtz and Hering still held quite similar views about the proximate mechanisms of depth perception, if not about its deep structures. Their schools, in their common commitment to component theories of color perception and punctiform analysis of the retinal image, always stood in closer agreement with each other than to other, rival approaches to these topics, both before and after them.

This narrative also reinforces the view that controversy, be it normal or anomalous, is nevertheless constitutive of deep change in science. At every stage of the Helmholtz–Hering dispute, partisans consciously exploited controversy and the potential for controversy, directing it to their own ends, intensifying it in one direction or against one adversary, minimizing it in another. Controversy influenced the partisans themselves and shaped the positions they espoused. Early chapters have shown that Helmholtz's views about spatial perception were developed between 1862 and 1866 in the heat of running criticism by Ewald Hering, and they argued that Helmholtz's particular positions were deeply shaped by those criticisms. They also contended that the strategic and rhetorical demands of controversy, as much or more than the actualities of the field, led Helmholtz to his radical and historically far-reaching dichotomization of perceptual studies along nativist-empiricist lines in 1867. Similarly, Hering's growing willingness from 1868 on to assume the nativist mantle represented in part a defiant acceptance of the very role Helmholtz had cast him for. The duplicity theory of vision, formulated by Kries in 1894, was equally a product of controversy. Neither its rationale, nor its timing, nor its motivation can be understood outside the context of the intense exchange that erupted in the early 1890s among König, Hillebrand, Kries, and Hering over monochromatism, the dark spectrum, and the specific brightnesses of colors. The duplicity theory in turn affected the controversy, largely by weakening the competitive position of Hering's school.

At every stage of the dispute, polemical exchanges functioned in part as a noisy, but oddly subtle negotiation between parties who rarely met face to face. Before 1867 Hering's papers sought explicitly to lever the great Helmholtz out of the projectionist (not the empiricist) camp; compromise positions proffered to Hering constituted a regular subtext of Kries' periodic reviews of the field. Polemical papers were thus written for two audiences and served a double purpose: to refute the opposition and win the allegiance of nonaligned members of the core set, and to tacitly negotiate terms of surrender, compromise, or ground-of-next-engagement with the opposition. Subtle negotiation is particularly explicit in Hering's less polemical papers, those addressed to nonaligned participants such as Volkmann, Donders, and Stumpf. Controversy was not the incidental result of a clash between two, autonomously unfolding research programs. Controversy was a tool of those programs, one that deeply affected their mutual development and was constitutive of their scientific activity.

The special interest of the Helmholtz–Hering controversy lies in the fact that in this case negotiation failed. The issues of the controversy were neither resolved nor successfully compromised, despite the repeated assertion by influential members of the core set that a basis for doing so was at hand. The dispute eludes understanding or classification in terms of the more common closure typologies that have proliferated in science studies. Throughout the period examined, the two schools disagreed fundamentally over what constituted the significant problems of vision research and what constituted solutions to them; their research practice was controversy- as much as theory-driven.

The story of the dispute has pointed to many elements that sustained the controversy. Chief among these was the polarization of the core set into two hostile schools. These schools were distinguished by their theoretical commitments, but as much or more by their geographical and institutional affiliations, styles of leadership, and—a factor the study has especially emphasized—the emotional ties and personal loyalties that they generated. The strong role played by the schools weakened the influence of nonaligned participants in the core set and undermined their attempts to negotiate compromise positions. The particular context of German academia in the late nineteenth century facilitated school formations of this kind. Nevertheless, the episode points to the larger significance of research schools as foci of change in science.

The controversy was also perpetuated by strong elements of incommensurability between the positions of the schools. Their spasmodic efforts at negotiation were frustrated at every turn by the real difficulties that the partisans encountered in understanding the concepts, models, and terminology of their opponents. The study suggested that this incommensurability had roots in real differences of perceptual sensitivity: that the two schools saw the sensory features of blacks, grays, and chromatic colors in subtly different ways. The study emphasized, however, the role of semantic incommensurability, while insisting at the same time that semantic incommensurability cannot be clearly separated from consciously adopted strategies of rhetoric and communication. In few if any scientific controversies of the nineteenth century was the struggle for semantic control so intense or so self-conscious as in the Helmholtz–Hering dispute. So fundamental was semantic control to Hering's program that he repeatedly rejected proposals that promised conceptual compromise at the price of terminological cooptation. The eclipse of Hering's program in the 1920s was marked less by the disappearance of his ideas from the international scientific literature than by the loss of his terminology, especially in the face of linguistic challenges posed by the new psychologists in Germany.

The outcome of the Helmholtz–Hering controversy was closely associated with its appeal to disciplinary interests and identities. Three of the four scientific disciplines mainly involved in vision research achieved disciplinary autonomy in Germany during the period of the controversy, and that with ironic consequences. The fragmentation of vision studies along disciplinary lines more and more overrode the pervasive but essentially interdisciplinary breach represented by the competing perspectives of Helmholtz and Hering. The issues of the controversy had limited significance for the therapeutic interests of ophthalmology, and by 1900 physics and physiology were moving toward more exclusive application of particular research methods that could address only a limited number of the issues. In psychology the phenomenological and Gestalt movements brought to the fore questions about vision quite different from those that Helmholtz and Hering had asked, and which mostly bypassed the central issues of their controversy. That controversy was too fundamental to disappear: it was reviewed and reformulated in textbook accounts deep into the twentieth century. But the issues of the controversy had been left suspended, no longer anchored to particular research agendas. Resolving the controversy or reaching a compromise ceased to be a pressing need in vision studies, even before the major partisans began to die off in the 1920s.

The Helmholtz–Hering dispute also points the moral that men and women, and not ideas, conduct scientific controversies. The reputations, personalities, idiosyncrasies, and rhetorical styles of the protagonists shaped the controversy as much or more than any empirical discoveries or constellation of interests. Of no participant was that more true than of the indomitable and indefatigable Ewald Hering, and scarcely less of the Olympian Helmholtz and the awe he inspired. By the same measure, the issues of the controversy cannot be readily extrapolated past the 1920s, when the personal continuity of the schools had already been broken or seriously attenuated. Post-1950 developments, which seemed on several fronts to mark a return to the views of Hering, were only ostensibly so. They were the creative products of different personalities, focal problems, methodologies, and in some cases epistemological assumptions. The eye's mind knew its history and drew upon it, but it made no historical return.

APPENDIX

TABLE 1

Scientific Literature on Physiological Optics, 1840–94

(per literature category, as a percentage of all literature per time interval)

Literature Category	Time Interval										
	1840 –44	1845 –49	1850 –54	1855 –59	1860 –64	1865 –69	1870 –74	1875 –79	1880 –84	1885 –89	1890 –94
I. Works on the whole, substantial parts, or general principles of physiological optics	2.1	2.8	1.3	0.3	0.3	2.6	1.1	1.6	1.0	0.4	0.4
II. Optical track and brain localization	—	—	—	—	—	—	—	1.2	4.3	6.0	5.0
III. Special literature on physiological optics											
1. Form of the visual organ											
1.1 Historical literature	—	—	—	—	—	—	—	0.3	—	—	—
1.2 Embryology. General, special, and comparative anatomy of the eyes of animals	3.1	0.7	0.3	0.3	—	0.7	0.8	0.5	1.5	3.3	3.4
1.3 General anatomy of the human eye	1.0	1.4	0.3	—	—	—	—	—	—	—	—
2. Sclera and cornea. Dimensions of the eye. Ophthalmometry. Interocular pressure	2.1	1.4	—	1.6	1.2	3.1	3.4	0.6	3.4	3.4	5.0
3. Uvea											
3.1 Anatomy and physiology of the iris, ciliary body, tapetum	—	—	1.3	3.5	0.6	3.8	0.7	1.3	1.9	3.4	1.6
3.2 Measurement of pupillary aperture	—	—	0.3	—	0.6	0.5	—	0.5	0.1	0.6	0.5
3.3 Anterior chamber	—	—	—	—	—	0.2	0.2	0.2	—	0.1	0.1
4. Retina and optic nerve	—	0.7	3.0	2.6	3.0	4.1	2.7	1.6	3.7	1.6	1.6
5. Crystalline lens	—	2.8	1.7	1.0	0.3	0.2	1.0	0.6	0.8	0.2	0.1
6. Aqueous and vitreous humour											
Vitreous body	2.1	3.5	1.3	—	—	0.7	0.4	0.1	0.4	0.2	0.3

Literature Category — Time Interval

Literature Category	1840 -44	1845 -49	1850 -54	1855 -59	1860 -64	1865 -69	1870 -74	1875 -79	1880 -84	1885 -89	1890 -94
7. Accessory structures	—	—	—	—	—	0.5	0.8	0.4	0.5	0.4	0.6
8. (Not used by König)											
9. Laws of refraction in systems of spherical surfaces											
9.1 & 9.2 Older literature, new literature	5.2	0.7	0.7	0.3	0.3	0.2	0.6	0.5	0.4	0.7	0.3
10. Refraction of rays in the eye											
10.1 Optical system of the eye	5.2	3.5	0.7	1.3	1.2	1.9	4.4	4.6	1.9	1.9	3.3
10.2 Measurement of the refractive indices	1.0	2.1	1.0	0.6	—	0.2	1.5	0.3	—	0.1	0.1
10.3 Visual field and the perimeter	—	—	—	0.3	0.3	1.7	2.1	1.2	2.4	2.2	1.8
11. Blur-circles on the retina											
11.1 & 11.2 Size and form of blur-circles. Older and new literature	1.0	1.4	2.7	0.6	—	—	0.4	0.4	0.4	0.4	1.1
11.3 Refraction and accommodation in general	—	—	0.3	—	1.5	3.3	1.0	1.5	1.9	0.5	1.1
11.4 Range of accommodation	—	—	0.7	2.6	3.0	1.0	0.4	1.1	0.4	1.3	1.1
11.5 Optometry, optometers, phacometers	—	—	—	—	1.8	1.0	1.0	2.7	1.4	1.9	1.0
11.6 Large-scale surveys of refraction and acuity	—	—	—	—	—	0.2	0.4	0.7	1.2	1.2	0.9
11.7 Spectacle scales and special forms of spectacles	—	—	—	—	0.3	1.0	2.8	0.9	0.5	0.6	0.7
11.8 Origin and treatment of refractive anomalies	—	—	0.7	—	—	1.4	0.4	1.0	2.7	3.4	6.6
11.9 Historical literature	—	—	—	—	—	0.5	—	0.1	0.3	0.1	0.4
12. Mechanism of accommodation											
12.1 Change of pupillary aperture (See 3.1 & 3.2)											
12.2 Accommodation in aphakia	—	—	—	—	—	—	1.1	0.1	0.1	0.3	0.3
12.3 Mechanism of accommodation	9.4	9.8	6.7	5.1	2.1	3.1	3.6	1.9	1.2	1.6	1.3

Section											
13. Chromatic dispersion in the eye	1.0	2.1	0.7	1.0	0.6	1.2	0.2	0.2	0.2	0.2	—
14. Monochromatic abnormalities											
14.1 Older literature	3.1	4.9	8.7	0.3	—	—	—	—	—	—	—
14.2 Regular astigmatism	—	—	—	—	6.3	7.6	1.9	1.0	3.0	3.6	4.7
14.3 Spherical aberration and faulty centering of the eye	—	—	—	—	—	0.2	—	0.1	0.3	0.4	0.8
14.4 Irregular astigmatism	—	—	—	—	—	1.0	0.2	0.4	0.4	0.8	0.4
15. Entoptical phenomena	2.1	4.2	2.3	2.2	2.1	0.7	1.3	0.2	1.0	0.7	0.4
16. Illumination of the interior of the eye and the ophthalmoscope											
16.1 Illumination of the interior of the eye and the ophthalmoscope	1.0	2.8	8.3	5.7	4.5	5.0	5.1	4.0	4.4	5.6	4.9
16.2 Skiagraphy, skiascopy, retinoscopy	—	—	—	—	—	—	0.4	0.3	1.0	3.6	3.3
16.3 Photography of the retina	—	—	—	—	0.2	0.2	—	—	—	0.4	0.4
17. Stimulation of the optic nerve											
17.1 Sympathetic response of other senses to visual stimulus	1.0	1.4	0.3	—	0.9	0.2	0.4	0.1	1.0	1.2	1.3
17.2 Mechanical stimulation	1.0	—	0.7	1.0	0.9	—	0.6	0.3	0.3	0.3	0.2
17.3 Electrical stimulation	—	0.7	—	—	—	0.4	0.4	—	0.2	0.2	0.3
18. On stimulation by light											
18.1 Optic disc or blindspot and the location of the light-sensitive layer	2.1	0.7	3.7	2.2	1.8	0.7	1.0	—	0.2	0.2	0.4
18.2 Processes in the retina and optic nerve triggered by a light stimulus—visual purple	—	—	—	—	—	0.2	1.0	7.8	2.5	2.3	1.2
18.3 Visual acuity—tests of acuity	4.2	1.4	1.3	1.0	2.1	2.4	3.0	3.4	3.3	3.8	3.5
19. The simple colors											
19.1 & 19.2 Older literature. Goethe and Newton	—	—	0.3	1.0	0.9	—	0.2	0.1	0.4	0.4	0.4

Literature Category

	Time Interval										
	1840 –44	1845 –49	1850 –54	1855 –59	1860 –64	1865 –69	1870 –74	1875 –79	1880 –84	1885 –89	1890 –94
19.3 Other physical color theories	—	4.2	0.7	0.3	—	—	—	—	—	—	—
19.4 Hue discrimination and limits of the visible spectrum	—	1.4	1.3	1.3	1.8	1.0	1.0	0.6	1.0	0.4	0.6
19.5 Color harmonies and comparison with tone intervals	—	—	1.3	1.3	—	0.2	0.4	0.4	—	0.1	0.1
19.6 Color sense of animals and various tribes. Historical and individual development of the color sense	—	—	—	0.3	0.3	0.7	0.4	6.3	4.0	1.0	0.8
20. The composite colors											
20.1 Older literature on normal color vision and theories of color	1.0	4.0	3.7	3.5	—	—	—	—	—	—	—
20.2 Older literature on color blindness	5.2	4.9	3.7	1.9	—	—	—	—	—	—	—
20.3 New literature on normal color vision and color blindness											
a) General discussions of color theories	—	—	—	—	—	0.5	1.0	1.0	0.7	0.1	0.4
b) Specific topics on normal and abmornal color vision	—	—	—	2.6	4.8	5.7	10.4	14.4	14.3	7.4	5.9
c) New theories of color vision	—	—	—	—	—	0.2	0.4	0.4	0.6	1.0	0.8
d) Peripheral color vision	—	—	—	—	—	—	1.5	0.8	0.3	0.5	0.9
e) Methods, apparatus, tests, etc. for investigation of color sense	—	—	—	—	—	0.2	0.8	2.9	4.3	2.9	1.8
f) Case histories of color blindness	1.0	—	—	0.3	0.3	0.2	0.6	1.3	1.5	0.6	1.6
g) Xanthopsia (santonin-effect), erythropia, chloropsia, and cyanopsia	1.0	—	0.7	1.9	2.1	1.0	0.8	0.4	1.2	1.9	1.1
h) Practical significance and incidence of color blindness	—	—	—	0.3	—	—	1.0	3.3	1.6	1.2	0.4
21. On the intensity of the light sensation											
21.1 Psychophysical law, adaptation, stimulus thresholds, intensity of the retinal self-light	3.1	0.7	—	1.3	1.2	0.2	2.5	2.2	2.8	4.2	3.1

21.2 Iso- and heterochromatic photometry	—	—	1.0	0.3	0.9	0.5	1.7	1.0	3.1	1.6	1.4
21.3 Dependence of acuity on level of illumination	—	—	—	0.3	0.3	—	0.2	0.8	0.4	0.7	0.2
21.4 Irradiation	2.1	0.7	4.0	2.2	1.2	2.2	1.0	0.5	0.2	0.2	—
22. Persistence of the light sensation	2.1	5.6	5.7	2.9	3.6	5.0	2.8	2.5	1.7	2.4	1.8
23. Changes in sensitivity to light	8.3	4.9	3.0	3.2	1.5	4.1	3.4	2.3	2.0	1.8	3.5
24. Contrast	3.1	1.4	1.3	3.8	5.1	2.2	2.3	1.3	1.1	1.3	1.1
25. Various subjective phenomena	1.0	6.3	3.0	1.9	1.8	0.7	0.6	0.4	1.0	0.9	0.5
26. On perceptions in general	—	0.7	0.3	0.6	2.7	0.5	0.6	0.8	0.6	0.5	0.8
27. Eye movements	8.3	4.9	1.0	2.2	3.3	3.3	8.7	4.5	1.1	1.9	3.1
28. The monocular visual field	2.1	1.4	3.3	3.5	2.7	1.7	0.2	1.4	1.0	1.0	1.6
29. Visual direction	2.1	1.4	1.3	1.3	2.7	1.9	1.1	1.3	1.2	1.7	1.0
30. Depth perception											
30.1 Monocular depth perception	2.1	—	1.7	1.6	2.4	3.6	0.4	0.3	0.4	1.3	0.6
30.2 Stereoscopy and binocular depth perception	3.1	0.7	8.0	15.3	7.4	6.7	4.0	1.5	1.4	1.6	1.8
31. Binocular double vision	5.2	2.8	2.0	6.1	10.4	3.6	4.5	2.5	1.8	2.2	3.1
32. Binocular rivalry	1.0	2.8	3.0	3.2	4.5	1.4	0.8	0.6	0.1	0.1	0.2
33. Critique of theories	—	1.4	0.7	2.2	3.0	1.2	1.5	1.1	0.4	0.8	1.7
Number of bibliographical items	96	143	300	314	336	419	529	1,008	1,352	1,354	1,145

TABLE 2

Scientific Literature on Physiological Optics, 1840–94, by Problem-Complex
(as a percentage of all literature per time interval, based on twelve-year moving averages)

Problem-Complex	1840 -44	1845 -49	1850 -54	1855 -59	1860 -64	1865 -69	1870 -74	1875 -79	1880 -84	1885 -89	1890 -94
					Time Interval						
I. General works	3.4	2.6	2.7	2.6	3.3	3.2	2.9	2.1	1.7	1.5	1.6
II. Anatomical and physiological studies not involving reports of perceptions	11.7	14.5	15.2	13.7	15.1	15.7	18.5	21.1	25.4	27.7	29.5
III. Dioptrics of the eye	25.1	23.8	18.6	17.3	19.0	21.8	20.9	19.2	19.6	21.7	23.3
IV. Color vision	12.6	12.1	13.6	12.1	11.3	13.3	23.4	28.4	25.7	20.8	15.9
V. Binocular vision, depth perception, eye movements	18.0	19.3	24.5	29.2	28.9	24.1	16.3	11.0	9.3	9.2	10.4
VI. Psychophysiology of vision (afterimages, contrast, adaptation, acuity)	29.3	27.8	25.5	25.2	22.5	22.0	18.1	18.2	18.4	19.1	19.3
Number of bibliographical items (moving averages)	120	180	252	316	356	428	652	963	1238	1284	1250

Notes

Chapter Two
Physiological Optics from Wheatstone to Helmholtz

1. For a detailed discussion of the König bibliography, its adequacy as a representative sample, and the assumptions implicit in the use of Tables 1 and 2 in the Appendix for historical inference, see Turner 1987a.

2. See the excellent treatment of these issues in Hatfield 1990, 67–164.

3. Brewster 1844. See also other articles by Brewster reprinted in Wade 1983, along with Wade's "Assessment," 301–28.

4. In practice Newton described his mix procedure as starting from a set of discrete points located at the center of the arcs corresponding to the color groupings red, yellow, green, and so forth. (the small circles just inside the circumference in Figure 2.3). The discrete number of binary hue mixtures possible under that limitation need not contain any complementary pairs, and Newton could not experimentally demonstrate the existence of any pair of complementary colors (Sherman 1981, 60–63). I am indebted to Richard Kremer for his advice on this question.

5. Sherman 1981, 15, 63, 60–70. See also Newton's own explanation of the phenomenon (Newton 1730, 150–54).

6. See Sherman's excellent survey of the history of color deficiency studies down to the 1850s (Sherman 1981, 117–52).

7. Each of these offered an example from what Richard Kremer has referred to as the two major types of color vision theories before Helmholtz and Maxwell: one class that saw the retinal receptors as passive transducers of incoming vibrations, and one that saw the receptors as discriminatory analyzers, tuned to particular frequencies of incoming light (Kremer 1993a).

Chapter Three
Helmholtz on Spatial Perception

1. On Helmholtz's life and career, see the three-volume study by Königsberger (1902–3), the abbreviated English translation by Königsberger (1906), Cahan 1989, and the excellent editors' introductions to several recent collections of correspondence (Cahan 1993a; Kirsten 1986; Kremer 1990). A major collection of scholarly articles on Helmholtz's work is Cahan 1993b.

2. These collections include Cahan 1993a; Kirsten 1986; Kremer 1990; and the many extracts of letters quoted in Königsberger 1902–3. The archive of the Deutsche Akademie der Wissenschaft in Berlin holds 1,641 items of Helmholtz correspondence, most of them letters to Helmholtz, as part of his scientific *Nachlaß*. I am grateful to officials of the archive for making portions of this collection available to me.

3. But see the important alternate interpretation advanced by Timothy Lenoir, which holds political and social consciousness to have powerfully influenced the

early scientific and philosophical work of Helmholtz and the 1847 school (Lenoir 1988a, 1988b, 1992, 1993).

4. Hatfield 1990, 109–65, 244–50; Köhnke 1986, 69–88; Ringer 1969, 295–304. A particularly vivid programmatic statement of this physiological and psychological reduction of Kant is Aubert 1865, iii–iv.

5. On this issue, see Coleman and Holmes 1988; Cranefield 1957; Kremer 1991, 1992; Lenoir 1988b; Nyhart 1986, 1987, 1991; and Tuchman 1986, 1993b.

6. To specify the position of the eye in the head, not only coordinates of ocular longitude and latitude are required, but also a third, torsional coordinate that specifies the rotation of some reference plane (thought of as fixed to the eyeball) from its initial orientation when the eye is in the primary position. The value of that coordinate at any tertiary position will depend not only upon that position, but also upon the convention adopted as to how the eye moves to reach that position. In 1863 Helmholtz defined one convention for establishing this third coordinate and called the coordinate value the *Raddrehungswinkel* or "angle of torsion." Neither his terminology nor his coordinate system distinguished between changes in the angle of torsion produced by cyclorotations—true rollings around the line of sight—and those produced by Listing rotations. This ambiguity subsequently caused much confusion, especially since other conventions were also widely used. See Hofmann 1925, 2:273–76; and the comments of Johannes Kries in *POS* 3:136–39. For a critique of Helmholtz's interpretation of this experiment, see Le Conte 1881, 164–76.

Chapter Four
Hering on Spatial Perception

1. The principal biographical sources are Kruta 1972; Hess 1918; Brücke 1928; Tschermak-Seysenegg 1934; and Garten 1918. Hering's personal papers were apparently destroyed during World War II, but the Hering family has kindly allowed me to consult the family genealogy, as well as surviving photographs and mementos. Fine discussions of Hering's work, although with little biographical information, are found in Hillebrand 1918 and Hurvich 1969. Also on Hering and his school, see Rothschuh 1973, 299–305; Lesky 1976, 480–84.

2. Hankel did, in fact, publish a detailed *analytic* discussion of the horopter, which was announced by Hering in the *Beiträge* with the statement that it was done at his request (Hankel 1864; Hering 1864a[25], i–v).

Chapter Five
The Nativist-Empiricist Controversy Begins

1. On Helmholtz's theory of unconscious inference and its relationship to that of other writers, see Hatfield 1990, 165–217. From the very large literature on Helmholtz's epistemology, see in addition to Hatfield, Hörz and Wollgast 1986; Heidelberger 1993; Moulines 1981; and Warren and Warren 1968.

2. See Hatfield's "Appendix A: Nativism-Empirism and Rationalism-Empiricism" for an excellent discussion of these positions and the terms for them (Hatfield 1990, 271–80). Hatfield prefers "empirism" to the more traditional "empir-

icism" as a translation of Helmholtz's *Empirismus*, since the former minimizes the danger of confusing a theory about the origin of spatial perception with the more general philosophical sense of "empiricism." But Helmholtz's rhetorical case against Hering depended heavily upon just that ambiguity, and so I have retained the traditional "empiricism" to better suggest that conflation of meanings.

3. Hatfield argues for nativist interpretations of the teachings of C. T. Tourtual (1802–65) on spatiality (Hatfield 1990, 144, 146–51). His account suggests that Tourtual regarded depth perception as a mental construction based on convergence movements and accommodation responses rather than retinal mechanisms per se.

Chapter Six
Helmholtz on Light and Color

1. This does, in fact, seem to have been Young's original meaning. Young's statement of his "theory," however, only amounted to several passing sentences. See Hargreave 1973; Sherman 1981, 1–19; Kremer 1993a.

2. See Maxwell 1855, 1860; Everitt 1974, 198–202; Boring 1942, 139–49; and esp. Sherman 1981, 153–222.

3. Strictly, the point W is the projection of the point in color space occupied by the mixed gray onto the color plane defined by the three primaries. W can be determined from knowing the *proportions* alone of the primaries in the mix. To know the position of the mixed-white point in color space, we must know its brightness relative to that of the primaries. The same applies to the position in color space of any mixed color. The determination involves the same considerations Helmholtz had addressed in the conclusion of his 1855 paper. Maxwell's techniques for making that determination are fascinating but irrelevant to the present discussion; see Maxwell 1855, 131–33 and *WAH* 2:66–70.

4. Helmholtz never acknowledged Maxwell's priority for the amended version of Young's theory, but rather wrote of himself and Maxwell as co-discoverers, who had independently "again directed attention" to a theory that had "gone unnoticed" since its enunciation by Thomas Young (*POS* 2:163). This niggardliness is sufficiently untypical of the mature Helmholtz as to lead some scholars to conclude that he did indeed come to the amended Young theory independently of Maxwell (cf. Kremer 1993a; Turner 1987b). Paul Sherman finds another puzzle in what he argues were Helmholtz's exaggerated claims about the obscurity into which Young's theory had fallen (Sherman 1981, 217–21).

5. Some these relationships are illustrated in Figure 6.6, which shows Helmholtz's spectral locus (with purples) located on the color plane inside a triangle VGR, the vertices of which correspond to Young's three primary sensations. On Helmholtz's interpretation of red color blindness, a red blind individual will lack the sensation R. All the hue sensations possible for such an individual will lie along the line VG. Imagine straight lines like CR and $C'R$ (called "confusion loci") passed through every point on VG and intersecting in R. Every such line will define a particular hue, presumably a mixture of green and violet, which will appear very bright for points on the spectral locus near VG and growing darker toward R to become totally black at R. One such straight line (like $C'R$) will

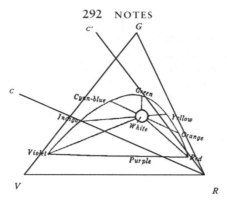

Fig. 6.6 Helmholtz's spectral locus of
1855, located inside a hypothetical triangle of fundamental sensations. On
Helmholtz's theory of color blindness,
all lines like CR and $C'R$ will be confusion loci for dichromats lacking the red
sensation. The red-orange-yellow-green
segment of the normal spectral locus will
lie approximately along a confusion
locus for these red blind dichromats.

closely coincide with the (almost straight) part of the spectral curve on which red,
orange, yellow, and some green colors are located for normals. The red blind
dichromat will see all these colors as of the same or very similar hue; the reds
should appear very dark, the yellows a highly saturated green. The confusion
locus passing through R and the white point will intersect the spectrum locus in
the blue-greens. The confusion loci of the green blind will pass through G and the
points of the line VR. These dichromats will be able to distinguish purples and
reds and see reds as very bright, but like the red blind they will confuse the red,
orange, and yellow spectral hues that lie near GR or a confusion locus that nearly
coincides with it. Analyses like this were soon to be the focus of very intense
controversy. The diagram is entirely heuristic.

Chapter Seven
Hering on Light and Color

1. Blue does appear to most observers to be a "simpler" color than violet,
which seems tinged with red. Postulating a blue fundamental, however, demands
that the spectral frequency response curve for the red receptor have a second peak
at short wavelengths to account for the reddish tinge of violets. Some held that
second peak to be physiologically improbable. Maxwell may have switched to a
blue fundamental as a result of his new colorimetric experiments with spectral
lights, in which he had determined the spectral locus (plus the interpolated purples) to be a triangle with three quite rounded vertices corresponding to the central greens, the extreme reds, and the extreme violets. Given that form, especially

for the violets, the choice of a blue fundamental allows the spectral locus to fit more snugly inside the triangle of the fundamental sensations. Choosing a violet fundamental requires a much larger triangle with fundamental sensations far removed from normal visual experience. Helmholtz was skeptical of Maxwell's results, probably because he believed Maxwell's apparatus permitted too much light dispersion. He had his student J. J. Müller make another determination of the spectral locus. Müller produced a locus that showed much less curvature in the extreme red and violet, thus supporting the plausibility of a violet fundamental sensation (PO5 2:165–67; Müller 1870; Preyer 1868, 329).

2. Hering always spoke of the "intensity" of the A- or the D-process, without specifying whether he meant the intensity of the associated sensation, the amount of accumulated product, or the rate at which the metabolic process was occurring. At the risk of anachronism, this historical treatment interprets intensity as reaction rate, which alone seems to yield a consistent picture of the model. Hering clearly did not think of assimilation as reuniting the parts of the visual substance previously separated by dissimilation. The visual substance is catabolized in dissimilation and restored by the assimilation of wholly new substance supplied by the blood.

3. Hering admitted that this neutral- or midgray seems anomalously dark, far closer to the blackest imaginable black than to the brightest imaginable white. But the anomaly is only apparent, Hering reasoned. If there were lights that could stimulate the A-process, as there are lights that stimulate the D-process, then we would be able to observe blacks far darker than those that are really accessible to us. In comparison to those blacks, the gray of the fully dark-adapted eye would seem a true midgray (Hering 1878/1874, 89).

4. Helmholtz had invoked the action of Fechner's law along the contour edge to explain why the blurring due to irradiation is not greater (PO5 2:188–89).

5. Hering meant that when his simple green and any spectral red are mixed, the pure red and green cancel and the yellow residue in the red is left. From this result supporters of the Young–Helmholtz theory falsely conclude that the yellow has been created; had they used "pure" green and the nonspectral "pure" red of the opponent process theory no yellow could be obtained. Hering's latter claim was soon acknowledged to be correct, but of course, the experimental outcome does not decide the theoretical question. On the Young–Helmholtz theory, Hering's nonspectral primary red stimulates the violet (or blue) receptor as well as the red one. Hence, mixing Hering's primary green and his primary red would naturally fail to produce yellow because the blue or violet contained in the mixture would cancel the complementary yellow that was created (cf. Hurvich and Jameson 1951).

Chapter Nine
The Nativist-Empiricist Debate, 1870–1925

1. A fourth front, ignored here, was the ongoing discussion of various geometrical, optical illusions.

2. Müller's horopter, a special case of the general horopter, is the circle defined by the fixation point and the optical centers of the two eyes, when the fixation

point lies in the median plane and also at eye level. The cylinder erected upon that circle was the vertical horopter, considered to be the locus of all vertical straight lines that would be seen single in the binocular field.

3. The manner and extent to which this locus differs from Müller's horopter circle (or the vertical horopter cylinder erected upon it) is now called the Hering–Hillebrand horopter deviation. A modern discussion of the problem is Reading 1983, 227–41.

4. If the breadth values of the retinal points are symmetrically distributed around the vertical meridian of each retina, then Hillebrand's conic locus reduces to Müller's horopter circle for all distances of C.

5. For the ensuing literature, see Hillebrand 1929, 130–39; Hofmann 1925, 2:411–66.

6. Greeff later retracted this extreme claim (Rivers 1900, 1134).

Chapter Ten
Color Vision Controversies, 1875–90

1. The evidence from unilaterals did not become any less confused as more were discovered and studied. For a sample of the later literature, see Holmgren 1881; König 1885b(10); and Hering 1890d(67).

2. Fick even asserted that there was only one color phenomenon known that the Young–Helmholtz theory, buttressed by displacement, could not explain. This was Fick's observation that for a fixed intensity, small colored fields lose their chromatic content entirely when their diameter becomes sufficiently small.

3. Hering's point is more easily understood by thinking of the superimposed valence curves of the two chromatic processes as they were frequently drawn by Hering's later followers (see Figure 14.2). "Pure blue" will, by definition, be excited at the point of the spectrum where the red-green valence curve crosses the abscissa and has zero value. Exhausting the retina for any color except pure blue or pure yellow will raise or depress the red-green valence curve with respect to the abscissa. Hence at the wavelength of the former pure blue, the red-green curve will no longer have zero value. In other words, the wavelength exciting any pure color will vary with the eye's state of adaptation.

4. Strictly A and A' are the same *functions* of Aa, $A'a'$, but this does not affect Kries' argument.

Chapter Eleven
Color Vision Controversies, 1890–1915

1. See the description of these theories in Parsons 1924; Boring 1942, 210–21; and the various writings of Christine Ladd-Franklin in Ladd-Franklin 1929.

2. Note that König's rhetoric subtly inverts the logic of his procedure: in fact, the assumption that dichromatism is a reduction form is necessary to the derivation of the three fundamental sensations of normal vision.

3. König's discussion implicitly adopts Fick's displacement hypothesis and uses it explicitly in its explanation of anomalous trichromats. König's data for the short-wavelength response were so uncertain as to prohibit an unambiguous

choice between blue and violet fundamentals. König initially adopted a blue fundamental, but on the basis of later research into blue blindness (tritanopia) he turned to a violet one (König 1897b[24]).

4. Hering pointed out that his pure and antagonistic colors must be complementary in König's terminology; hence König's fundamental green and red cannot be "pure" in Hering's theory (Hering 1887e[52], 44). König accepted this correction, acknowledging Hering's *dankenswerthe Freundlichkeit* in pointing out his error (König 1892[21], 318).

5. For a light that stimulates only one of the chromatic processes Hering's formula for the brightness is $(W + .5C) / (W + B + C)$; his formula for purity is $C / (B + W + C)$. W and B are the rates of assimilative and dissimilative activity in the black-white substance. C (though Hering is not precise about this) is the weight (*Gewicht*): the total psychophysical activity in the process and hence $A - D$ (or $A + D$ if the antagonistic sensations are understood to have opposite signs). The "weight" corresponds to the quality sometimes called "chroma" today. From these formulas it can be seen that the chromatic element in a sensation does influence the total brightness, but its contribution is small in comparison to the whiteness and it is the same for all hues for a given weight.

6. As König noted, that assumption also implies that Newton's mixture law will no longer be valid near the Purkinje threshold. König had, in fact, been routinely reporting small deviations from Newton's law for several years prior to this encounter. In a rare display of unanimity, both Kries and Hering (both of whom had built theoretical arguments on the inviolability of the law) had ignored or rejected these reports.

7. Tschermak and Hess also conceded to Helmholtz's students that macular absorption cannot explain the separate classes of red and green blindness (Tschermak 1902, 798; Hess 1922).

8. Christine Ladd-Franklin made the same observation, also in König's laboratory, and it occasioned a lasting priority dispute between her and Ebbinghaus (Ladd-Franklin 1892a,b; 1898, 195). Hering dismissed the result as due to macula absorption of yellow and its variation with intensity, as well as to various experimental errors committed by Ebbinghaus.

9. By modern measurements the rod-free area of the fovea is very close to the size measured by König as dichromatic. The dichromatism of the fovea, although discredited during the disputes of the 1890s, was rediscovered in 1944 (Willmer 1944). Elements of König's theory, including his association of the blue sensation with the visual purple and the location of one or more receptor substances in the epithelium, resurface in twentieth-century color theories; see Willmer 1943a,b; and Le Grand 1968, 456–58.

Chapter Twelve
The Roots of Incommensurability

1. In fact, at the end of his career Hering denied that colors could legitimately be called "sensations." In common language, sensations denote something perceived in or on one's body, while colors are always localized outside the body. See Hering 1964/1905, 4–6.

2. Consider the elaborate theory of color vision advanced in 1896 by Göttingen psychologist Georg Elias Müller (Müller 1896–97). Müller's theory adopted many basic principles from Hering's, so that E. G. Boring could say of it that it is "so well known now as often to be called Hering's theory, which it includes" (Boring 1942, 213). Müller hypothesized that equilibrium in the black-white process of the retina (which he understood differently from Hering) produces no sensation, just as equilibrium in the chromatic processes does not. The *Eigengrau* we see in the dark-adapted eye is a "brain gray" imposed in higher cortical centers. This hypothesis, Müller believed, completed the symmetry between the black-white sensations and those of red-green and blue-yellow. But Müller purchased theoretical symmetry at the price of Hering's understanding of black. On Müller's theory the retinal gray imposed upon the brain gray is proportional to $I_w - I_b$, the difference of the intensities of the black-making and white-making physiological activities. This allows the grays in the black-white series to function overall as an intensity series with respect to brightness. Hering had envisioned the retinal gray as determined by the *ratio* I_w/I_b, so that, as Hering understood the distinction, the series does not behave as an intensity series. Müller was convinced that the principles of psychophysics required the brightness sensation to be associated with absolute levels of physiological action, not with ratios.

Chapter Thirteen
Controversy and Disciplinary Structure

1. *ZfdPuPdS* 1(1890):1–4, on 2.

2. For more on line element theory, and especially on the unexpected results obtained by Helmholtz, see Stiles 1972; Le Grand 1968, 480–85; Peddie 1922; Wassermann 1978, 82; Turner 1982b, 152–54.

3. For descriptions of this apparatus, see König 1886(15), 93–95; König 1892(21), 217–23; *PO2*;350–57; Kries *PO5* 2:395–98; and the references in König and Dieterici 1884(6), 61. For German colorimeters other than those of Hering and Helmholtz, see Kries *PO5* 2:98.

4. Hering's son Heinrich Ewald collaborated with C. S. Sherrington on studies of the reflex (Hering and Sherrington 1897; Rothschuh 1973, 316–18).

5. Pfetsch 1972, 32–33; Eulner 1970; Fahrenbach 1983, 1987. I am indebted to Sabine Fahrenbach for kindly sending me a copy of her dissertation on the disciplinary establishment of ophthalmology in Germany.

Chapter Fourteen
In Search of Denouement: The Twentieth Century

1. See their autobiographical article (Hurvich and Jameson 1989) and Dorothea Jameson's unpublished manuscript (Jameson 1981). I am very grateful to Dorothea Jameson for a copy of this paper.

2. Erwin Schrödinger had published a similar set of curves derived theoretically from a transformation of König's data (Schrödinger 1926, 478). Svaetichin produced a set based on his microelectrode readings (Svaetichin 1956; Figure 14.1). The technique employed by Hurvich and Jameson to produce these heuris-

tically powerful representations could readily have been used by Hering and his students in the nineteenth century. That they did not do so suggests again Hering's personal indifference to graphical methods and his principled animosity to color-mixture measurements. Hurvich and Jameson portray their method as innovative and controversial at the time, in that they accepted the validity of observer-responses "redder/greener than" or "same hue/different hue" as well as the conventionally approved "same field/different field" or "brighter than/darker than" (Hurvich and Jameson 1989, 186). For a discussion of this methodological distinction, which goes back to the confrontations of Hering and Kries, see Brindley 1970, 132–38.

3. The furor raised in the early 1960s by Edwin Land, his retinex theory of color perception, and the two-color projection demonstrations on which it was based may have impressed on skeptical specialists how unexpectedly powerful and instantaneous the effects of simultaneous color contrast could be (Hardin 1988, 187–93; Judd 1960).

References and Abbreviations

Abbreviations

AAPwM   *Archiv für Anatomie, Physiologie und wissenschaftliche Medicin.* Ed. Karl Reichert and Emil du Bois-Reymond.

AfO   *Archiv für Ophthalmologie.*

BksGW   *Berichte der Königlichen Sächsischen Gesellschaft der Wissenschaften. Mathematisch-Physische Classe.*

CPMaxwell   James Clerk Maxwell. *The Collected Papers of James Clerk Maxwell.* Ed. W. D. Niven. 2 vols. Cambridge: Cambridge University Press, 1890. Reprint. New York: Dover, 1965. Citations of individual articles give page references to *CPMaxwell.*

DSB   *Dictionary of Scientific Biography.* Ed. Charles S. Gillispie. 16 vols. New York: Charles Scribner's Sons, 1970–80.

ErgebPhysiol   *Ergebnisse der Physiologie. Abt. II: Biophysik und Psychophysik.*

GesAbhKönig   Arthur König. *Gesammelte Abhandlungen zur Physiologischen Optik.* Leipzig: J. A. Barth, 1903. Citations of individual articles by König in the text give the item number and page references in *GesAbhKönig.*

GesSchFick   Adolf Fick. *Gesammelte Schriften von Adolf Fick.* 4 vols. Würzburg: Stahel'sche Verlag, 1903.

JOSA   *Journal of the Optical Society of America.*

Lotos   *Lotos, Jahrbuch für Naturwissenschaft.* Neue Folge.

Pflüger   *Archiv für die gesammte Physiologie des Menschen und der Tiere.* Ed. Eduard Friedrich Wilhelm Pflüger.

PO1–PO5   Hermann L. F. von Helmholtz. *Handbuch der Physiologischen Optik*, 3 pts. 1st German edition: Leipzig: L. Voss, 1856, 1860, 1866, reissued as a whole with supplements 1867. Cited here as *PO1.* 2d German edition: Ed. Arthur König. Hamburg and Leipzig: L. Voss, 1896, issued in 17 parts, 1886–96. Cited here as *PO2.* 3d German edition: Ed. A. Gullstrand, J. von Kries, and W. Nagel. Hamburg and Leipzig: L. Voss, 1910. Incorporates the text of the first German edition, with extensive supplementary material by the editors. Cited here as *PO3.* 1st English edition: *Helmholtz's Treatise on Physiological Optics.* Ed. James P. C. Southall. 3 vols. in 2. New York: Optical Society of America, 1924–25. A translation of the text and supplementary material of *PO3,* with notes by the American editor. Cited here as *PO4.* Reprint edition of P04: 3 vols. in 2. New York: Dover, 1962. Cited here as *PO5.*

Poggendorff	*Annalen der Physik und Chemie.* Ed. J. C. Poggendorff.
SbAkadBerlin	*Sitzungsberichte der Akademie der Wissenschaften in Berlin.*
SbAkadWien	*Sitzungsberichte der Kaiserlichen Akademie der Wissenschaften in Wien. Mathematisch-naturwissenschaftliche Classe.*
SbWürzburg	*Sitzungsberichte der physikalisch-medizinischen Gesellschaft zu Würzburg.*
SSS	*Social Studies of Science.*
Virchow's Archiv	*Archiv für pathologische Anatomie und Physiologie und für klinische Medizin.* Ed. Rudolf Virchow.
VuR	Hermann L. F. von Helmholtz. *Vorträge und Reden von Hermann von Helmholtz . . .* 5th ed. 2 vols. Braunschweig: Friedrich Vieweg und Sohn.
WAH	Hermann L. F. von Helmholtz. *Wissenschaftliche Abhandlungen.* 3 vols. Leipzig: J. A. Barth, 1895. Citations of articles by Helmholtz in the text give the volume number and page references to their appearance in *WAH.* The citation also includes the item number assigned to the work in the chronological list of Helmholtz's publications appearing in *WAH* 3:608–36.
WAHer	Karl Ewald Konstantin Hering. *Wissenschaftliche Abhandlungen von Ewald Hering.* Ed. Sächsische Akademie der Wissenschaft zu Leipzig. 2 vols. Leipzig: Georg Thieme, 1931. No consecutive pagination. Articles by Hering are cited in the text by year of publication and the item number assigned to them in *WAHer.* The pages cited refer to the original appearance of the article; articles are reprinted in *WAHer* with the same page numbers. For example, Hering 1864b(27), 34–41. *WAHer* retains the pagination of the originals and has no consecutive pagination. Works by Hering cited in the text are also listed individually in the bibliography by year of appearance.
ZADAW	Zentrales Archiv der Deutschen Akademie der Wissenschaft (Berlin).
ZfdPuPdS	*Zeitschrift für die Physiologie und Psychologie der Sinnesorgane.* (After 1907: Abteilung I: *Zeitschrift für Psychologie* and Abteilung II: *Zeitschrift für die Physiologie der Sinnesorgane.*)

References

Abney, William. 1914. *Researches in Colour Vision and the Trichromatic Theory.* London: Longmans, Green.

Ash, Mitchell G. 1980. "Academic Politics in the History of Science: Experimental Psychology in Germany, 1879–1941." *Central European History* 13:255–86.

———. 1982. *The Emergence of Gestalt Theory: Experimental Psychology in Germany, 1890–1920.* Ph.D. diss., Harvard University.

———. 1985. "Gestalt Psychology: Origins in Germany and Reception in the United States." In *Points of View in the Modern History of Psychology*, ed. C. Buxton, 295–344. San Diego: Academic Press.

———. 1991. "Gestalt Psychology in Weimar Culture." *History of the Human Sciences* 4:395–415.

———. Forthcoming. *Holism and the Quest for Objectivity: Gestalt Psychology in German Culture*. New York: Oxford University Press.

Aubert, Hermann. 1865. *Physiologie der Netzhaut*. Breslau: E. Morgenstern.

———. 1876. *Grundzüge der physiologischen Optik*. Handbuch der gesammten Augenheilkunde, ed. A. Graefe and T. Saemisch, 2 (pt. 2): 393–696. Leipzig: Wilhelm Engelmann.

Barlow, H. B., C. Blackmore, and J. D. Pettigrew. 1967. "The Neural Mechanism of Binocular Depth Perception." *Journal of Physiology* 193:327–42.

Becker, Otto. 1871–88. 7 unpublished letters to Helmholtz. ZADAW. Cited by item number and date.

———. 1879. "Ein Fall von angeborener einseitiger totaler Farbenblindheit." *AfO* 25 (Abt. 2): 205–12.

Ben-David, Joseph. 1960. "Scientific Productivity and Academic Organisation." *American Sociological Review* 25:828–43.

Ben-David, Joseph, and Randall Collins. 1966. "Social Factors in the Origins of a New Science: The Case of Psychology." *American Historical Review* 31:451–72 (with a critique by Dorothy Ross).

Ben-David, Joseph, and Avraham Zloczower. 1962. "Universities and Academic Systems in Modern Society." *European Journal of Sociology* 3:62–84.

Bevilacqua, Fabio. 1993. "Helmholtz's *Ueber die Erhaltung der Kraft*: The Emergence of a Theoretical Physicist." In Cahan 1993b, 291–333.

Biagioli, Mario. 1990. "The Anthropology of Incommensurability." *Studies in History and Philosophy of Science* 21:183–209.

Bielschowsky, Alfred. 1900. "Untersuchungen über das Sehen der Schielenden." *AfO* 50 (Abt. 2): 406–510.

———. 1907. "Die neueren Anschauungen über Wesen und Behandlung des Schielens." *Beiheft zur "Medizinischen Klinik"* 3:311–42.

———. 1945. *Lectures on Motor Anomalies*. Hanover, N.H.: Dartmouth College Publications.

Blackmore, John T. 1972. *Ernst Mach: His Work, Life, and Influence*. Berkeley: University of California Press.

Bohn, Johann Conrad. 1865. "Ueber das Farbensehen und die Theorie der Mischfarben." *Poggendorff* 200:87–118.

Boring, Edwin G. 1942. *Sensation and Perception in the History of Experimental Psychology*. New York: Appleton-Century-Crofts.

———. 1950. *A History of Experimental Psychology*. 2d ed. New York: Appleton-Century-Crofts.

Borscheid, Peter. 1976. *Naturwissenschaft, Staat und Industrie in Baden (1848–1914)*. Stuttgart: Ernst Klett Verlag.

Bourdieu, Pierre. 1991. *Language and Symbolic Power*. Trans. Gino Raymond and Matthew Adamson. Ed. John B. Thompson. Cambridge: Harvard University Press.

Brentano, Franz. 1924. *Psychologie vom empirischen Standpunkt*, 2 vols. Leipzig: Felix Meiner. (1st ed. 1874)

Breuer, Joseph. 1868. "Die Selbsteuerung der Athmung durch den Nervus vagus." *SbAkadWien* 58 (Abt. 2): 909–37.

———. 1970/1868. "Self-Steering of Respiration through the *Nervus Vagus*." Trans. of Breuer 1868, by Elisabeth Ullmann. In Porter 1970, 365–94.

Brewster, David. 1844. "On the Law of Visible Position in Single and Binocular Vision, and on the Representation of Solid Figures by the Union of Dissimilar Plane Pictures on the Retina." *Transactions of the Royal Society of Edinburgh* 15:349–68. Reprinted in Wade 1983, 93–114.

Brindley, G. S. 1970. *Physiology of the Retina and Visual Pathway*. 2d ed. London: Edward Arnold. (1st ed. 1960)

Brodhun, Eugen. 1893. "Die Gültigkeit des Newtonschen Farbenmischungsgesetzes bei dem sog. grünblinden Farbensystem." *ZfdPuPdS* 5:323–34.

Brodhun, Eugen, and Otto Lummer. 1905. "Experimentelles über das Sehen im Dunkeln und Hellen (Hypothesen über die Ursache der Farbenblindheit." *Verhandlungen der Deutschen Physikalischen Gesellschaft* 6:62–77.

Brown, P. K., and G. Wald. 1964. "Visual Pigments in Single Rods and Cones of the Human Retina." *Science* 144:45–51.

Brozek, Josef, and Horst Gundlach, eds. 1987. *G. T. Fechner and Psychology*. Passau: Passavia Universitätsverlag.

Brücke, Ernst. 1841. "Ueber die stereoscopischen Erscheinungen und Wheatstone's Angriff auf die Lehre von den identischen Stellen der Netzhäute." *Archiv für Anatomie und Physiologie* Jg. 1841, 459–76.

———. 1851. "Untersuchungen über subjective Farben." *Poggendorff* 84:418–48.

———. 1873. *Vorlesungen über Physiologie*. 2 vols. Wien: Wilhelm Braumüller.

Brücke, Ernst Theodor von. 1928. "Hering, Ewald." In *Deutsches Biographisches Jahrbuch. Ueberleitungsband II: 1917–1920*, 258–63. Berlin: Deutsche Verlags-Anstalt.

Brunner, Emil. 1908. "Ein Abänderungsvorschlag zu Hering's Theorie der Gegenfarben." *European Journal of Physiology* 123:370–76.

Brush, Stephen G. 1978. *The Temperature of History: Phases of Science and Culture in the Nineteenth Century*. New York: Bart Franklin.

Buchwald, Jed Z. 1993. "Electrodynamics in Context: Object States, Laboratory Practice, and Anti-Romanticism." In Cahan 1993b, 334–73.

Budge, Julius Ludwig. 1855. 1 letter to Helmholtz. *ZADAW*.

Cahan, David. 1989. *An Institute for an Empire: The Physikalisch-Technische Reichsanstalt 1871–1918*. Cambridge: Cambridge University Press.

———, ed. 1993a. *Letters of Hermann von Helmholtz to His Parents, 1837–1846*. Stuttgart: Franz Steiner Verlag. Text citations to letters in this collection also include the item number (e.g., Cahan 1993, 43–48 [no. 5]).

———, ed. 1993b. *Hermann von Helmholtz and the Foundations of Nineteenth-Century Science*. Berkeley/Los Angeles: University of California Press.

———. 1993c. "Helmholtz and the Civilizing Power of Science." In Cahan 1993b, 559–602.

Caneva, Kenneth L. 1978. "From Galvanism to Electrodynamics: The Transformation of German Physics and Its Social Context." *Historical Studies in the Physical Sciences* 9:63–160.

———. 1993. *Robert Mayer and the Conservation of Energy.* Princeton: Princeton University Press.

Carterette, Edward C., and Morton P. Friedman, eds. 1975. *Seeing.* New York: Academic Press.

Cattell, J. McKeen. 1898. "Review of *Handbuch der physiologischen Optik . . .*" *Science* 8 (n.s.): 794–96.

Classen, August. 1863. *Ueber das Schlussverfahren des Sehactes.* Rostock: G. B. Leopold.

———. 1865(?)–67. Two unpublished letters to Helmholtz. *ZADAW.* Cited by item number and date.

———. 1876. *Physiologie des Gesichtssinnes zum ersten Mal begründet auf Kant's Theorie der Erfahrung.* Braunschweig: F. Vieweg und Sohn.

Cohn, Hermann. 1879. *Die Arbeiten des Herrn Professor Holmgren über Farbenblindheit und seine Kampfesweise. Antwort.* Breslau: E. Morgenstern.

Coleman, William, and Frederic L. Holmes, eds. 1988. *The Investigative Enterprise: Experimental Physiology in Nineteenth-Century Medicine.* Berkeley: University of California Press.

Collins, Harry M. 1979. "The Investigation of Frames of Meaning in Science: Complementarity and Compromise." *Sociological Review* 27:703–18.

———. 1981. "Stages in the Empirical Programme of Relativism." *SSS* 11:3–10.

———. 1983. "The Sociology of Scientific Knowledge: Studies of Contemporary Science." *Annual Review of Sociology* 9:265–86.

———. 1985. *Changing Order: Replication and Induction in Scientific Practice.* London: SAGE.

Committee on Colorimetry of the Optical Society of America. 1953. *The Science of Color.* New York: Thomas Y. Crowell.

Conze, Werner, and Jürgen Kocka, eds. 1985. *Bildungsbürgertum im 19. Jahrhundert.* Part 1: *Bildungssystem und Professionalisierung in internationalen Vergleichen.* Stuttgart: Ernst Klett Verlag.

Cranefield, Paul F. 1957. "The Organic Physics of 1847 and the Biophysics of Today." *Journal of the History of Medicine and Allied Sciences* 12:407–23.

———. 1966. "Freud and the 'School of Helmholtz.'" *Gesnerus* 23:35–39.

Danziger, Kurt. 1980. "Wundt and the Two Traditions of Psychology." In *Wilhelm Wundt and the Making of a Scientific Psychology*, ed. R. W. Reiber, 73–88. New York: Plenum.

De Valois, R. L. 1965. "Analysis and Coding of Color Vision in the Primate Visual System." *Cold Spring Harbor Symposium on Quantitative Biology* 30:567–79.

De Valois, R. L., and K. K. De Valois. 1975. "Neural Coding of Color." In Carterette and Friedman 1975, 117–66.

Derrington, A. M., J. Krauskopf, and P. Lennie. 1984. "Chromatic Mechanisms in Lateral Nucleus of Macaque." *Journal of Physiology* 357:241–65.

Diamond, Solomon. 1980. "Wundt before Leipzig." In *Wilhelm Wundt and the Making of a Scientific Psychology*, ed. R. W. Reiber, 3–70. New York: Plenum.

Dodwell, P. C. 1975. "Contemporary Theoretical Problems in Seeing." In Carterette and Friedman 1975, 57–77.

Donders, Franciscus Cornelis. 1856–88. 31 unpublished letters to Helmholtz. *ZADAW*. Cited by item number and date.

———. 1860. "Beiträge zur Kenntniss der Refractions- und Accommodationsanomalien." *AfO* 6:62–106.

———. 1863. "Die Refractionsanomalien des Auges und ihre Folgen." *AfO* 3:327–86.

———. 1866. *Die Anomalien der Refraction und Accommodation des Auges.* Wien: Wilhelm Braumüller.

———. 1867. "Das binoculare Sehen und die Vorstellung von der dritten Dimension." *AfO* 13:1–48.

———. 1871. "Die Projection der Gesichtserscheinungen nach den Richtungslinien." *AfO* 27:1–68.

———. 1872. "Ueber angeborene und erworbene Association." *AfO* 18:153–64.

———. 1881. "Ueber Farbensysteme." *AfO* 26:155–223.

———. 1884. "Noch einmal die Farbensysteme." *AfO* 30 (Abt. 1): 15–90.

Dor, Henri. 1872. "Ueber Farbenblindheit. Einwendungen gegen die Young-Helmholtz'sche Theorie." *Mittheilungen der Naturforschenden Gesellschaft in Bern.* Jg. 1872, 7–23.

Du Bois-Reymond, Emil. 1870. "Leibnizische Gedanken in der neueren Naturwissenschaften (1870)." In his *Vorträge über Philosophie und Gesellschaft*, ed. Siegfried Wollgast, 25–44. Berlin: Akademie Verlag, 1974.

———. 1896. *Gedächtnisrede auf Hermann von Helmholtz, aus den Abhandlungen der königl. preuss. Akademie der Wissenschaften zu Berlin vom Jahre 1896.* Berlin: Georg Reimer.

Du Bois-Reymond, Estelle, ed. 1927. *Zwei grosse Naturforscher des 19. Jahrhunderts. Ein Briefwechsel zwischen Emil du Bois-Reymond und Karl Ludwig.* Leipzig: J. A. Barth.

Dunlap, Knight. 1922. *The Elements of Scientific Psychology.* London: Henry Kimpton.

Ebbinghaus, Hermann. 1893. "Theorie des Farbensehens." *ZfdPuPdS* 5:145–238.

———. 1919. *Grundzüge der Pyschologie.* 4th ed. Leipzig: Veit & Comp. (1st ed. 1897)

Eccles, John Carew. 1979. *Sherrington, His Life and Thought.* Berlin: Springer International, 1979.

Einthoven, Willem. 1902. "Die Accommodation des menschlichen Auges." *ErgebPhysiol* 1:680–96.

Engelhardt, H. Tristram, Jr., and Arthur L. Caplan, eds. 1987a. *Scientific Controversies: Case Studies in the Resolution and Closure of Disputes in Science and Technology.* London: Cambridge University Press.

———. 1987b. "Introduction: Patterns of Controversy and Closure." In Engelhardt and Caplan 1987a, 1–26.

Engelmann, Theodor W. 1903. "Vorwort." In Arthur König, *Gesammelte Abhandlungen zur Physiologischen Optik*, v–viii. Leipzig: J. A. Barth.

Epstein, William. 1988. "Has the Time Come to Rehabilitate Gestalt Theory?" *Psychological Research* 50:2–6.

Eulner, Hans-Heinz. 1970. *Die Entwicklung medizinischer Specialfächer an den Universitäten des deutschen Sprachgebiets.* Stuttgart: Enke Verlag.

Everitt, C.W.F. 1974. "Maxwell, James Clerk." *DSB* 9:198–230.

Exner, Franz. 1918. "Einige Versuche und Bemerkungen zur Farbenlehre." *SbAkadWien* 127 (Abt. 2a): 1829–64.

———. 1919. "Zur Kenntnis des Purkinje'schen Phänomens." *SbAkadWien* 128 (Abt. 2a): 71–84.

———. 1921. "Zur Frage nach der spezifischen Helligkeit der Farben." *ZfdPuPdS* 52 (Abt. 2): 157–64.

Exner, Sigmund. 1868–91. 7 unpublished letters to Helmholtz. *ZADAW.* Cited by item number and date.

———. 1868. "Ueber einige neue subjective Gesichtserscheinungen." *Pflüger* 1:375–94.

———. 1885. "Ueber eine neue Urtheils-Täuschung . . ." *Pflüger* 37:520–23.

———. 1887. "Gegenbemerkung, eine neue Urtheiltäuschung im Gebiete des Gesichtssinnes' betreffend." *Pflüger* 40:323–30.

Fahrenbach, Sabine. 1983. *Zur Herausbildung der Ophthalmologie als eigenständige Wissenschaftsdisziplin in Preußen unter Berücksichtigung der Wechselwirkung zwischen Disziplinbildungsprozeß und der Tätigkeit der wissenschaftlichen Schuls A. V. Graefes.* Ph.D. diss., Wilhelm-Pieck-Universität Rostock.

———. 1987. "Die Herausbildung der Ophthalmologie in Preussen und die wissenschaftliche Schule Albrecht von Graefes (1828–1870." In Guntau and Leitko 1887a, 315–27.

Falkenstein, Lorne. 1990. "Was Kant a Nativist?" *Journal of the History of Ideas* 51:573–97.

Fechner, Gustav Theodor. 1838. "Ueber die subjectiven Complementärfarben." *Poggendorff* 44:221–45, 513–35.

———. 1840. "Ueber die subjectiven Nachbilder und Nebenbilder." *Poggendorff* 50:193–221, 427–70.

———. 1860a. "Ueber die Contrastempfindung." *BksGW* 12:71–145.

———. 1860b. *Elemente der Psychophysik.* 2 vols. Leipzig: Breitkopf & Härtel.

———. 1861. "Ueber einige Verhältnisse des binocularen Sehens." *BksGW* 5:227–65.

Fick, Adolf Eugen. 1864. *Lehrbuch der Anatomie und Physiologie der Sinnesorgane.* Lahr: M. Schauenburg.

———. 1873. "Zur Theorie der Farbenblindheit." *Verhandlungen der physikalisch-medizinischen Gesellschaft zu Würzburg* 5 (Neue Folge): 158–63. Also in *GesSchFick* 3:426–31.

———. 1879. *Dioptrik. Nebenapparate des Auges. Lehre von der Lichtempfindung.* Handbuch der Physiologie, ed. Ludimar Hermann, 3 (pt. 2): 1–234. Leipzig: F.C.W. Vogel.

———. 1890. "Zur Theorie des Farbensinnes bei indirektem Sehen." *Pflüger* 47:247–57. Also in *GesSchFick* 3:461–71.

———. 1900. "Kritik der Hering'schen Theorie der Lichtempfindung." *SbWürzburg* Jg. 1900, 9–14. Also in *GesSchFick* 3:481–86.

Fischer, F. P. 1924. "Ueber Stereoskopie im indirekten Sehen." *Pflüger* 204:247–60.

Forman, Paul. 1971. "Weimar Culture, Causality, and Quantum Theory, 1918–1927: Adaptation by German Physicists and Mathematicians to a Hostile Intellectual Environment." *Historical Studies in the Physical Sciences* 3:1–116.

Freudenthal, Gad. 1984. "The Role of Shared Knowledge in Science: The Failure of the Constructivist Programme in the Sociology of Science." *SSS* 14:185–95.

Fruton, Joseph S. 1990. *Contrasts in Scientific Style: Research Groups in the Chemical and Biochemical Sciences*. Philadelphia: American Philosophical Society.

Funke, Otto. 1863. *Lehrbuch der Physiologie für akademische Vorlesungen und zum Selbstudium*. 4th ed. 2 vols. Leipzig: Leopold Voss.

Gardner, Howard. 1985. *The Mind's New Science: A History of the Cognitive Revolution*. New York: Basic Books.

Garten, Siegfried. 1918. "Ewald Hering zum Gedächtnis." *Pflüger* 170:501–22.

———. 1920. "Herings Farbenmischapparat für spektrale Lichter." *Zeitschrift für Biologie* 72:89–100.

Gehler, Johann Samuel Traugott. 1787–96. *Physikalisches Wörterbuch oder Versuch einer Erklärung der vornehmsten Besgriffe und Kunstwörter der Naturlehre . . .* 6 vols. Leipzig: Schwickertschen Verlag.

Geison, Gerald L. 1978. *Michael Foster and the Cambridge School of Physiology: The Scientific Enterprise in Late Victorian Society*. Princeton: Princeton University Press.

———. 1981. "Scientific Change, Emerging Specialties, and Research Schools." *History of Science* 19:20–40.

Gibson, James J. 1950. *The Perception of the Visual World*. Boston: Houghton Mifflin.

———. 1966. *The Senses Considered as Perceptual Systems*. London: Allen & Unwin.

———. 1982. *Reasons for Realism: Selected Essays of James J. Gibson*. Ed. Edward Reed and Rebecca Jones. Hillsdale, N.J.: Lawrence Erlbaum Associates.

Gilgen, Albert R. 1982. *American Psychology since World War II: A Profile of the Discipline*. Westport, Conn.: Greenwood Press.

Goldstein, Eugen. 1921. "Helmholtz. Erinnerungen eines Laboratoriumspraktikanten." *Die Naturwissenschaften* 9:708–11.

Gooding, David, Trevor Pinch, and Simon Schaffer, eds. 1989. *The Uses of Experiment: Studies in the Natural Sciences*. Cambridge: Cambridge University Press.

Graefe, Albrecht von. 1870. *Sehen und Sehorgan. Vortrag, gehalten in der Singakademie am 23. März 1867*. 2d ed. Berlin: Carl Habel. (1st ed. 1867)

———. 1935. *Die Briefe Albrecht von Graefe's an F. C. Donders (1852–1870)*. Ed. H.J.M. Weve and G. ten Doesschate. Stuttgart: Ferdinand Enke Verlag.

Graefe, Alfred Karl. 1897. *Das Sehen der Schielenden. Eine ophthalmologisch-physiologische Studie*. Wiesbaden: J. F. Bergmann.

Graham, C. H. 1951. "Visual Perception." In Stevens 1951, 868–920.

Granit, Ragnar. 1947. *Sensory Mechanisms of the Retina, with an Appendix on Electroretinography*. London: Oxford University Press.

Grassmann, Hermann Günther. 1853. "Zur Theorie der Farbenmischung." *Poggendorff* 89:69–84.

Greeff, Richard. 1892. "Untersuchungen über binokulares Sehen mit Anwendung des Heringschen Fallversuchs." *ZfPuPdS* 3:21–47.

Guntau, Martin, and Hubert Laitko, eds. 1987a. *Der Ursprung der modernen Wissenschaften. Studien zur Entstehung wissenschaftlicher Disziplinen.* Berlin: Akademie Verlag.

———. 1987b. "Entstehung und Wesen wissenschaftlicher Disziplinen." In Guntau and Laitko 1987a, 17–92.

Hankel, Hermann. 1864. "Mathematische Bestimmung des Horopters." *Poggendorff* 122:575–88.

Hardin, C. L. 1988. *Color for Philosophers: Unweaving the Rainbow.* Indianapolis: Hackett.

Hargreave, David. 1973. *Thomas Young's Theory of Color Vision: Its Roots, Development, and Acceptance by the British Scientific Community.* Ph.D. diss., University of Wisconsin.

Hartline, Haldan K. 1938. "The Response of Single Optic Nerve Fibres of the Vertebrate Eye to Illumination of the Retina." *American Journal of Physiology* 121:400–415.

Hartline, Haldan K., and Floyd Ratliff. 1957–58. "Spatial Summation of Inhibitory Influences in the Eye of Limulus, and the Mutual Interaction of Receptor Units." *Journal of General Physiology* 41:1049–66.

Hatfield, Gary. 1990. *The Natural and the Normative: Theories of Spatial Perception from Kant to Helmholtz.* Cambridge: MIT Press.

———. 1993. "Helmholtz and Classicism: The Science of Aesthetics and the Aesthetics of Science." In Cahan 1993b, 522–58.

Hecht, Selig. 1928. "On the Binocular Fusion of Colors and Its Relation to Theories of Color Vision." *Proceedings of the National Academy of Sciences* 14:237–41.

———. 1930. "The Development of Thomas Young's Theory of Color Vision." *JOSA* 20:231–70.

Heidelberger, Michael. 1993. "Force, Law, and Experiment: The Evolution of Helmholtz's Philosophy of Science." In Cahan 1993b, 461–97.

Heine, Ludwig. 1900. "Sehschärfe und Tiefenwahrnehmung." *AfO* 50:146–73.

Hering, Ewald. 1861. *Vom Ortssinne der Netzhaut.* Pt. 1 of *Beiträge zur Physiologie,* 1–80. Leipzig: Wilhelm Engelmann. (*WAHer* 25)

———. 1862. *Von den identischen Netzhautstellen.* Pt. 2 of *Beiträge zur Physiologie,* 81–170. Leipzig: Wilhelm Engelmann. (*WAHer* 25)

———. 1863a. *Vom Horopter.* Pt. 3 of *Beiträge zur Physiologie,* 171–224. Leipzig: Wilhelm Engelmann. (*WAHer* 25)

———. 1863b. "Ueber W. Wundt's Theorie des binocularen Sehens." *Poggendorff* 119:115–30. (*WAHer* 26)

———. 1863c. "Ueber Dr. A. Classen's 'Beitrag zur physiologischen Optik.'" *Virchow's Archiv* 26:560–72. (*WAHer* 27)

———. 1864a. *Allgemeine geometrische Auflösung des Horopterproblems. Von den Bewegungen des menschlichen Auges.* Pt. 4 of *Beiträge zur Physiologie,* 225–86. Leipzig: Wilhelm Engelmann. (*WAHer* 25)

———. 1864b. "Zur Kritik der Wundt'schen Theorie des binocularen Sehens." *Poggendorff* 122:476–81. (*WAHer* 28)

Hering, Ewald. 1864c. "Das Gesetz der identischen Sehrichtungen." *AAPwM* Jg. 1864: 27–51. (*WAHer* 29)

———. 1864d. "Die sogenannte Raddrehung des Auges in ihre Bedeutung für das Sehen bei ruhendem Blicke." *AAPwM* Jg. 1864: 278–85. (*WAHer* 30)

———. 1864e. "Bemerkungen zu Volkmann's neuen Untersuchungen über das Binocularsehen." *AAPwM* Jg. 1864: 303–19. (*WAHer* 31)

———. 1865a. *Vom binocularen Tiefsehen. Kritik einer Abhandlung von Helmholtz über den Horopter.* Pt. 5 of *Beiträge zur Physiologie,* 287–358. Leipzig: Wilhelm Engelmann. (*WAHer* 25)

———. 1865b. "Die Gesetze der binocularen Tiefenwahrnehmung." *AAPwM* Jg. 1865: 79–97, 152–65. (*WAHer* 32)

———. 1865c. "Gegenbemerkungen über die Form des Horopters." *Poggendorff* 124:638–41. (*WAHer* 33)

———. 1868a. *Die Lehre vom binocularen Sehen.* Leipzig: Wilhelm Engelmann. (*WAHer* 34)

———. 1868b. "Bemerkungen zu der Abhandlung von Donders über das binoculare Sehen." *AfO* 14:1–12. (*WAHer* 35)

———. 1868c. "Die Selbststeuerung der Athmung durch den Nervus vagus. Mittheilung über eine von Dr. Joseph Breuer in physiologischen Institute der k. k. Josephsakademie ausgeführte Untersuchungen." *SbAkadWien* 57 (Abt. 2): 672–77 (IV. 10). (*WAHer* 10) Also see Hering 1970.

———. 1869. "Ueber die Rollung des Auges um die Gesichtslinie." *AfO* 15:1–16. (*WAHer* 36)

———. 1870. "Ueber das Gedächtnis als eine allgemeine Funktion der organisierten Materie. (Vortrag, Wien 1870)." In Hering 1921, 5–32.

———. 1872. "Zur Lehre vom Lichtsinne. I. Ueber successive Lichtinduction." *SbAkadWien* 66 (Abt. 3): 5–24. (*WAHer* 37)

———. 1874a. "Zur Lehre vom Lichtsinne. II. Ueber simultanen Lichtcontrast." *SbAkadWien* 68 (Abt. 3): 186–201. (*WAHer* 38)

———. 1874b. "Zur Lehre vom Lichtsinne. III. Ueber simultane Lichtinduction und über successiven Contrast." *SbAkadWien* 68 (Abt. 3): 229–44. (*WAHer* 39)

———. 1874c. "Zur Lehre vom Lichtsinne. IV. Ueber die sogenannte Intensität der Lichtempfindung und über die Empfindung des Schwarzen." *SbAkadWien* 69 (Abt. 3): 85–104. (*WAHer* 40)

———. 1874d. "Zur Lehre vom Lichtsinne. V. Grundzüge einer Theorie des Lichtsinnes." *SbAkadWien* 69 (Abt. 3): 179–217. (*WAHer* 41)

———. 1874e. *Zur Lehre vom Lichtsinne. Sechs Mittheilungen an die kaiserl. Akademie der Wissenschaften in Wien.* Wien: Carl Gerold's Sohn, 1872–74. Reprint by installment of Hering 1872; 1874a,b,c,d; 1875.

———. 1875. "Zur Lehre vom Lichtsinne. VI. Grundzüge einer Theorie des Farbensinnes." *SbAkadWien* 70 (Abt. 3): 169–204. (*WAHer* 42)

———. 1876. "Zur Lehre von der Beziehung zwischen Leib und Seele. I. Ueber Fechner's psychophysisches Gesetz." *SbAkadWien* 72 (Abt. 3): 310–48.

———. 1877. "Grundzüge einer Theorie des Temperatursinns." *SbAkadWien* 75 (Abt. 3): 101–35. (*WAHer* 24)

————. 1878/1874. *Zur Lehre vom Lichtsinne. Sechs Mittheilungen an die kaiserl. Akademie der Wissenschaften in Wien*. 2d ed. Wien: Carl Gerold's Sohn. Reprint of Hering 1874e.

————. 1879a. *Der Raumsinn und die Bewegungen des Auges*. Handbuch der Physiologie, ed. Ludimar Hermann, 3 (pt. 1): 341–601. Leipzig: F.C.W. Vogel.

————. 1879b. *Der Temperatursinn*. Handbuch der Physiologie, ed. Ludimar Hermann, 3 (pt. 2): 415–48. Leipzig: F.C.W. Vogel.

————. 1880. "Zur Erklärung der Farbenblindheit aus der Theorie der Gegenfarben." *Lotos* 1:76–107. (*WAHer* 43)

————. 1882. "Kritik einer Abhandlung von Donders 'Ueber Farbensysteme.'" *Lotos* 2:69–101. (*WAHer* 44)

————. 1884. "Ueber die spezifischen Energien des Nervensystems. Vortrag, Prag 1884." In Hering 1921, 33–52.

————. 1885a. "Ueber individuelle Verschiedenheiten des Farbensinnes." *Lotos* 6:142–98. (*WAHer* 45)

————. 1885b. "Bemerkungen zu A. König's Kritik einer Abhandlung über individuelle Verschiedenheiten des Farbensinnes." *Centralblatt für praktische Augenheilkunde* 9:327–32. (*WAHer* 46)

————. 1886. "Ueber Sigmund Exner's neue Urtheilstäuschung auf dem Gebiete des Gesichtssinnes." *Pflüger* 39:159–70. (*WAHer* 47)

————. 1887a. "Ueber Newton's Gesetz der Farbenmischung." *Lotos* 7:177–268. (*WAHer* 48)

————. 1887b. "Ueber Holmgren's vermeintlichen Nachweis der Elementarempfindungen des Gesichtssinnes." *Pflüger* 40:1–20. (*WAHer* 49)

————. 1887c. "Ueber die Theorie des simultanen Contrastes von Helmholtz. I." *Pflüger* 40:172–91. (*WAHer* 50)

————. 1887d. "Ueber die Theorie des simultanen Contrastes von Helmholtz. II." *Pflüger* 41:1–29. (*WAHer* 51)

————. 1887e. "Beleuchtung eines Angriffes auf die Theorie der Gegenfarben." *Pflüger* 41:29–46. (*WAHer* 52)

————. 1887f. "Ueber den Begriff, 'Urteilstäuschung' in der physiologischen Optik und über die Wahrnehmung simultaner und successiver Heiligkeitsunterschiede." *Pflüger* 41:91–106. (*WAHer* 53)

————. 1887g. "Ueber die Theorie des simultanen Contrastes von Helmholtz. III." *Pflüger* 41:358–67. (*WAHer* 54)

————. 1888a. "Zur Theorie der Vorgänge in der lebendigen Substanz. Vortrag, Prag 1888." In Hering 1921, 53–104.

————. 1888b. "Eine Verrichtung zur Farbenmischung, zur Diagnose der Farbenblindheit und zur Untersuchung der Contrasterscheinungen." *Pflüger* 42:119–44. (*WAHer* 55)

————. 1888c. "Ueber die von v. Kries wider die Theorie der Gegenfarben erhobenen Einwände. I. Ueber die Unabhangigkeit der Farbengleichungen von der Erregbarkeitsänderung des Sehorgans." *Pflüger* 42:488–506. (*WAHer* 56)

————. 1888d. "Ueber die Theorie des simultanene Contrastes von Helmholtz. IV. Die subjective Trennung des Lichtes in zwei complementäre Portionen." *Pflüger* 43:1–21. (*WAHer* 57)

Hering, Ewald. 1888e. "Ueber die von v. Kries wider die Theorie des Gegen-farben erhobenen Einwände. II. Ueber successiver Lichtinduction und soge-nannte negative Nachbilder." *Pflüger* 43:264–88. (*WAHer* 58)

———. 1888f. "Ueber die von v. Kries wider die Theorie der Gegenfarben er-hobenen Einwände. III. Ueber die sogenannten Ermüdungsserscheinungen." *Pflüger* 43:329–46. (*WAHer* 59)

———. 1888g. "Berichtigung." *AfO* 34 (Abt. 4): 272–73. (*WAHer* 61)

———. 1889a. "Vorbemerkungen von E. Hering zur Abhandlung: 'Ueber die specifische Helligkeit der Farben von Dr. Franz Hillebrand.'" *SbAkadWien* 98 (Abt. 3): 70–73. (*WAHer* 60)

———. 1889b. "Ueber die Hypothesen zur Erklärung der peripheren Farbenblindheit." *AfO* 35 (Abt. 4): 63–83. (*WAHer* 62)

———. 1890a. "Beitrag zur Lehre vom Simultankontrast." *ZfdPuPdS* 1:18–28. (*WAHer* 64)

———. 1890b. "Eine Methode zur Beobachtung des Simultanencontrastes." *Pflüger* 47:236–42. (*WAHer* 65)

———. 1890c. "Zur Diagnostik der Farbenblindheit." *AfO* 36 (Abt. 1): 217–33. (*WAHer* 66)

———. 1890d. "Die Untersuchung einseitiger Störungen des Farbensinnes mit-tels binocularer Farbengleichungen." *AfO* 36 (Abt. 3): 1–23. (*WAHer* 67)

———. 1890e. "Prüfung der sogenannten Farbendreiecke mit Hülfe des Farben-sinns excentrischer Netzhautstellen." *Pflüger* 47:417–38. (*WAHer* 68)

———. 1891a. "Untersuchungen eines total Farbenblinden." *Pflüger* 49:563–608. (*WAHer* 69)

———. 1891b. "Ueber Ermüdung und Erholung des Sehorgans." *AfO* 37 (Abt. 3): 1–36. (*WAHer* 70)

———. 1892. "Bemerkungen zu E. Fick's Entgegnung auf die Abhandlung über Ermüdung und Erholung des Sehorgans." *AfO* 38 (Abt. 3): 252–58. (*WAHer* 71)

———. 1893a. "Offener Brief an Prof. H. Sattler." *AfO* 39 (Abt. 2): 274–90. (*WAHer* 72)

———. 1893b. "Ueber den Einfluss der Macula lutea auf spectrale Farben-gleichungen." *Pflüger* 54:277–312. (*WAHer* 73)

———. 1894a. "Ueber einen Fall von Gelb-Blaublindheit." *Pflüger* 57:308–32. (*WAHer* 74)

———. 1894b. "Ueber angebliche Blaublindheit des Fovea centralis." *Pflüger* 59:403–14. (*WAHer* 75)

———. 1895a. "Ueber das sogenannte Purkinje'sche Phänomen." *Pflüger* 60:519–42. (*WAHer* 76)

———. 1895b. "Ueber angebliche Blaublindheit der Zapfen-Sehzellen." *Pflüger* 61:106–112. (*WAHer* 77)

———. 1898. "Untersuchungen an Totalfarbenblinden." *Pflüger* 71:105–27. (*WAHer* 78)

———. 1899a. "Zur Theorie der Nerventätigkeit. Akademischer Vortrag, Leipzig 1898." In Hering 1921, 105–31.

———. 1899b. "Ueber die Grenzen der Sehschärfe." *BksGW* (Naturwissen-schaftlicher Teil) Jg. 1899: 16–24. (*WAHer* 79)

———. 1899c. "Ueber die anomale Localisation der Netzhautbilder bei Strabismus alternans." *Deutschen Archiv für klinische Medizin* 64:15–32. (*WAHer* 80)

———. 1902/1870. *On Memory and the Specific Energies of the Nervous System.* 3d ed. Chicago: Open Court. Translation and reprint of Hering 1870 and 1888.

———. 1905–11. *Grundzüge der Lehre vom Lichtsinn.* Berlin: Julius Springer. Published in installments 1905, 1907, and 1911. Reprinted in *Graefe-Saemischs Handbuch der gesamten Augenheilkunde,* 2d ed., 3:1–294. Berlin: Julius Springer, 1925. Also see Hering 1964.

———. 1906. "Antwortrede, gehalten auf der 33. Versammlung der Ophthalmologischen Gesellschaft, Heidelberg 1906." In Hering 1921, 133–40.

———. 1915. "Das Purkinjesche Phänomen in zentralen Bezirke des Sehfeldes." *AfO* 90:1–12. (*WAHer* 84)

———. 1921. *Fünf Reden.* Ed. H. E. Hering. Leipzig: Wilhelm Engelmann.

———. 1942/1879. *Spatial Sense and Movements of the Eye.* Trans. Carl A. Radde. Baltimore: American Academy of Optometry. (Trans. of Hering 1879a)

———. 1964/1905. *Outlines of a Theory of the Light Sense.* Ed. and trans. Leo M. Hurvich and Dorothea Jameson. Cambridge: Harvard University Press. (Trans. of Hering 1905–11)

———. 1970/1868c. "Self-Steering of Respiration Through the *Nervus vagus.*" Trans. Elisabeth Ullmann. In Porter 1970, 359–64. (Trans. of Hering 1868c)

———. 1977/1868. *The Theory of Binocular Vision. (1868).* Ed. and trans. Bruce Bridgemann. Commentary by Lawrence Stark. New York/London: Plenum. (Trans. of Hering 1868a).

Hering, Ewald, and A. Brückner. 1903. "Ueber die von der Farbenempfindlichkeit unabhängige Aenderung der Weissempfindlichkeit. Nach Versuchen von A. Brückner und E. Hering." *Pflüger* 94:533–54. (*WAHer* 82)

Hering, H. E., and C. S. Sherrington. 1897. "Ueber Hemmung der Contraction willkürlicher Muskeln bei elektrischer Reizung der Grosshirnrinde." *Pflüger* 68:222–28.

Hermann, Ludimar, ed. 1862–99. *Grundriß der Physiologie des Menschen.* 12 editions, 1862–99. Mostly Berlin: August Hirschwald. (Title varies.)

Hess, Carl von. 1893. "Ueber die Unvereinbarkeit gewisser Ermüdungserscheinungen des Sehorgans mit der Dreifasertheorie." *AfO* 39 (Abt. 2): 45–70.

———. 1889. "Ueber den Farbensinn bei indirectem Sehen." *AfO* 35 (Abt. 4): 1–62.

———. 1890. "Ueber die Tonänderungen der Spectralfarben durch Ermüdung der Netzhaut mit homogenem Lichte." *AfO* 36 (Abt. 1): 1–32.

———. 1897. "Experimentelle Untersuchungen über die Nachbilder bewegter leuchtender Punkte." *AfO* 44 (Abt. 3): 445–80.

———. 1918a. "Ewald Hering. Ein Nachruf." *Archiv für Augenheilkunde* 83:89–97.

———. 1918b. "Ewald Hering." *Die Naturwissenschaften* 6:305–8.

———. 1922. "Farbenlehre." *ErgebPhysiol* 20:1–107.

Hess, Carl von, and Hugo Pretori. 1894. "Messende Untersuchungen über die Gesetzmässigkeit des simultanen Helligkeits-Contrastes." *AfO* 40:1–24.

Hillebrand, Franz. 1889. "Ueber die specifische Helligkeit der Farben. Beiträge zur Psychologie der Gesichtsempfindungen." *SbAkadWien* 98 (Abt. 3): 70–122.

———. 1893. "Die Stabilität der Raumwerte auf der Netzhaut." *ZfdPuPdS* 5:1–59.

———. 1894. "Das Verhältnis von Accommodation und Konvergenz zur Tiefenlokalisation." *ZfdPuPdS* 7:97–51.

———. 1910. "Die Heterophorie und das Gesetz der identischen Sehrichtungen." *ZfdPuPdS* 54 (Abt. 1): 1–55.

———. 1918. *Ewald Hering. Ein Gedenkwort der Psychophysik*. Berlin: Springer.

———. 1920. "Purkinjesches Phänomen und Eigenhelligkeit." *ZfdPuPdS* 51 (Abt. 2): 46–95.

———. 1922a. "Zur Theorie der stroboskopischen Bewegungen." *ZfdPuPdS* 88 (Abt. 1): 209–72; 90 (Abt. 1): 1–66.

———. 1922b. "Grundsätzliches zur Theorie der Farbenempfindungen." *ZfdPuPdS* 53 (Abt. 2): 129–33.

———. 1929. *Lehre von den Gesichtsempfindungen auf Grund hinterlassener Aufzeichnungen*. Ed. Franziska Hillebrand. Vienna: Springer.

Hippel, Arthur von. 1880. "Ein Fall von einseitiger, congenitaler Roth-Grünblindheit bei normalen Farbensinn des anderen Auges." *AfO* 26 (Abt. 2): 176–86.

———. 1881. "Ueber einseitige Farbenblindheit." *AfO* 27 (Abt. 3): 47–55.

Hirschberg, Julius. 1985–88. *The History of Ophthalmology*. 5 vols. in 8. Bonn: J. P. Wayenborgh. Trans. of Hirschberg, *Geschichte der Augenheilkunde*, multiple vols. Berlin: Springer, 1899–1911.

Hochberg, Julian E. 1962. "Nativism and Empiricism in Perception." In *Psychology in the Making: Histories of Selected Research Problems*, ed. Leo Postman, 255–330. New York: Alfred A. Knopf.

———. 1988. "Visual Perception." In *Stevens' Handbook of Experimental Psychology*, ed. Richard C. Atkinson et al., 2 vols., 1:195–276. 2d ed. New York: John Wiley & Sons.

Hofmann, Franz Bruno. 1902. "Die neueren Untersuchungen über das Sehen der Schielenden." *ErgebPhysiol* 1:801–46.

———. 1918. "Ewald Hering." *Münchener Medizinische Wochenschrift* 65 (Nr. 20, 14 May 1918): 539–42.

———. 1925. *Die Lehre vom Raumsinn des Auges*. 2 vols. Berlin: Julius Springer, 1920, 1925.

Hofmann, Franz Bruno, and Alfred Bielschowsky. 1900. "Ueber die der Willkür entzogenen Fusionsbewegungen der Augen." *Pflüger* 80:1–40.

Holmes, Frederic L. 1986. "The Formation of the Munich School of Metabolism." In Coleman and Holmes 1988, 179–210.

Holmes, Frederic L., and Gerald L. Geison, eds. 1993. *Research Schools*. OSIRIS, vol. 8. Chicago: University of Chicago Press.

Holmgren, Frithiof. 1879. *Die Arbeiten des Herrn Professor Cohn über Farbenblindheit. Eine kritische Erwiderung*. Upsala: Berling.

———. 1881a. "How Do the Colour-Blind See the Different Colours? Introductory Remarks." *Proceedings of the Royal Society of London* 31:302–6.

————. 1881b. 1 unpublished letter to Helmholtz. *ZADAW*.

————. 1889. "Studien über die elementaren Farbenempfindungen." *Skandanavisches Archiv für Physiologie* 1 (1889): 152–83; 3 (1892): 253–94.

Homer, William Innes. 1964. *Seurat and the Science of Painting*. Cambridge, Mass.: MIT Press.

Hood, D. C., and M. A. Finkelstein. 1983. "A Case for the Revision of Textbook Models of Color Vision: The Detection and Appearance of Small Brief Lights." In Mollon and Sharpe 1983, 375–84.

Hörz, Herbert, and Siegfried Wollgast. 1986. "Hermann von Helmholtz und Emil du Bois-Reymond." In Kirsten 1986, 11–66.

Hoyningen-Huene, Paul. 1990. "Kuhn's Conception of Incommensurability." *Studies in History and Philosophy of Science* 21:481–92.

————. 1993. *Reconstructing Scientific Revolutions: Thomas S. Kuhn's Philosophy of Science*. Trans. Alexander T. Levine. Chicago: University of Chicago Press.

Hubel, David H., and Torsten Wiesel. 1963. "Receptive Fields of Cells in Striate Cortex of Very Young, Visually Inexperienced Kittens." *Journal of Neurophysiology* 26:994–1002.

————. 1965. "Receptive Fields and Functional Architecture in Two Nonstriate Visual Areas (18 and 19) of the Cat." *Journal of Neurophysiology* 28:229–89.

————. 1968. "Receptive Fields and Functional Architecture of Monkey Striate Cortex." *Journal of Physiology* 195:215–43.

Huerkamp, Claudia. 1985. *Der Aufstieg der Aerzte im 19. Jahrhundert. Vom gelehrten Stand zum professionellen Experten: Das Beispiel Preussens*. Göttingen: Vandenhoeck & Ruprecht.

Hughes, H. Stuart. 1962. *Ostwald Spengler: A Critical Estimate*. 2d ed. New York: Charles Scribner.

Hurvich, Leo M. 1969. "Hering and the Scientific Establishment." *American Psychologist* 24:497–514.

————. 1981. *Color Vision*. Sunderland, Mass.: Sinauer Associates.

Hurvich, Leo M., and Dorothea Jameson. 1951. "The Binocular Fusion of Yellow in Relation to Color Theories." *Science* 114:199–202.

————. 1957. "An Opponent-Process Theory of Color Vision." *Psychological Review* 64:384–404.

————. 1966. *The Perception of Brightness and Darkness*. Boston: Allyn and Bacon.

————. 1974. "Opponent Processes as a Model of Neural Organization." *American Psychologist* 29:88–112.

————. 1989. "Leo M. Hurvich and Dorothea Jameson." In *A History of Psychology in Autobiography*, ed. Gardner Lindzey, multiple vols., 8:156–206. Stanford: Stanford University Press.

Hyslop, J. H. 1888. "On Wundt's Theory of Psychic Synthesis in Vision." *Mind* (old series) 13:499–526.

————. 1891. "Helmholtz's Theory of Space-Perception." *Mind* (old series) 16:54–79.

Jaensch, Erich R. 1909. *Zur Analyse der Gesichtswahrnehmungen. Experimentell-psychologische Untersuchungen nebst Anwendung auf die Pathologie des Sehens*. ZfdPuPdS, Abt. 1, Ergänzungsband 4. Leipzig: J. A. Barth.

Jaensch, Erich R. 1911. *Ueber die Wahrnehmung des Raumes . . . . ZfdPuPdS,* Abt. 1, Ergänzungsband 6. Leipzig: J. A. Barth.

———. 1920. "Ueber Grundfragen der Farbenpsychologie." *ZfdPuPdS* 8 (Abt. 1): 257–65.

———. 1921. "Ueber den Nativismus in der Lehre von der Raumwahrnehmung." *ZfdPuPdS* 52 (Abt. 1): 229–34.

Jaensch, Erich R., and E. A. Müller. 1920. "Ueber die Wahrnehmung farbloser Helligkeiten und den Helligkeitskontrast." *ZfdPuPdS* 83 (Abt. 1): 266–341.

Jaensch, Erich R., and F. Reich. 1921. "Ueber den Aufbau der Wahrnehmungswelt und ihre Struktur im Jugendalter. II. Ueber die Lokalisation im Sehraum." *ZfdPuPdS* 86 (Abt. 1): 278–367.

Jahn, Theodore Louis. 1946. "Color Vision and Color Blindness: A Mechanism in Terms of Modern Evidence." *JOSA* 36:595–97.

James, William. 1890. *The Principles of Psychology.* 3 vols. New York: Holt. Reprint. Cambridge: Harvard University Press, 1981.

Jameson, Dorothea. 1981. "Color Vision in 1948: Issues and Origins." Unpublished MS, written for a symposium held at the University of Pennsylvania in honor of Leo M. Hurvich, March 1981.

Jameson, Dorothea, and Leo M. Hurvich. 1961. "Complexities of Perceived Brightness." *Science* 133:174–79.

Javal, Lous-Emile. 1867–68. 10 unpublished letters to Helmholtz. *ZADAW.* Cited by item number and date.

———. 1896. *Manuel théorique et pratique du strabisme.* Paris: G. Masson.

Jaynes, Julian. 1971. "Fechner, Gustav Theodor." *DSB* 4:556–59.

Jeismann, Karl-Ernst. 1974. *Das preussische Gymnasium in Staat und Gesellschaft. Die Entstehung des Gymnasiums als Schule des Staates und der Gebildeten, 1787–1817.* Stuttgart: Ernst Klett Verlag.

Jones, Lloyd A. 1953. "Introduction." In Committee on Colorimetry 1953, 3–15.

Judd, Dean B. 1951. "Basic Correlates of the Visual Stimulus." In Stevens 1951, 811–87.

———. 1960. "Appraisals of Land's Work on Two-Primary Color Projections." *JOSA* 50 (no. 3): 254–68.

Julesz, Bela. 1962. "Visual Pattern Discrimination." *IRE Transactions on Information Theory* 8:84–92.

———. 1964. "Binocular Depth Perception Without Familiarity Cues." *Science* 145:356–62.

———. 1971. *Foundations of Cyclopean Perception.* Chicago: University of Chicago Press.

Jungnickel, Christa, and Russell McCormmach. 1986. *The Intellectual Mastery of Nature: Theoretical Physics from Ohm to Einstein.* 2 vols. Chicago: University of Chicago Press.

Karsten, Gustav. 1851–53. 4 unpublished letters to Helmholtz. *ZADAW.* Cited by item number and date.

Katz, David. 1911. *Die Erscheinungsweisen der Farben und ihre Beeinflussung durch die individuelle Erfahrung. ZfdPuPdS,* Abt. 1, Ergänzungsband 7. Leipzig: J. A. Barth.

———. 1935. *The World of Colour.* London: Kegan Paul. (Trans. of Katz 1911)

————. 1952. "Katz, David." In *History of Psychology in Autobiography*, ed. Edwin G. Boring et al., 4:189–212. Worchester, Mass.: Commonwealth Press.

Kirsten, Christa, ed. 1986. *Dokumente einer Freundschaft: Briefwechsel zwischen Hermann von Helmholtz und Emil Du Bois-Reymond, 1846–1894*. Berlin: Akademie Verlag. Text citations of letters in this collection also include the item number.

Koertling, Walther. 1968. *Die deutsche Universität in Prag. Die letzten hundert Jahre ihrer Medizinischen Fakultät*. Schriftenreihe der Bayerischen Landesärztekammer, vol. 11. Bonn: Bayerische Landesärztekammer.

Kohler, Robert E. 1982. *From Medical Chemistry to Biochemistry: The Making of a Biomedical Discipline*. Cambridge: Cambridge University Press.

Köhnke, Klaus Christian. 1986. *Entstehung und Aufstieg des Neukantianismus. Die deutsche Universitätsphilosophie zwischen Idealismus und Positivismus*. Frankfurt am Main: Suhrkamp.

König, Arthur. 1883–90. 11 unpublished letters to Helmholtz. ZADAW. Cited by item number and date.

————. 1884. "Zur Kenntniss dichromatischer Farbensysteme." *Poggendorff* 22:567–78. (*GesAbhKönig* 11–22, no. 5)

————. 1885a. "Zur Kritik einer Abhandlung von Herrn E. Hering: Ueber individuelle Verschiedenheiten des Farbensinnes." *Centralblatt für praktische Augenheilkunde* 9:260–65. (*GesAbhKönig* 37–43, no. 8)

————. 1885b. "Ueber einen Fall pathologisch entstandener Violetblindheit." *Verhandlung der physikalischen Gesellschaft in Berlin* Jg. 1885: 65–69. (*GesAbhKönig* 46–49, no. 10)

————. 1886. " 'Ueber die neuere Entwicklung von Thomas Young's Farbentheorie,' vortragen vor . . . der B.A.A.S. zu Birmingham am 3. Sept. 1886." *GesAbhKönig* 88–107, no. 15.

————. 1887. "Ueber Newton's Gesetz der Farbenmischung und darauf bezügliche Versuche des Hrn. Eugen Brodhun." *SbAkadBerlin* (31. März 1887), 311–17. (*GesAbhKönig* 108–15, no. 16)

————. 1888a. "Experimentelle Untersuchungen über die psychophysische Fundamentalformel in Bezug auf den Gesichtssinn. (In Gemeinschaft mit Dr. Eugen Brodhun)." *SbAkadBerlin* (26. Juli 1888), 917–31. (*GesAbhKönig* 116–34, no. 17)

————. 1888b. "Experimentelle Untersuchungen über die psychophysische Fundamentalformel in Bezug auf den Gesichtssinn (In Gemeinschaft mit Dr. Eugen Brodhun). Zweite Mittheilung." *SbAkadBerlin* (27. Juni 1889), 135–39. (*GesAbhKönig* 135–39, no. 18)

————. 1891a. "Ueber den Helligkeitswerth der Spectralfarben bei verschiedener absoluter Intensität (Nach gemeinsam mit R. Ritter ausgeführten Versuchen." In König 1891b, 309–88. (*GesAbhKönig* 144–213, no. 20)

————. 1891b. *Beiträge zur Psychologie und Physiologie der Sinnesorgane, Hermann von Helmholtz als Festgruß zu seinem siebzigsten Geburtstage dargebracht*. Ed. A. König. Hamburg: Leopold Voss.

————. 1892. "Die Grundempfindungen in normalen und anomalen Farbensystemen und ihre Intensitätsvertheilung im Spectrum (In Gemeinschaft mit Conrad Dieterici)." *ZfdPuPdS* 4:241–347. (*GesAbhKönig* 124–321, no. 21)

König, Arthur. 1893. "Review of H. Blümmer 'Die Farbenbezeichnungen bei den römischen Dichtern,'" *Berliner Studien für klassische Philologie und Archäologie* 13 (Pt. 3): 231–32." *ZfdPuPdS* 5:350–51. (*GesAbhKönig* 440–41, no. 32)

———. 1894a. "Eine bisher noch nicht beobachtete Form angeborener Farbenblindheit (Pseudo-Monochromasie)." *ZfdPuPdS* 7:161–71. (*GesAbhKönig* 322–32, no. 22)

———. 1894b. "Ueber die lichtempfindliche Schicht in der Netzhaut des menschlichen Auges (In Gemeinschaft mit Dr. Joh. Zumft)." *SbAkadBerlin* (24. Mai 1894), 439–42. (*GesAbhKönig* 333–37, no. 23)

———. 1894c. "Ueber die menschlichen Sehpurpur und seine Bedeutung für das Sehen." *SbAkadBerlin* (21. Juni 1894), 577–98. (*GesAbhKönig* 338–63, no. 24)

———. 1895a. "Ein kurzes Wort zur Entgegnung und Berichtigung." *Pflüger* 60:230–32. (*GesAbhKönig* 364–66, no. 25)

———. 1895b. "Ueber die Anzahl der unterscheidbaren Spectralfarben und Helligkeitsstufen." *ZfdPuPdS* 8:375–80. (*GesAbhKönig* 367–72, no. 26)

———. 1896. "Quantitative Bestimmungen an complementären Spectralfarben." *SbAkadBerlin* (30. Juli 1896), 945–49. (*GesAbhKönig* 373–77, no. 27)

———. 1897a. "Die Abhängigkeit der Sehschärfe von der Beleuchtungsintensität." *SbAkadBerlin* (13. Mai 1897), 559–75. (*GesAbhKönig* 378–95, no. 28)

———. 1897b. "Ueber 'Blaublindheit.'" *SbAkadBerlin* (8. Juli 1897), 718–31. (*GesAbhKönig* 396–415, no. 24)

———. 1897c. "Die Abhängigkeit der Farben- und Helligkeitsgleichungen von der absoluten Intensität." *SbAkadBerlin* (29. Juli 1897), 871–82. (*GesAbhKönig* 416–29, no. 30)

———. 1897d. "Bemerkungen über angeborene totale Blindheit." *ZfdPuPdS* 20:425–34. (*GesAbhKönig* 430–39, no. 31)

König, Arthur, and Conrad Dieterici. 1884. "Ueber die Empfindlichkeit des normalen Auges für Wellenlängenunterschiede des Lichtes." *Poggendorff* 22:579–89. (GesAbhKönig 23–33, no. 6)

———. 1886. "Die Grundempfindungen und ihre Intensitäts-Vertheilung im Spectrum." *SbAkadBerlin* (29. Juli 1886), 805–29. (*GesAbhKönig* 60–87, no. 14)

Koenigsberger, Leo. 1902–3. *Hermann von Helmholtz.* 3 vols. Braunschweig: F. Vieweg und Sohn.

———. 1906. *Hermann von Helmholtz.* Ed. and trans. Frances A. Welby. Oxford: Clarendon Press, 1906. Reprint. New York: Dover, 1965.

Koffka, Kurt. 1919. "Ueber den Einfluß der Erfahrung auf die Wahrnehmung." *Die Naturwissenschaften* 7:597–605.

Kraul, Margret. 1984. *Das deutsche Gymnasium 1780–1980.* Frankfurt am Main: Suhrkamp Verlag.

Krauskopf, John, David R. Williams, and David W. Heeley. 1982. "Cardinal Directions in Color Space." *Vision Research* 22:1123–31.

Kremer, Richard L., ed. 1990. *Letters of Hermann von Helmholtz to His Wife, 1847–1859.* Stuttgart: Franz Steiner Verlag.

———. 1991. "Between *Wissenschaft* and Praxis: Experimental Medicine and the Prussian State, 1807–1850." In Schubring 1991, 155–70.

———. 1992. "Building Institutes for Physiology in Prussia: Interests, Rhetoric and Models." In *The Laboratory Revolution in Medicine*, ed. Andrew Cunningham and Perry Williams, 72–109. Cambridge: University Press.

———. 1993a. "Innovation Through Synthesis: Helmholtz and Color Research." In Cahan 1993b, 205–58.

———. 1993b. "From Psychophysics to Phenomenalism: Mach and Hering on Color Vision." In *The Invention of Physical Science. Intersections of Mathematics, Theology, and Natural Philosophy since the Seventeenth Century: Essays in Honor of Erwin N. Hiebert*, ed. Mary Jo Nye, Joan Richards, and Roger Stuewer, 147–74. Boston Studies in the Philosophy of Science, vol. 139. Norwell, Mass.: Kluwer.

Kries, Johannes von. 1882. "Die Gesichtsempfindungen und ihre Analyse." *AAPwM Supplement-Band* (Physiologische Abt.): 1–178.

———. 1887a. "Zur Theorie der Gesichtsempfindungen." *AAPwM* Jg. 1887: 113–19.

———. 1887b. "Entgegnung an Herrn E. Hering." *Pflüger* 41:389–97.

———. 1888. "Nochmalige Bemerkung zur Theorie der Gesichtsempfindungen." *AAPwM* Jg. 1888: 380–88.

———. 1892. "Ueber die Beziehung der Physik und der Physiologie. Rede gehalten bei der Einweihung des physikalischen und physiologischen Instituts der Universität Freiburg i. B. am 14. Mai 1891." *Berichte der Naturforschenden Gesellschaft zu Freiburg im Bresgau* 6:1–17.

———. 1894. "Ueber den Einfluss der Adaptation auf Licht- und Farbenempfindung und über die Funktion der Stäbchen." *Berichte der Naturforschenden Gesellschaft zu Freiburg im Breisgau* 9:61–70.

———. 1896. "Ueber die Funktion der Netzhautstäbchen." *ZfdPuPdS* 9:81–123.

———. 1897a. "Ueber das Purkinje'sche Phänomen und sein Fehlen auf der Fovea Centalis." *Centralblatt für Physiologie* 10:1–3.

———. 1897b. "Ueber Farbensysteme." *ZfdPuPdS* 13:473–324.

———. 1899. "Kritische Bemerkungen zur Farbentheorie." *ZfdPuPdS* 19:175–91.

———. 1905. "Die Gesichtsempfindungen." In *Handbuch der Physiologie des Menschen*, ed. W. Nagel, 3:109–282. Braunschweig: F. Vieweg und Sohn.

———. 1910. "Appendices" in *PO3*, 497–534; also *PO5* 3: 560–652.

———. 1921. "Helmholtz als Physiolog." *Die Naturwissenschaften*. 9 (Heft 35, 31. Aug. 1921): 673–93.

———. 1923. *Allgemeine Sinnesphysiologie*. Leipzig: F.C.W. Vogel.

———. 1925. "Kries, Johannes von." In *Die Medizin der Gegenwart in Selbstdarstellungen*, ed. L. R. Grote, multiple vols., 4:124–87. Leipzig: Felix Meiner.

Kries, Johannes von, and Friedrich Küster. 1879. "Ueber angeborne Farbenblindheit." *AAPwM* (Physiologische Abt.) Jg. 1879: 513–24.

Kries, Johannes von, and Willibald Nagel. 1896. "Ueber den Einfluß von Lichtstärke und Adaptation auf das Sehen der Dichromaten (Grünblinden)." *ZfdPuPdS* 12:1–38.

———. 1900. "Weitere Mittheilungen über die functionelle Sonderstellung des Netzhautcentrums." *ZfdPuPdS* 23:161–86.

Kroh, Ostwald. 1921. "Ueber Farbenkonstanz und Farbentransformation." *ZfdPuPdS* 52 (Abt. 1): 181–216, 235–73.

Kröncke, Karl. 1921. "Zur Phänomenologie der Kernfläche des Sehraums." *ZfdPuPdS* 52 (Abt. 1): 217–28.

Kruta, Vladislav. 1972. "Hering, Karl Ewald Konstantin." *DSB* 7:299–301.

———. 1976. "Weber, Ernst Heinrich." *DSB* 14:199–201.

Kuffler, Stephen W. 1953. "Discharge Patterns and Functional Organization of Mammalian Retina." *Journal of Neurophysiology* 16:37–68.

Külpe, Oswald. 1893. *Grundriß der Psychologie*. Leipzig: Wilhelm Engelmann.

Kuhn, Thomas S. 1962. *The Structure of Scientific Revolutions*. Chicago/London: University of Chicago Press.

———. 1970. *The Structure of Scientific Revolutions*. 2d ed. Chicago/London: University of Chicago Press.

———. 1974. "Second Thoughts on Paradigms." In Kuhn 1977, 293–319.

———. 1977. *The Essential Tension: Selected Studies in Scientific Tradition and Change*. Chicago/London: University of Chicago Press.

———. 1979. "Metaphor in Science." In *Metaphor and Thought*, ed. Andrew Ortony, 409–19. Cambridge: Cambridge University Press.

———. 1981. "What Are Scientific Revolutions?" Occasional Papers (Center for Cognitive Science), no. 18. Cambridge, Mass.: MIT Press. Reprinted in *The Probabilistic Revolution*, ed. L. Krüger, L. J. Daston, and M. Heidelberger. Vol. 1, *Ideas in History*, 7–23. Cambridge, Mass.: MIT Press, 1987.

———. 1983. "Commensurability, Comparability, Communicability." In *PSA 1982*, ed. P. D. Asquith and Tom Nickles, 2:669–88, 712–16. East Lansing: Philosophy of Science Association.

Kundt, August. 1863. "Untersuchungen über Augenmaaß und optische Täuschungen." *Poggendorff* 120:118–58.

Ladd, George Trumbull. 1908. *Outlines of Physiological Psychology: A Text-Book of Mental Science*. New York: Charles Scribner's Sons.

Ladd-Franklin, Christine. 1892a. "Eine neue Theorie der Lichtempfindungen." *ZfdPuPdS* 4:211–21. Also in Ladd-Franklin 1929, 219–30.

———. 1892b. "A New Theory of Light-Sensation." *Proceedings of the International Congress of Experimental Psychology, London*. Also in Ladd-Franklin 1929, 66–71.

———. 1893. "On Theories of Light-Sensation." *Mind* 2 (new series): 473–79. Also in Ladd-Franklin 1929, 72–91.

———. 1895. "Normal Night-Blindness of the Fovea: Disproof of the König Theory of Colour." *Psychological Review* 2:137–46.

———. 1898. "The Extended Purkinje Phenomenon (for White Lights)." *Psychological Review* 5:309–13. Also in Ladd-Franklin 1929, 193–97.

———. 1916. "On Colour Theories and Chromatic Sensations: A Criticism of Parsons' *Colour Vision*." *Psychological Review* 23:237–53. Also in Ladd-Franklin 1929, 132–48.

———. 1924. "The Nature of Colour-Sensations." Appendix to *PO4* and *PO5*; see *PO5* 2:455–68. Also in Ladd-Franklin 1929, 148–64.

———. 1929. *Colour and Colour Theories*. New York: Harcourt, Brace.

Lakatos, Imre, and Arthur Musgrave, eds. 1970. *Criticism and the Growth of Knowledge*. Cambridge: Cambridge University Press.

Laudan, Larry. 1982. "Two Puzzles about Science: Reflections on Some Crises in the Philosophy and Sociology of Science." *Minerva* 20:253–68.

La Vopa, Anthony J. 1988. *Grace, Talent, and Merit: Poor Students, Clerical Careers, and Professional Ideology in Eighteenth-Century Germany.* New York: Cambridge University Press.

Le Grand, Yves. 1968. *Light, Colour and Vision.* 2d ed. Trans. R.W.G. Hunt et al. London: Chapman and Hall.

Leary, David E. 1982. "Immanuel Kant and the Development of Modern Psychology." In Woodward and Ash 1982, 17–42.

Leber, Theodor. 1873. "Ueber die Theorie der Farbenblindheit und über die Art und Weise, wie gewisse, der Untersuchungen von Farbenblinden entnommene Einwände gegen die Young–Helmholtz'sche Theorie sich mit derselben vereinigen lassen." *Klinische Monatsblätter für Augenheilkunde* Jg. 1873: 467–73.

———. 1884. "Die Ophthalmologie seit 1870." *AfO* 30 (Abt. 1): 1–14.

Le Conte, Joseph. 1881. *Sight: An Exposition of the Principles of Monocular and Binocular Vision.* London: C. Kegan Paul.

Lemaine, Gerard, Roy MacLeod, Michael Mulkay, and Peter Weingart, eds. 1976. *Perspectives on the Emergence of Scientific Disciplines.* The Hague: Mouton.

Lenoir, Timothy. 1982. *The Strategy of Life: Teleology and Mechanics in Nineteenth-Century German Biology.* Dordrecht: Reidel.

———. 1988a. "Science for the Clinic: Science Policy and the Formation of Carl Ludwig's Institute in Leipzig." In Coleman and Holmes 1988, 139–78.

———. 1988b. "Social Interests and the Organic Physics of 1847." *Science in Reflection. The Israel-Boston Colloquium: Studies in History, Philosophy, and Sociology of Science* 3:169–91.

———. 1992. "Laboratories, Medicine and Public Life in Germany 1830–1849: Ideological Roots of the Institutional Revolution." In *The Laboratory Revolution in Medicine*, ed. Andrew Cunningham and Perry Williams, 14–71. Cambridge: University Press.

———. 1993. "The Eye as Mathematician: Clinical Practice, Instrumentation, and Helmholtz's Construction of an Empiricist Theory of Vision." In Cahan 1993b, 109–53.

Lesky, Erna. 1976. *The Vienna Medical School of the 19th Century.* Trans. L. Williams and I. S. Levij. Baltimore: Johns Hopkins University Press.

Levelt, W.J.M. 1968. *On Binocular Rivalry.* Paris: Mouton.

Liebermann, Paul von. 1910. "Beitrag zur Lehre von der binokularen Tiefenlokalisation." *ZfdPuPdS* 44 (Abt. 2): 428–43.

Linksz, Arthur. 1952. *Vision.* Vol. 2 of *Physiology of the Eye.* 3 vols. New York: Grune & Stratton.

Lipps, Theodor. 1885. *Psychologische Studien.* Leipzig: Dürr.

———. 1892. "Die Raumanschauung und die Augenbewegungen." *ZfdPuPdS* 3:123–71.

Listing, Johann Benedikt. 1845. *Beitrag zur physiologische Optik.* In Göttingische Studien, Jg. 1845. Reprinted in *Ostwald's Klassiker der Exakten Wissenschaften*, ed. Otto Schwarz, no. 147. Leipzig: Wilhelm Engelmann, 1905.

———. 1854. "Mathematische Discussion des Ganges der Lichtstrahlen im Auge zur Dioptrik des Auges." In Wagner 1854, 4:451–504.

Lummer, Otto. (See Brodhun and Lummer.)

Mach, Ernst. 1866. "Ueber die Wirkung der räumlichen Vertheilung des Lichtreizes auf die Netzhaut." *SbAkadWien* 52 (Abt. 2): 303–22.

———. 1959/1897. *The Analysis of Sensations and the Relation of the Physical to the Psychical.* Trans. C. M. Williams. New York: Open Court, 1897. Reprint. New York: Dover, 1959.

Marks, W. B., W. H. Dobelle, and E. F. MacNichol, Jr. 1964. "Visual Pigments of Single Primate Cones." *Science* 143:1181–82.

Marriott, F.H.C. 1976. "Colour Vision." In *Visual Function in Man,* ed. Hugh Davidson, 477–586. New York: Academic Press.

Maxwell, James Clerk. 1855. "Experiments on Colour, as Perceived by the Eye." *Transactions of the Royal Society of Edinburgh* 21:275–98. (*CPMaxwell* 1:126–54)

———. 1856. "On the Theory of Colours in Relation to Colour-Blindness . . . in a Letter to Dr. G. Wilson." *Transactions of the Royal Scottish Society of Arts* 4:394–400. (*CPMaxwell* 1:119–25)

———. 1860. "On the Theory of Compound Colours, and the Relations of the Colours of the Spectrum." *Philosophical Transactions of the Royal Society of London* 150:57–84. (*CPMaxwell* 1:410–44 and plates)

———. 1972. "On Colour Vision." *Proceedings of the Royal Institution of Great Britain* 6:260–71. (*CPMaxwell* 2:267–79)

———. 1990. *The Scientific Letters and Papers of James Clerk Maxwell,* ed. P. M. Harman. Vol. 1, *1846–1862.* Cambridge: Cambridge University Press.

McClelland, Charles E. 1980. *State, Society, and University in Germany, 1700–1914.* Cambridge: Cambridge University Press.

McDougall, William. 1903. "The Nature of Inhibitory Processes within the Nervous System." *Brain* 26 (pt. 2): 156–66.

———. 1908. *Physiological Psychology.* 2d ed. London: Richard Clay and Sons.

———. 1912. *Psychology, the Study of Behavior.* London: Williams and Norgate.

Meissner, Georg. 1854. *Beiträge zur Physiologie des Sehorgans.* Leipzig: Wilhelm Engelmann.

Meyer, Heinrich. 1855. "Ueber Contrast- oder Complementärfarben." *Poggendorff* 95:170–71.

Meyering, Theo C. 1981. *Naturalistic Epistemology: Helmholtz and the Rise of a Cognitive Theory of Perception.* Ph.D. diss., University of California–Berkeley.

———. 1989. *Historical Roots of Cognitive Science.* Norwell, Mass.: Kluwer.

Miller, Stephen J. H. 1984. *Parsons' Diseases of the Eye.* 17th ed. Edinburgh: Churchill Livingstone.

Mischel, Theodore. 1970–71. "Wundt and the Conceptual Foundations of Psychology." *Philosophy and Phenomenological Research* 31:1–26.

Mollon, J. D., and L. T. Sharpe, eds. 1983. *Colour Vision: Physiology and Psychophysics.* London: Academic Press.

Monakow, C. von. 1902. "Ueber den gegenwärtigen Stand der Frage nach der Lokalisation im Grosshirn." *ErgebPhysiol* 1:534–665.

Morell, J. B. 1972. "The Chemist Breeders: The Research Schools of Liebig and Thomas Thomson." *Ambix* 9:1–46.

Moulines, Carlos-Ulises. 1981. "Hermann von Helmholtz: A Physiological Approach to the Theory of Knowledge." In *Epistemological and Social Problems of the Sciences in the Early Nineteenth Century*, ed. H. Jahnke and M. Otte, 65–73. Dordrecht: D. Reidel.

Mügge, Felix. 1911. "Ueber anomale Sehrichtungsgemeinschaft bei Strabismus convergens." *AfO* 79:1–41.

Müller, Georg Elias. 1873. *Zur Theorie der sinnlichen Aufmerksamkeit. Inauguraldissertation . . . Göttingen.* Leipzig: A. Adelmann.

———. 1896–97. "Zur Psychophysik der Gesichtsempfindungen." *ZfdPuPdS* 10 (1896): 1–82; 14 (1897): 1–76, 161–96.

Müller, Johannes. 1837, 1840. *Handbuch der Physiologie des Menschen für Vorlesungen.* 2 vols. Coblenz: J. Hülscher.

Müller, Johann Jacob. 1869. 1 unpublished letter to Helmholtz. *ZADAW.*

———. 1870. "Zur Theorie der Farben." *Poggendorff* 139:411–31, 593–614.

———. 1871. "Ueber den Einfluss der Raddrehung der Augen auf die Wahrnehmung der Tiefdimension." *BksGW* 23:125–34.

Mulligan, Joseph F. 1989. "Hermann von Helmholtz and His Students." *American Journal of Physics* 57:68–74.

Nagel, Albrecht. 1861. *Das Sehen mit zwei Augen und die Lehre der identischen Netzhautstellen.* Leipzig: C. F. Winter.

———. 1869. *Der Farbensinn. Populär-wissenschaftlicher Vortrag, im November 1868 zu Tübingen gehalten.* Berlin: Lüderitz.

Nagel, Willibald. 1909. "The Adaptation of the Eye for Different Intensities of Light." Appendix to *PO3, PO4,* and *PO5;* see *PO5* 2:313–43.

Newton, Isaac. 1730. *Opticks, or a Treatise on the Reflections, Refractions, Inflections & Colours of Light.* 4th ed. London. Reprint. New York: Dover, 1952.

Nyhart, Lynn. 1986. *Morphology and the German Universities, 1866–1900.* Ph.D. diss., University of Pennsylvania.

———. 1987. "The Disciplinary Breakdown of German Morphology, 1870–1900." *Isis* 78:365–89.

———. 1991. "Physiology and the Sciences of Animal Life in Germany, 1845–1870." Department of the History of Science. University of Wisconsin. Photocopy.

Olesko, Kathryn M., ed. 1989. *Science in Germany: The Intersection of Institutional and Intellectual Issues.* OSIRIS, vol. 5. Philadelphia: Sheridan Press.

———. 1991. *Physics as a Calling: Discipline and Practice in the Königsberg Seminar for Physics.* Ithaca: Cornell University Press.

Olesko, Kathryn M., and Frederic L. Holmes. 1993. "Experiment, Quantification, and Discovery: Helmholtz's Early Physiological Researches, 1843–50." In Cahan 1993b, 50–108.

Optical Society of America. 1966. "Fifty-Year History of the Optical Society of America." *JOSA* 56:1–68.

Panum, Peter Ludwig. 1858. *Physiologische Untersuchungen über das Sehen mit Zwei Augen.* Kiel: Schwersche Buchhandlung.

———. 1859. "Die Scheinbare Grösse der gesehenen Objecte." *AfO* 5:1–36.

Parsons, John Herbert. 1924. *An Introduction to the Study of Colour-Vision.* 2d ed. Cambridge: University Press.

Pastore, Nicholas. 1973. "Helmholtz's 'Popular Lectures on Vision.'" *Journal of the History of the Behavioral Sciences* 9:190–202.

———. 1974. "Reevaluation of Boring on Kantian Influence, Nineteenth-Century Nativism, Gestalt Psychology and Helmholtz." *Journal of the History of the Behavioral Sciences* 10:375–90.

Pauli, Wolfgang. 1902. *Der kolloidale Zustand und die Vorgänge in der lebendigen Substanz.* Braunschweig: F. Vieweg und Sohn.

Peddie, W. 1922. *Colour Vision: A Discussion of the Leading Phenomena and Their Physical Laws.* London: Edward Arnold.

Peritz, Georg. 1909. "Biochemie des Zentralnervensystems." In *Handbuch der Biochemie des Menschen und der Tiere*, ed. Carol Oppenheimer, 2.2:316–22. Jena: Gustav Fischer.

Petyt, K. M. 1980. *The Study of Dialect: An Introduction to Dialectology.* Boulder: Westview Press.

Pfetsch, Frank R. 1972. "Die Institutionalisierung medizinischer Fachgebiete im deutschen Wissenschaftssystem." In *Innovation und Widerstände in der Wissenschaft*, ed. Frank Pfetsch and Avraham Zloczower, 3–90. Düsseldorf: Bertelsmann.

Pickering, Andrew. 1984. *Constructing Quarks: A Sociological History of Particle Physics.* Chicago: University of Chicago Press.

———. 1989. "Living in the Material World." In Gooding et al. 1989, 1–28.

———. 1990. "Knowledge, Practice and Mere Construction." *SSS* 20:682–729.

Porter, Ruth, ed. 1970. *Breathing: Hering–Breuer Centenary Symposium.* London: J. & A. Churchill.

Prelli, Lawrence J. 1989. *A Rhetoric of Science: Inventing Scientific Discourse.* Columbia: University of South Carolina Press.

Pretori, Hugo, and Moriz Sachs. 1895. "Messende Untersuchungen des farbigen Simultancontrastes." *Pflüger* 60:71–90.

Preyer, William Thierry. 1868. "Ueber anomale Farbenempfindungen und die physiologischen Grundfarben." *Pflüger* 1:299–329.

———. 1870. *Die fünf Sinne des Menschen. Eine populäre Vorlesung. Gehalten im akademischen Rosensaal in Jena am 9. Februar 1870.* Leipzig: Fues's Verlag.

———. 1870–88. 4 unpublished letters to Helmholtz. *ZADAW.* Cited by item number and date.

———. 1884. *Die Seele des Kindes. Beobachtungen über die geistige Entwicklungen des Menschen in dem ersten Lebensjahren.* 2d ed. Leipzig: L. Fernau. (1st ed. 1881)

———. 1895. *Die Seele des Kindes.* 4th ed. Leipzig: Grieben's Verlag.

Pyenson, Lewis. 1983. *Neohumanism and the Persistence of Pure Mathematics in Wilhelmian Germany.* Philadelphia: American Philosophical Society.

Raehlmann, Eduard. 1873. "Beiträge zur Lehre vom Daltonismus und seiner Bedeutung für die Young'sche Farbentheorie." *AfO* 19 (Abt. 3): 86–106.

———. 1891. "Physiologisch-psychologische Studien über die Entwicklung der Gesichtswahrnehmungen bei Kindern und bei operierten Blindgeborenen." *ZfdPuPdS* 2:53–96.

Raehlmann, Eduard, and Ludwig Witkowski. 1877. "Ueber atypische Augenbewegungen." *AAPwM* Jg. 1877: 454–71.

Reading, R. W. 1983. *Binocular Vision: Foundations and Applications.* Boston: Butterworths.

Recklinghausen, Friedrich Daniel von. 1859. "Netzhautfunctionen." *AfO* 5 (Abt. 2): 127–79.

———. 1860. "Zur Theorie des Sehens." *Poggendorff* 110:65–92.

Reed, Edward S. 1988. *James J. Gibson and the Psychology of Perception.* New Haven: Yale University Press.

Richter, Manfred. 1951. "Ueber einige neuere Theorien des Farbensehens." *Klinische Monatsblätter für Augenheilkunde* 118:240–59.

———. 1860. "Zur Theorie des Sehens." *Poggendorff* 110:65–92.

Riese, Reinhard. 1977. *Die Hochschule auf dem Wege zum wissenschaftlichen Grossbetrieb. Die Universität Heidelberg und das badische Hochschulwesen (1860–1914).* Stuttgart: Ernst Klett Verlag.

Riese, Walther, and George E. Arrington, Jr. 1963. "The History of Johannes Müller's Doctrine of the Specific Energies of the Senses: Original and Later Versions." *Bulletin of the History of Medicine* 37:179–83.

Ringer, Fritz K. 1969. *The Decline of the German Mandarins: The German Academic Community 1890–1933.* Cambridge: Harvard University Press.

Rivers, W.H.R. 1900. "Vision." In *Text-Book of Physiology,* ed. E. A. Schäfer, 2:1026–1148. Edinburgh: York J. Pentland.

Rood, Ogden N. 1879. *Modern Chromatics, with Applications to Art and Industry.* London: C. Kegan Paul.

Rose, Edmund. 1865. "Die Farbenkrankheiten im Abriss." *Poggendorff* 126:68–87.

Roth, Paul, and Robert Barrett. 1990. "Deconstructing Quarks." *SSS* 20:579–632.

Rothschuh, Karl E. 1973. *History of Physiology.* Ed. and trans. Guenter B. Risse. Huntington, N.Y.: Robert E. Krieger.

Royce, Josiah. 1911. *Outlines of Psychology: An Elementary Treatise with Some Practical Application.* New York: Macmillan.

Rudwick, Martin J. S. 1985. *The Great Devonian Controversy: The Shaping of Scientific Knowledge among Gentlemanly Specialists.* Chicago: University of Chicago Press.

Sachs, Moriz. 1881. "Ueber die specifische Lichtabsorption des gelben Fleckes der Netzhaut." *Pflüger* 50:574–86.

———. 1897. "Ueber das Sehen der Schielenden." *AfO* 43:597–612.

Schenck, Friedrich. 1903. "Zum Andenken an A. Fick." *GesSchFick* 1:3–42.

———. 1905. "Dioptrik und Accommodation des Auges." In *Handbuch der Physiologie des Menschen,* ed. Willibald Nagel, 3:30–90. Braunschweig: F. Vieweg und Sohn.

Schirmer, Rudolf. 1873. "Ueber erworbene und angeborene Anomalien des Farbensinnes." *AfO* 19 (Abt. 2): 194–235.

Schorske, Carl E. 1980. *Fin-de-siecle Vienna: Politics and Culture.* New York: Alfred A. Knopf.

Schrödinger, Erwin. 1926. "Ueber das Verhältnis der Vierfarben- zur Dreifarben-theorie." *SbAkadWien* 134 (Abt. 2a): 471–90.

Schubring, Gert. 1983. *Die Entstehung des Mathematiklehrerberufs im 19. Jahrhundert. Studien und Materialien zum Prozess der Professionalisierung in Preussen (1910–1870)*. Weinheim und Basel: Beltz Verlag.

———, ed. 1991. *'Einsamkeit und Freiheit' Neu Besichtigt. Universitätsreformen und Disziplinenbildung in Preussen als Modell für Wissenschaftspolitik im Europa des 19. Jahrhunderts*. Stuttgart: Franz Steiner Verlag.

Schultze, Max. 1858–72. 7 unpublished letters to Helmholtz. *ZADAW*. Cited by number and date.

———. 1866. *Zur Anatomie und Physiologie der Retina*. Bonn: Max Cohen und Sohn.

Segall, Marshall H., Donald T. Campbell, and Melville Herskovits. 1966. *The Influence of Culture on Visual Perception*. Indianapolis: Bobbs-Merrill.

Servos, John W. 1993. "Research Schools and Their Histories." In Holmes and Geison 1993.

Shapin, Steven, and Simon Schaffer. 1985. *Leviathan and the Air-Pump: Hobbes, Boyle, and the Experimental Life*. Princeton: Princeton University Press.

Sheehan, James J. 1978. *German Liberalism in the Nineteenth Century*. Chicago/London: University of Chicago Press.

Sherman, Paul D. 1981. *Colour Vision in the Nineteenth Century: The Young-Helmholtz-Maxwell Theory*. Bristol: Adam Hilger.

Siemens-Helmholtz, Ellen von, ed. 1929. *Anna von Helmholtz. Ein Lebensbild in Briefen*. 2 vols. Berlin: Verlag für Kulturpolitik.

Spengler, Ostwald. 1926. *Form and Actuality*. Vol. 1 of *The Decline of the West*. 2 vols. Trans. Charles Francis Atkinson. New York: Alfred A. Knopf. (1st German ed. 1918)

Stern, Fritz. 1961. *The Politics of Cultural Despair: A Study in the Rise of the Germanic Ideology*. Berkeley: University of California Press.

Stevens, S. S., ed. 1951. *Handbook of Experimental Psychology*. New York: John Wiley & Sons.

Stichweh, Rudolf. 1984. *Zur Entstehung des modernen Systems wissenschaftlicher Disziplinen. Physik in Deutschland 1740–1890*. Frankfurt am Main: Suhrkamp.

Stiles, W. S. 1972. "The Line Element in Colour Theory: A Historical Review." In *Colour Metrics: Proceedings of the Helmholtz Memorial Symposium on Color Metrics . . .*, ed. J. J. Vos et al., 1–25. Soesterberg: AIC/Holland.

———. 1978. *Mechanisms of Colour Vision: Selected Papers of W. S. Stiles, F.R.S., with an Introductory Essay*. London: Academic Press.

Stilling, Jakob. 1879. "Ueber den Stand der Farbenfrage." *Archiv für Augenheilkunde* 8:18–37.

———. 1910. "Ueber Entstehung und Wesen der Anomalien des Farbensinnes." *ZfdPuPdS* 44:371–427.

Stout, George F. 1929. *A Manual of Psychology*. 4th ed., rev. by C. A. Mace. London: W. B. Clive.

Stumpf, Carl. 1873. *Ueber den psychologischen Ursprung der Raumvorstellung*. Leipzig: S. Hirzel.

———. 1895. "Hermann von Helmholtz and the New Psychology." *Psychophysical Review* 2:1–12.

Stumpf, Carl, and H. Rupp. 1927. "Franz Hillebrand." *ZfdPuPdS* 102 (Abt. 1): 1–5.

Sully, James. 1878. "The Question of Visual Perception in Germany." *Mind* (old series) 3:1–23, 167–95.

———. 1886. *Teacher's Handbook of Psychology*. New York: D. Appleton.

Svaetichin, Gunnar. 1956. "Spectral Response Curves from Single Cones." *Acta Physiologica Scandinavica* 39 (Supp. 134): 17–46.

Swazey, Judith P. 1975. "Sherrington, Charles Scott." *DSB* 12:395–403.

Taylor, James G. 1962. *The Behavioral Basis of Perception*. New Haven: Yale University Press.

Titchener, Edward Bradford. 1902. *An Outline of Psychology*. Rev. ed. New York: Macmillan.

Tonn, Emil. 1894. "Ueber die Gültigkeit des Newtonschen Farbenmischungsgesetzes." *ZfdPuPdS* 7:279–304.

Trendelenburg, Wilhelm. 1961. *Der Gesichtssinn. Grundzüge der physiologischen Optik*. 2d. rev. ed., ed. Manfred Monjé, Ingeborg Schmidt, and Eric Schutz. Berlin: Springer Verlag. (1st ed. 1943)

Troland, Leonard Thompson. 1922a. *The Present State of Visual Science*. Bulletin of the National Research Council of the National Academy of Sciences, vol. 5, pt. 2, no. 27. Washington, D.C.: National Research Council.

———. 1922b. "Report of the Committee on Colorimetry." *JOSA* 6:527–96.

———. 1929. "Visual Phenomena and Their Stimulus Correlations." In *The Foundations of Experimental Psychology*, ed. Carl Murchison, 169–215. Worchester: Clark University Press.

Tschermak-Seysenegg, Armin. 1898. "Ueber die Bedeutung der Lichtstärke und des Zustandes des Sehorgans für farblose optische Gleichungen." *Pflüger* 70:297–328.

———. 1899. "Ueber anomale Sehrichtungsgemeinschaft der Netzhaut bei einem Schielenden." *AfO* 47 (pt. 3): 508–50.

———. 1900. "Beitrag zur Lehre vom Längshoropter (Nach Beobachtungen von Dr. Kiribuchi)." *Pflüger* 81:328–48.

———. 1902. "Die Hell-Adaptation des Auges und die Funktion der Stäbchen und Zapfen." *ErgebPhysiol* 1:695–800.

———. 1932. *Der exakte Subjektivismus in der neuen Sinnesphysiologie*. 2d rev. ed. Wien and Leipzig: Emil Haim. (1st ed. Berlin: Springer, 1921)

———. 1934. "Zu Ewald Herings 100. Geburtstag. Gedenkrede, gehalten an der Universität Köln." *Münchener medizinische Wochenschrift* 83:1230–33.

———. 1942. *Einführung in die physiologische Optik*. Berlin: Springer.

Tuchman, Arleen. 1986. "From the Lecture to the Laboratory: The Institutionalization of Scientific Medicine at the University of Heidelberg." In Coleman and Holmes 1988, 65–99.

———. 1993a. "Helmholtz and the German Medical Community." In Cahan 1993b, 17–49.

———. 1993b. *Science, Medicine,and the State in Germany: The Case of Baden, 1815–1871*. New York: Oxford University Press.

Turner, R. Steven. 1971. "The Growth of Professorial Research in Prussia, 1818–1848—Causes and Context." *Historical Studies in the Physical Sciences* 3:137–82.

———. 1972. "Helmholtz, Hermann von." *DSB* 4:241–53.

———. 1980a. "The *Bildungsbürgertum* and the Learned Professions in Prussia, 1770–1830: The Origins of a Class." *Histoire Sociale—Social History* 13:105–35.

———. 1980b. "The Prussian Universities and the Concept of Research." *Internationales Archiv für Sozialgeschichte der deutschen Literatur* 5:68–93.

———. 1982a. "Justus von Liebig versus Prussian Chemistry: Reflections on the Rise of the Institute System in Germany." *Historical Studies in the Physical Sciences* 13:129–62.

———. 1982b. "Helmholtz, Sensory Physiology, and the Disciplinary Development of German Psychology." In *The Problematic Science: Psychology in Nineteenth-Century Thought*, ed. William R. Woodward and Mitchell G. Ash, 147–66. New York: Praeger.

———. 1986. "Toward a Disciplinary Order of Sciences." *Minerva* 24:495–502.

———. 1987a. "Paradigms and Productivity: The Case of Physiological Optics, 1840–94." *SSS* 17:35–68.

———. 1987b. "Fechner, Helmholtz, and Hering on the Interpretation of Simultaneous Contrast." In Brozek and Gundlach 1987, 137–50.

———. 1987c. "The Great Transition and the Social Patterns of German Science." *Minerva* 25:56–76.

———. 1993a. "Consensus and Controversy: Helmholtz on the Visual Perception of Space." In Cahan 1993b, 154–204.

———. 1993b. "Vision Studies in Germany: Helmholtz versus Hering." In Holmes and Geison 1993.

Uhthoff, W. 1891. "Untersuchungen über das Sehenlernen eines siebenjährigen blindgeborenen und mit Erfolg operierten Knaben." In König 1891b, 113–72.

Ullmann, Elisabeth. 1970. "About Hering and Breuer." In Porter 1970, 3–15.

Verworn, Max. 1915. *Allgemeine Physiologie. Ein Grundriß der Lehre vom Leben.* 6th ed. Jena: Gustav Fischer.

Vitz, Paul C., and Arnold B. Glimcher. 1984. *Modern Art and Modern Science: The Parallel Analysis of Vision.* New York: Praeger.

Vogel, Stephan. 1993. "Sensation of Tone, Perception of Sound, and Empiricism: Helmholtz's Physiological Acoustics." In Cahan 1993b, 259–90.

Volkmann, Alfred Wilhelm. 1846. "Sehen." In Wagner 1854, 3.1:264–351.

———. 1856–71. 22 unpublished letters to Helmholtz. *ZADAW*. Cited by item number and date.

———. 1859. "Die stereoskopischen Erscheinungen in ihrer Beziehung zu der Lehre von den identischen Netzhautpunkten." *AfO* 5 (Abt. 2): 1–100.

———. 1863. *Physiologische Untersuchungen im Gebiete der Optik.* Leipzig: Breitkopf und Härtel.

Vries, H. de. 1946. "On the Basic Sensation Curves of Three-Color Theory." *JOSA* 36:121–26.

Wade, Nicholas J., ed. 1983. *Brewster and Wheatstone on Vision.* London: Academic Press.

Wagner, Rudolf, ed. 1854. *Handwörterbuch der Physiologie mit Rücksicht auf physiologische Pathologie*, 4 vols. in 5. Braunschweig: F. Vieweg und Sohn, 1842 (pt. 1), 1844 (pt. 2), 1846 (pt. 3.1), 1846 (pt. 3.2), 1854 (pt. 4).

Ward, James. 1918. *Psychological Principles*. Cambridge: University Press.

Wardhaugh, Ronald. 1986. *An Introduction to Sociolinguistics*. New York: Basil Blackwell.

———. 1987. *Languages in Competition: Dominance, Diversity, and Decline*. New York: Basil Blackwell.

Warren, Richard M., and Roslyn P. Warren. 1968. "Introduction." In *Helmholtz on Perception: Its Physiology and Development*, ed. Richard M. Warren and Roslyn P. Warren, 3–23. New York: John Wiley & Sons.

Wasserman, G. S. 1978. *Color Vision: An Historical Introduction*. New York: John Wiley & Sons.

Wertheimer, Max. 1912. "Experimentelle Studien über das Sehen von Bewegungen." *ZfdPuPdS* 61 (Abt. 1): 161–265.

———. 1923. "Bemerkungen zu Hillebrands Theorie der stroboskopischen Bewegungen." *Psychologische Forschung* 3:106–23.

Westman, Robert L., et al. 1978. "The Rational Explanation of Historical Discoveries (Panel Discussion)." In *Scientific Discoveries: Case Studies*, ed. Thomas Nickles, 21–49. Dordrecht/Boston: D. Reidel.

Wheatstone, Charles. 1838. "Contributions to the Physiology of Vision—Part the First: On some Remarkable, and hitherto Unobserved, Phenomena of Binocular Vision." *Philosophical Transactions of the Royal Society* 28:371–94. Reprinted in Wade 1983, 65–93.

Wiesel, T. N., and D. H. Hubel. 1966. "Spatial and Chromatic Interactions in the Lateral Geniculate Body of the Rhesus Monkey." *Journal of Neurophysiology* 29:1115–56.

Wiesflecker, Hermann, ed. 1978. *Ernst Wilhelm von Brücke. Briefe an Emil Du Bois-Reymond*. Publicationen aus dem Archiv der Universität Graz, vol. 811. Graz: Akademische Druck.

Willey, Thomas E. 1978. *Back to Kant: The Revival of Kantianism in German Social and Historical Thought, 1860–1914*. Detroit: Wayne State Press.

Willmer, E. N. 1943a. "Observations on the Physiology of Colour Vision." *Nature* 151:212–15.

———. 1943b. "Physiology of Colour Vision." *Nature* 151:632–35.

———. 1944. "Colour of Small Objects." *Nature* 153:774–75.

Woodward, William. 1978. "From Association to Gestalt: The Fate of Hermann Lotze's Theory of Spatial Perception, 1846–1920." *Isis* 69:572–82.

———. 1982. "Wundt's Program for the New Psychology: Vicissitudes of Experiment, Theory, and System." In Woodward and Ash 1982, 167–97.

Woodward, William R., and Mitchell Ash, eds. 1982. *The Problematic Science: Psychology in Nineteenth-Century Thought*. New York: Praeger.

Worth, Claud Alley. 1915. *Squint: Its Causes, Pathology, and Treatment*. 4th ed. Philadelphia: P. Blakiston's Son, 1915.

Wundt, Wilhelm. 1862a. *Beiträge zur Theorie der Sinneswahrnehmung*. Leipzig/ Heidelberg: C. F. Winter. Reprinted in *The Origins of Psychology: A Collection of Early Writings*, ed. Wolfgang G. Bringmann, 4:109–206, and 5: (entire). New York: Alan R. Liss, 1977.

Wundt, Wilhelm. 1862b. "Ueber binoculares Sehen." *Poggendorff* 192:617–26.

———. 1863a. "Ueber Dr. E. Hering's Kritik meiner Theorie des Binocularsehens." *Poggendorff* 196:172–76.

———. 1863b. *Vorlesungen über die Menschen- und Thierseele.* 2 vols. Leipzig: Leopold Voss.

———. 1888. "Die Empfindung des Lichts und der Farben. Grundzüge einer Theorie der Gesichtsempfindungen." *Philosophische Studien* 4:311–89.

———. 1920. *Erlebtes und Erkanntes.* Stuttgart: Alfred Krönser.

Zloczower, Avraham. 1972. "Konjunktur in der Forschung." In *Innovation und Widerstände in der Wissenschaft*, ed. Frank Pfetsch and Avraham Zloczower, 91–151. Düsseldorf: Bertelsmann.

Zoth, Oscar. 1905. "Augenbewegungen und Gesichtswahrnehmungen." In *Handbuch der Physiologie des Menschen*, ed. W. Nagel, 3:283–436. Braunschweig: F. Vieweg und Sohn.

Index

abathic surface, 167
Abney, William, 263
accommodation and convergence, 12, 61, 91–92, 169
adaptation: and experimental practice, 243; on opponent process theory, 133, 190
afterimages. *See* contrast, successive
Allen, Grant, 177
animals, observations and experiments on, 244–45; and the nativist-empiricist debate, 160; and neurophysiological studies, 266–67, 272–73
anomalous dichromatism, 185
anomalous retinal correspondence. *See* correspondence
art, experimentation with spatial representation in, 175
Ash, Mitchell, 274
Aubert, Hermann, 141, 158, 228, 231; on color theory, 115, 178; critique of projection, 68

barycentricity in color mixing, 193; Helmholtz on, 98; Newton on, 28, 289n.4
Becker, Otto, 179, 205
Berkeley, George, 13
Bezold, Wilhelm, 141, 145
Biagioli, Mario, 231
Bielschowsky, Alfred, 141, 142; on etiology and treatment of strabismus, 250–51; on strabismus and anomalous correspondence, 171
binocular disparity. *See* stereopsis
binocularity, 14. *See also* stereopsis
biogen hypothesis, 247
bite-bar, 52
black: critiques of Hering's theory of, 194, 220–23; Hering on, 126–27. *See also* brightness, white
blind individuals with sight restored, 77, 162
blindspot, retinal, 75
Bohn, Conrad, 118
Boll, Franz, 206

Boltzmann, Ludwig, 152
Boring, Edwin G., 271
Bourdieu, Pierre, 230
Brentano, Franz, 252, 255
Breuer, Josef, 55, 120–21
Brewster, David, 41, 95, 194; his color theory, 30; and projection theory, 14–15
brightness: chromatic contribution to, 202–5; critiques of Hering's theory of, 194, 221; Helmholtz on defining and measuring, 98–99; Hering on, 132, 202–3, 220–21, 293n.3, 295n.5; Hering's perception of dependent upon differential sensitivity, 222; Hering's school's understanding of as tacit knowledge, 224; in sensory compounds, 223; on Young's theory, 202
Brodhun, Eugen, 141, 145, 148
brown, 221
Brücke, Ernst Wilhelm von, 36, 38, 39, 41, 105, 109, 111, 141, 145, 152, 156, 226; adoption of Young's theory, 115; career, 147; defence of identity, 17; relationship to Helmholtz, 147; role in the controversy, 147
Brücke, Ernst T., 141, 142
Brückner, Arthur, 151
Budge, Julius, 119

Cahan, David, 152
Caneva, Kenneth, 239
Cattell, J. McKeen, 264
Cheselden case, 77
Chevreul, Michel, 109
chromatic fading, 29, 108
Classen, August, 60, 63, 81, 88, 232; and binocular localization, 20
Cohn, Hermann, 178–79
Collins, Harry, 6, 139, 154
color blindness: and color triangle, 291–92n.5; and displacement hypothesis, 178; Donders on, 184; Henri Dor on, 118; explained by Young's theory, 102–4, 118; Helmholtz on, 106–7; history before Maxwell and Helmholtz, 28–29; Kries on, 181–82; Maxwell on, 102–4; periph-

color blindness (cont.)
eral, 119, 186; public interest in, 177–78;
Rose on, 118; and santonin effect, 118;
Schirmer on, 119; unilaterals and, 179–
80. See also dichromats; monochromats

color circle, Newton's, 27–28, 289n.4

color constancy: Katz and Jaensch on, 253;
on opponent process theory, 133; unconscious inference in (Helmholtz), 111

color equations: in König's work, 197;
Maxwell's, 101–4; persistence with adaptation, 188, 189–93

color mixing: additive and subtractive mixtures, 96, 105; binocular, 79; experimental methods, 96, 100, 113–14, 238;
Grassmann's laws of, 97; Helmholtz on,
95–99; Newton's law of, 287–88. See
also colorimetry

color triangle, 26, 102–4, 200–201, 291–
92n.5

color vision studies: consolidation as a field
around midcentury, 30–31; 113–14; in
England, 263; history before Maxwell
and Helmholtz, 26–31; instrumentation
in, 113–14; methods of the physicist in,
114, 237–39; microelectrode studies and,
266–67; physicalist tradition in twentieth
century, 266; proliferation of theories in
1890s, 196; terminological standardization, 114

colored shadows experiment, 110

colorimeters, 238; Helmholtz-König, 240;
Hering, 240–41; as reflecting the theory
and experimental style of the schools,
242–43

colorimetry: 220, 233, 238, 240–43; contributions of König to, 197; Helmholtz on,
105–6; Maxwell on, 99–104, 291n.3. See
also color mixing; colorimeters

complementary colors: Grassmann on, 97;
Helmholtz on, 96

cones. See rods and cones

contrast, successive: explained on opponent
process theory, 129; Helmholtz's explanation by retinal fatigue and Young's theory, 107–8; Hering's critique of exhaustion theory, 123–26; Hering's students
on, 223; used to confirm extraspectral nature of fundamental sensations, 108

contrast, simultaneous, 109, 194; explained
on the opponent process theory, 129;
Helmholtz's explanation of by uncon-

scious inference, 108–13; Hering's critique of inferential explanations, 123,
185; Katz and Jaensch on, 253; Kries on,
181; twentieth-century studies of, 271–
72

controversy, the Helmholtz-Hering: agreement on major experimental outcomes,
234; and disciplinary interests, 235–57,
279; experimental constraints on in the
1860s, 60; and the fragmentation of vision studies, 256–57; over the horopter,
58–60; incommensurability in, 7, 218–
34, 278–79; intractability of, 218, 278;
lack of clear denouement, 261–76; loses
character of school controversy, 261–62;
negotiations in, 278; ophthalmologists
in, 247–51; overview of, 3–5, 70, 94,
177, 196, 218, 276–80; polarization of,
154, 278; psychologists in, 251–56; public nature of, 154; as school controversy,
6, 140, 278; shared assumptions of the
antagonists, 69, 135, 181, 233, 277; shift
to achromatic perception in the 1890s,
214; struggle for semantic control of,
226–31, 279. See also controversy, scientific; nativist-empiricist controversy

controversy, scientific: as constitutive of scientific change, 6, 7, 93–94, 277; and disciplinary interests, 235; Laudan on, 276–
77

core point of visual space, 65

core surface of visual space, 65

core set: concept of, 6, 139, 154, 278;
Helmholtz partisans, 142–48; and the
Helmholtz-Hering controversy, 7, 140–
42, 278; Hering partisans, 141–43; Hering's partisans divided on his concept of
brightness, 224; nonaligned participants,
153–54, 278; psychologists in, 251–56

correspondence, retinal, 15, 16, 18, 63, 65,
226; anomalous, 78–79, 168–72; empiricist explanations of, 78; and retinal incongruity, 44–45. See also identity,
theory of

Cramer, Antonie C., 12

Dalton, John, 28

depth perception: absolute and relative, 13,
63–64; empirical cues in, 13–14. See also
localization; projection, theory of;
stereopsis

depth values, retinal: binocular and monocular, 81–82; crucial experiment on, 84–86; debate over the stability of, 162–68; defined by Hering, 65–66; Helmholtz's critique of monocular, 81–86; indistinguishable from disparities, 86; monocular defined, 82; rejection by Kries, 173; versus experiential factors, 82–84

deuteranopes See dichromats

developmental stages: and visual capacity, 161; and strabismus, 250–51

dichromats: defined by Maxwell, 102–4; distinct groups of, 182, 184, 185, 194, 234; König's determination of response curves and fundamental sensations of, 198–202; Kries on, 216; protanope-deuteranope terminology, 184; visual experiences of, 104, 107, 180, 182, 183, 220. See also color blindness

Dieterici, Conrad, 141, 145, 146, 148; collaboration with König, 197

dioptrics, 11–12

displacement hypothesis, 178, 182, 216; criticized by Hering, 185–86

dominator-modulator theory, 267

Donders, Franciscus, 39, 141, 142, 152, 197, 198, 228, 231, 232, 247, 278; on accommodation and convergence, 169; on color vision, 183–84; on Donders' Law, 22; and nativism, 158; as nonaligned participant, 153

Donders' Law, 22, 50–51, 72, 91

double eye, 62

double images: localization of, 61; on projection theory, 19–20; on theory of identity, 15–16

double white, 2

Dove, Heinrich, 17, 105

Du Bois-Reymond, Emil, 42, 36, 38, 39, 41, 55, 56, 74, 141, 161, 232; on the nativist-empiricist controversy, 158

duplicity theory, 277; described, 211; and foveal adaptation, 213; and monochromatism, 213; Purkinje phenomenon in, 213–14; reception of, 215, 216; response of Hering's school to, 215

easiest orientation, principle of, 50–51

Ebbinghaus, Hermann, 141, 154, 252, 255; his color theory, 207; critique of König and Dieterici, 206; his key experiment, 206, 212

ecological realism, 275

elementary sensations (König), 197

empiricist theory of spatial localization: in America, 263–64; defined by Helmholtz, 76; in England, 262–63; Helmholtz's defense of, 80–88; Helmholtz's early views on, 69–71; history of according to Helmholtz, 81; methodological precepts of, 75–76; reception of, 156–57; retinal correspondence in, 78; and twentieth-century perception theory, 275–76

entoptical shadows, 12, 209

equal innervations, Hering's law of, 89–91

Exner, Franz, 141, 238; critique of opponent process theory, 228–29

Exner, Sigmund, 118, 141, 145, 148, 152, 185; attacked by Hering, 227

eye movements: anatomical limitations on, 72–73; coordinates of, 22, 290n.6; divergences, 72, 92; equal innervations, 89–91; fusional cyclorotations, 72, 92; Helmholtz disagrees with Wundt over, 69; Helmholtz on involuntary cyclorotations, 73; inadequate as cues to localization (Hering), 61; ocular muscles in, 91; the will as cue to visual direction, 77. See also Donders Law; Listings Law

Fechner, Gustav Theodor, 105, 109, 226, 237, 251; critique of Helmholtz, 112; ideas used by Helmholtz, 108; influence on Hering, 57; on simultaneous contrast, 110–11, 117

Fichte, Immanuel Hermann, 40

Fichte, Johann Gottlieb, 26, 40

Fick, Adolf, 141, 145, 232; attacked by Hering, 185–86; career, 147; critique of Hering's theory of brightness, 221; and displacement hypothesis, 178; on Young's theory, 115, 180

Fick, Eugene, 184

fin de siècle mood, 174

Fischer, F. P., 171

Fleischl von Marxow, Ernst, 141

fovea: alleged blue blindness of, 209; in duplicity theory, 212–14; uncertainty over rod-free area, 211, 295n.9

fundamental sensations: Donders on, 184; S. Exner on, 117; as extra-spectral, 102; Helmholtz on, 106–7, 117, 292–93n.1; König's deduction of, 197–202; Maxwell on, 117, 292–93n.1; Maxwell deduces from evidence of dichromats, 102–4;

fundamental sensations (*cont.*)
J. J. Müller on, 117, 118, 292–93n.1; number of, 189–93, 200; Preyer on, 117
fusion, binocular, 15, 79; contour relationships in, 16; mechanism of, 249; physiological versus psychological explanations of, 23–26; Volkmann on, 18; Volkmann-Panum dispute about, 24

Garten, Siegfried, 141, 142, 149, 224, 240, 241, 262
Gauss, Karl Friedrich, 12
Geiger, Lazarus, 177
Geison, Gerald, 143
Gestalt psychology, 271; and the Helmholtz-Hering dispute, 254–56
Gibson, James J., 274, 276
Goethe, Johann Wolfgang, 28, 194
Goldstein, Eugen, 152
Graefe, Albrecht von, 17, 48, 156, 247
Graefe, Alfred, 141; on strabismus and anomalous correspondence, 170
Granit, Regnar, 267, 272
Grassmann, Hermann Günther, 97
gray: brain gray, 296n.2; midgray in opponent-process theory, 129; as a nuanced series, 130; as a qualitative series, 126
Greeff, Richard, 169

half images: localization of, 84. *See also* double images
Hankel, Hermann, 58
Hartline, H. K., 272
Hatfield, Gary, 290n.2, 291n.3
Hecht, Selig, 266
Hegel, Georg Wilhelm Friedrich, 26, 40, 87
Helmholtz, Hermann Ludwig Ferdinand von, 10, 12, 22, 56, 93, 200, 271, 274, 279–80; adopts Young's theory, 104–5; career, 3, 35–37; character and personality, 38–40; on color blindness, 106–8, 119; on color vision, 104–8; concession to nativism, 77; critique of Brewster, 95; critique of Hering's theory of brightness, 221; critique of monocular depth values, 81–86; critique of nativism, 76, 80–87; critique of opponent process theory, 193–95; empiricist theory, 43, 69–71; epistemological views, 74–75, 156; establishes Listing's Law, 48; on evolution and spatial localization, 159; and functional explanation, 59; and the *Handbook of*

Physiological Optics, 10,37, 42, 73–88, 104–14, 193–95, 264; on the horopter, 41–48; on the horopter deviation, 165–66; and the horopter dispute, 58–60; initial rejection of Young's theory, 96; intellectual formation, 40–41; leadership style, 151–53; and line-element theory, 237–38; and Maxwell, 291n.4; needles/thread-triple experiment, 46–47, 66, 71; and ophthalmology, 247; perceives Hering as a threat, 73–74; political views, 39, 289n.7; recruited by Hering, 68; repudiates projection, 69; on simultaneous contrast, 108–13; social origins of, 35, 56; as teacher, 148; views in America, 264
Hering, Heinrich Ewald, 55
Hering, Karl Ewald Konstantin, 44, 51, 75, 87, 93, 212, 272, 279–80; attacks on the Helmholtz school, 184–86; attitude to Helmholtz, 68–69; becomes more nativist in outlook, 92; and *Beiträge zur Physiologie,* 54–55, 60; career, 3, 54–56; character and personality, 56; on classes of color theories, 187–89; collaboration with Josef Breuer, 120–21; his colorimeter, 240–41; critique of empiricism, 91, 122–23, 127; critique of König's theory, 210–11; critique of physicalist assumptions by Helmholtz school, 188–89; critique of reductionism, 245–46; critique of terminology of Helmholtz's school, 227–28; critique of unconscious inference, 127; critique of Wundt, 61; critique of Young's theory, 134; determines spectral luminosity curve for monochromats, 204; on displacement hypothesis, 185–86; emotional ties to students, 150; on evolution and memory, 57–58, 91, 120, 159, 226–27; his experimental style, 238–39; on extended theory of identity, 62, 63, 68; on eye movements, 157–58; on Helmholtz's needles/thread-triple experiment, 66; on the horopter, 58–60; on identical visual directions, 62; intellectual formation, 56–57; leadership style of, 149–51; on light and color, 115–35, 293n.2; on mix space, 187; as nationalist, 55, 150; *On the Theory of the Light Sense,* 121; phenomenological approach, 126, 135; philosophy of the organism, 57–58, 62, 120–21, 135, 245; physiologi-

cal-psychological method, 122–23, 135; poses as bilingual, 232; projection, 60–62, 68; and psychologists, 151; reform program for physiological optics, 60; rejects Kries' NeoKantian understanding of spatiality, 229–30; reply to Donders, 187–88; reply to Kries, 189–93, 294n.3; reply to Helmholtz, 89–93; response to duplicity theory, 212, 215; retreat from the theory of retinal depth values, 157; social origins, 56; on specific nerve energies, 120, 245–46; on strabismus and anomalous correspondence, 169; strategy for the reform of physiological optics, 68; success in placing students, 151; and terminology, 226; and *Theory of Binocular Vision*, 89–91; ties to ophthalmological community, 248; views in America, 264; views in twentieth-century Germany, 265

Hermann, Ludimar, 159; adoption of Young's theory, 115; growing acceptance of nativism, 172; growing acceptance of opponent process theory, 215; influenced by Schultze, 117

Hess, Carl von, 141, 142, 215, 223, 224, 239, 262, 295n.7; on central scotoma in monochromats, 213; on foveal adaptation, 213; and peripheral color blindness, 186; recollections of Hering, 150–51

Hillebrand, Franz, 141, 142, 151, 162, 215, 218, 221, 224, 239, 251, 262; career, 143; critique of Wertheimer, 255–56; critique of Young's theory, 204; emotional tie to Hering, 150; on the Phi phenomenon, 255; rejects Kries' NeoKantian understanding of the spatial sense, 230–31; semantic strategies of, 227; on specific brightness of colors, 202–5; on stability of retinal depth values, 162–68, 294n.4

Hippel, Arthur von, 141; his unilateral, 179–80

Hofmann, Franz, 141, 142, 262; draws nativist conclusions from strabismus evidence, 172; on Gestalt psychology, 256; on Hering's terminology, 227; on strabismus and anomalous correspondence, 170–71

Hillebrand, Franziska, 150, 175, 215

Holmgren, Frithiof, 141, 142, 184; and color blindness, 177; dispute with Cohn, 178–79; on Hippel's unilateral, 179

horopter, 65; definition of around 1850, 21; as defined by Tschermak-Seysenegg, 166; function of, 21–22, 46; and the ground-plane, 47–48; Helmholtz on, 41–48; Hering on, 58; Johannes Müller on, 293–94n.2; point- and line-, 44–45; problem of before Helmholtz, 21–22; in theory of retinal space values, 64; vertical, 163. *See also* abathic surface

horopter deviation, the Hering-Hillebrand: described, 163–65, 294n.3; Helmholtz's explanation of, 165–66; Tschermak-Seysenegg on, 166

Hubel, David H., 273

hue cancelation technique, 269, 296–97n.2

Humboldt, Alexander von, 36

Hurvich, Leo: career, 268; continues Hering's program, 268–71. *See also* Jameson, Dorothea

identical visual directions, Hering's law of: described, 62–63; Helmholtz's critique of, 72; relation to space values, 65

identity, theory of, 15, 62, 68; Brücke's defense of, 17; Hering's extension of, 63–64; versus projection, 17–20. *See also* correspondence

illusions, geometrical, 75, 76

incommensurability, 219, 278; function in scientific change, 231; limits of, 233; of perception, 222, 279; of program, 219–20, 279; of semantics, 224–25, 279; tied to disciplinary interests, 231

infants, observations on: and the nativist-empiricist debate, 92, 160–61; by Preyer, 160–61; by Raehlmann, 161–62

interests: affective, 6, 235; cognitive, 235; sociodisciplinary, 6, 8, 235, 279

intrinsic self-light of the retina, 107, 222

Jaensch, Erich, 141, 154, 231; on contrast, 253; critique of Hillebrand, 253–54; on the 'new nativism,' 254; on spatial perception, 253–54; and transformation theory, 253–54

James, William, 263

Jameson, Dorothea: career, 268; continues Hering's program, 268–71. *See also* Hurvich, Leo

Javal, Louis-Emile, 141, 142; on strabismus and anomalous correspondence, 170–71

Julesz, Bela, 272

Kant, Immanuel, 23, 71, 76, 81, 156; and Helmholtz, 88, 156; and Hering, 88; and nativism, 88; psychological readings of, 14, 40; on spatiality, 14. *See also* NeoKantianism

Karsten, Gustav, 42

Katz, David, 141, 154, 231, 264; on Hering and Helmholtz, 253; and phenomenology of color, 253

Koffka, Kurt, 274; on the nativist-empiricist dispute, 254–56

Köhler, Wolfgang, 274

König, Arthur, 10, 141, 145, 184, 214, 220, 232, 234, 238, 262; career, 145–46; his color theory of 1894, 207–10; his colorimeter, 240; contributions to colorimetry, 197, 202; critique of Hering, 200; critique of rival color theories, 209; determination of the fundamental sensations, 197–202, 294n.3; measures the spectral absorption curve of visual purple, 207; on monochromats, 205–6; reception of his work, 202; responds to specific brightness of colors, 205–6

Koster, Felix, 214

Kremer, Richard, 39, 105

Kries, Johannes von, 140, 141, 145, 148, 188, 203, 214, 215, 221, 226, 232, 247, 255, 264; attacks on opponent process theory, 189–93, 216, 246; career, 146–47; concessions to nativists, 172–73; defense of terminology of the Helmholtz school, 228; defense of Young's theory, 180–82, 215–16; and duplicity theory, 211–14; on evolution and spatial localization, 159–60; on eye movements, 173; on horopter deviation, 167; on König's work, 202, 210; negotiations with Hering's school, 229; and NeoKantianism, 175; research program on foveal vision, 214; responses to Tschermak, 213; on strabismus and anomalous correspondence, 173; urges return to Kantian understanding of the spatial sense, 230

Kuhn, Thomas S.: on incommensurability, 7, 219, 222, 224; linguistic turn of, 225; on pre-paradigm state, 11

Kühne, Wilhelm, 207, 212

Külpe, Ostwald, 252

Kundt, August Adolph, 164

Kundt's illusion: described, 164; Helmholtz's explanation of, 167; Hering's explanation of, 164

Ladd-Franklin, Christine, 141, 142, 154, 196, 202, 209, 218, 228; criticizes Hering's theory of brightness, 221; criticizes König's theory, 210, 246; demonstrates foveal blindness of monochromats, 207; dispute with Ebbinghaus, 295n.8

Land, Edwin, 297n.3

Leber, Theodor, 141, 145, 148; and displacement hypothesis, 178

Liebermann, Paul: on the abathic surface, 167; on the horopter deviation, 167

Lincke, Maria Antonie, 55

line element, theory of the, 237–38

Lipps, Theodor, 141, 154, 252

Listing, Johann Benedikt, 12, 23, 237, 248

Listing's Law, 72; eye's conformity to experientially acquired, 50; controversy over departures from, 53; deduced from principle of easiest orientation, 50–51; determined by musculature, 91; Helmholtz's establishment of, 48–53; stated, 23

local signs, 25, 64

localization, 13; two- and three-dimensional distinguished, 25. *See also* depth values; projection, theory of

Lotze, Hermann, 66, 77

Ludwig, Carl, 41, 38, 55, 56

Lummer, Otto, 141, 145, 148, 214

luster, stereoscopic, 42, 71, 110; as proof of empiricism (Helmholtz), 79–80

McDougall, William: critique of the energetics of Hering's physiological model, 246–47, 263

Mach, Ernst, 140, 141, 142, 175, 237, 272; critique of Young's theory, 117–18

macula pigmentation and absorption, 185; adequacy to explain dichromat classes, 194, 295n.7

Magnus, Hugo, 177

Marxow, Fleischl von, 145, 148

Mauthner, Ludwig, 178

Maxwell, Clerk, 105, 108, 117, 237; accepts Young's theory, 101; on color blindness, 102–4; and origins of colorimetry, 99–104

Meissner, Georg, 17, 48, 52, 69, 248; on the

empirical horopter, 21; on Listing's Law, 23
Meyer, Heinrich, 105, 111
Meyer's experiment: described, 111; Helmholtz's interpretation of, 112
mix space (Hering), 187–88
Mohl, Anna von, 37
monochromats: explained by the duplicity theory, 213; explained by opponent process theory, 204; König's determination of luminosity curve of, 198, 234; not a reduction form of ordinary vision, 200. *See also* color blindness
Morrell, J. B., 143
Müller, Georg E., 140, 141, 151, 252, 265; critique of Hering's physiological model, 246–47; and empiricism, 156; theory of brightness compared to Hering's, 296n.2; theory of color vision, 196, 265
Müller, Heinrich, 12, 209
Müller, Johann Jacob, 118, 141, 145, 262
Müller, Johannes, 17, 20, 26, 28, 36, 42, 71, 76, 81, 88, 105, 120, 246; on the horopter, 21; influence on Hering, 56–57; as a two-dimensional nativist, 89

Nagel, Albrecht, 17, 24, 81; on binocular localization, 19–20; on color theory, 117; on the horopter, 21–22
Nagel, Willibald, 141, 210, 214, 215, 262
narrative reconstruction: of Helmholtz-Hering controversy, 261, 265, 271; history as, 261
nativist theory of spatial localization: in America, 263; ascendance in Germany after 1900, 172–75; described by Helmholtz, 76; in England, 263; Hering on, 70; history of according to Helmholtz, 81; and psychologists, 252; reception of, 158; and twentieth-century perception theory, 275–76
nativist-empiricist controversy, 158–59; and anomalous retinal correspondence, 168–72; and developmental issues, 159–62; before the *Handbuch*, 23–26, 69–73; in the *Handbuch*, 73–87; before Helmholtz and Hering, 23–26; and the new psychology, 251–55; as originating with Helmholtz and Hering, 70–88, 94; and stability of retinal depth values, 162–68; in the twentieth century, 271–75

Naturphilosophen, 41, 87
NeoKantianism, 174–75, 229–30
Newton, Isaac, 27–28
normal surface, 22
nuancing of colors (Hering), 131

ophthalmology and ophthalmologists: and the Helmholtz-Hering controversy, 247–51; institutionalization of, 247
ophthalmometer, 12
ophthalmoscope, 36, 42, 247
opponent process theory of vision, 55, 128–34; adaptation and, 190–91; in America, 264; assimilation in, 128–29; brightness, 129, 293n.2; chromatic processes, 133; color triangle in, 131; confirmed by microelectrode studies in twentieth century, 267–68; critique by Fick, 180; critique by Helmholtz, 193–95; critique by Kries, 180–82, 189–93; critique of physiological plausibility, 246–47; dissimilation in, 128; Donders on, 183; and work of Hurvich and Jameson, 268–71; mathematical equivalence to Young's, 194; metabolic model of (Hering), 128–30; and monochromatism, 204; opponent colors, 130; simultaneous contrast in, 129; successive contrast in, 129; visual contours in, 129; visual substance in, 128–30, 132
optical valences (Hering), 187–88, 191–92
Osann, Gottfried, 110

Panum, Peter Ludwig, 17, 24, 26, 75, 81; and sensory circles, 18
Parsons, John Herbert, 263
perception theory in twentieth century: cognitive science and, 274; compared to the positions of Helmholtz and Hering, 275–76; 'direct' theories in, 274–75; neurophysiological direction in, 273. *See also* empiricist theory of spatial localization; nativist theory of spatial localization
Pflüger, Eduard, 178
Phi phenomenon, 254–56
physics and physicists: and vision research, 237–39
physiological optics: disciplines in, 6, 8; growth of, 10–11; interest in binocularity during the 1850s, 17; relationship to psychology, 244, 255; in twentieth century,

physiological optics (*cont.*)
8; unification of at midcentury, 11–13, 30–31. *See also* color vision studies; vision studies
physiology and physiologists: institutionalization of, 244; retreat from psychophysical methods, 244–45; and vision research, 243–47
pigment epithelium: as light-sensitive on König's theory, 209
Plateau, Joseph, 105, 108, 109
Prelli, Lawrence, 87
Pretori, Hugo, 223, 227, 239
Prévost, Alexandre, 21
Preyer, Thierry William, 141, 156; on color blindness, 119; on fusion mechanism, 250; on visual development of the infant, 160–61
primary colors, 26,30; Helmholtz on, 96. *See also* fundamental sensations
primary position: redefined by Helmholtz, 52
projection, theory of: critique by Hering, 60–62; explained, 14–15; Panum on, 18; projection surfaces in, 19–20; and stability of retinal depth values, 163; versus the theory of identity, 17–20
protanopes. *See* dichromats
psychology and psychologists: Gestalt, 254–56; and the Helmholtz-Hering dispute, 154, 251–56; institutionalization of, 251; phenomenological, 253–54; and vision research, 251. *See also* Hurvich, Jameson
psychophysical law, 57, 237, 246
Purkinje, Jan Evangelista, 28, 105
Purkinje phenomenon, 108, 205, 211, 212; and duplicity theory, 213–14; Hering on, 214; König's explanation of, 205
purple, 98–99

radial fibres, 116
Raehlmann, Edward, 141, 148; on color blindness, 118; on organic development and spatial perception, 161–62
Recklinghausen, Friedrich von, 17, 44; on the horopter and normal surface, 22; on Listing's Law, 23
reduction hypothesis: and color blindness, 102–4, 106; Donders on, 183–84; König's defense of, 200

retina, 12, 182; Hering on, 132, 190
retinal incongruity: defined, 44; explanations of, 44; Hering rejects significance of, 59
rhetorical strategies, 5–6; in the *Handbuch*, 80–81; Helmholtz's, 52–53, 74, 94, 194–95; Hering's, 92–93, 121–22; logic of, 87
Ringer, Fritz, 39
Ritter, Carl, 205
rivalry, retinal, 79
Rivers, W.H.R., 215, 263
rods and cones, 12, 211; cone photopigments identified, 267–68; Helmholtz on, 105; and rod-free area of fovea, 295n.9; Schultze on, 115–16; visual purple in rods, 207
Rollet, Alexander, 17
Rood, Ogden, 264
Rose, Edmund, and color blindness, 118
Royce, Josiah, 263
Rudwick, Martin: and concept of the core set, 6, 139, 154; on constitutive nature of controversy in scientific change, 6, 93

Sachs, Moriz, 141, 142, 223, 224, 227, 239; on strabismus and anomalous correspondence, 170, 175
santonin effect. *See* color blindness
Sattler, Hubert, 142, 151, 248
saturation: Hering's critique of, 226; of monochromatic lights, 98; on Young's theory, 102
Schelling, Friedrich W. J., 26, 40
Schirmer, Rudolf, on color blindness, 119
Schöler, Heinrich, 178
schools: criteria for success of, 143–44; epideictic function of publication in Hering's, 232; explanatory priorities in, 220; of Helmholtz, 148–49; of Hering, 144–45; as intellectual alignments, 144–45; of König, 148–49; as linguistic communities, 231–33; as loci of speciation, 232; as research groups, 143; research program of Helmholtz's, 113; response of Hering's to duplicity theory, 213; strategy of noncommunication pursued by Helmholtz's; as transdisciplinary constellations, 256–57
Schrödinger, Erwin, 263
Schultze, Max, 115–17
Seebeck August, 28, 106

self-regulation of the organism (Hering), 55, 121, 263
sensation-perception distinction, 14, 43, 67, 225, 273, 275; Hering on, 127
Sherrington, Charles Scott, 263
Siemens, Werner von, 37, 40
simultaneous light induction (Hering), 125
space values, retinal, 63–67. *See also* depth values
specific brightness of colors, 202–5, 212; refutes Young's theory (Hillebrand), 204
specific nerve energies, 29, 42, 57, 106, 246
spectral locus: Helmholtz on, 98–99; König's determination of, 197–202; Maxwell on, 102–3
spectral luminosity curve: form for dark spectrum, 207; form for monochromats, 204
spectral response curves, 106, 197–202
Spencer, Herbert, 159
Spengler, Ostwald, and spatial perception, 174
stereopsis, 13, 43, 64; early disputes over, 71; muscle kinesthesia as key to, 77; neurophysiological basis of, 272; physiological versus psychological explanations of (before Helmholtz and Hering), 23–26; twentieth-century studies of, 272; vertical disparities in, 72
stereoscope, 14–15, 24
Stiles, Walter S., 266
Stilling, Jakob, 141, 178, 179, 238
strabismus, 78, 168–72; debates over etiology and treatment, 249–51
Stumpf, Carl, 141, 154, 232, 252, 278; moderate nativism of, 158
successive light induction (Hering), 125
Svaetichin, Gunnar, 267

temperature sense, 55
Traube-Hering pressure waves, 121
trichromatic theory. *See* Young's theory
Troland, Leonard Thompson, 256–57, 262, 263
Tschermak-Seysenegg, Armin, 141, 215, 224, 226, 242, 262, 295n.7; career, 143; on the duplicity theory, 213; on exact subjectivism, 239; on the horopter deviation, 166; reverence for Hering, 150; on strabismus and anomalous correspondence, 171

unconscious inference, 71, 74–75; interpreted as associations, 252
unilaterals, 179–80, 294n.1

veiling of colors (Hering), 223
Velten, Olga von, 36, 39, 42
Verworn, Max, defense of Hering's physiological model, 247
Vieth, Gerhard U. A., 21
Virchow, Rudolf, 177
vision studies: disciplinary status of, 235–36; experimental methods in, 238; fragmentation of, 256–57, 261–65; instruments in, 240–43; ophthalmology and ophthalmologists in, 247–51; physics and physicists in, 237–39; physiology and physiologists in, 243–47; psychology and psychologists in, 251–56; transformation around 1850, 69, 277; in twentieth century, 261–76. *See also* physiological optics
visual purple, 206–9; role in duplicity theory, 211–12; role in König's theory, 207–10; spectral absorption curve of, 207
visual space (Hering), 62
visual yellow, 206–7, 208
Volkmann, Alfred W., 17, 22, 24, 29, 39, 44, 53, 60, 69, 70, 92, 146, 278; and the psychological theory of fusion, 18; on Young's theory, 29–30

Wagner, Ernst, 54
Weber, Ernst Heinrich, 57
Wertheimer, Max, 274; and Phi phenomenon, 254; reply to Hillebrand, 256
Westman, Robert, 93
Wheatstone, Charles, 14, 17, 237
Wheatstone's stereogram, 16, 18, 20, 61, 79
white: role of inference in visual assessment of, 111. *See also* brightness
white valence curve: compared to luminosity distribution curve, 204; determined by Hillebrand, 204
Wiesel, Torsten, 273
Wilson, George, 102
Worth, Claud Alley, 249
Wundt, Wilhelm, 17, 44, 49, 52, 60, 66, 69, 77, 81, 141, 151, 196, 252, 262, 263, 271; and binocular localization, 20; on color theory, 115; his empiricist account of spatial perception, 25–26; on Listing's

Wundt, Wilhelm (*cont.*)
   Law, 23; as nonaligned participant, 153;
   relationship to Helmholtz, 152; on unconscious inference, 26, 74

Young, Thomas, 29, 105
Young's theory, 220, 234; adoption by
   Helmholtz, 104–6; adoption by Maxwell,
   101–4; in America, 264; defended by
   Donders, 183–84; defended by Fick,
   180–81; defended by Kries, 180–82; explanation of color blindness, 106–8; Hering on, 134; initial rejection by
   Helmholtz, 96; nerve fibres in, 106, 113;
   reception after 1860, 115–20; as understood by Maxwell, 101–2; Volkmann on,
   29–30
zone theory, 196, 216; contemporary critiques of two-zone models, 271; established in twentieth century, 265–71;
   Helmholtz on, 194–95; Hering and Hillebrand reject, 229; Hurvich and Jameson
   on, 269; Kries and Donders on, 182–83;
   in twentieth-century Germany, 265
Zoth, Oskar, 141, 142, 175
Zumft, Johannes, 209